To Candice Pellegrino
a most dedicated
professional

BLACKWELL'S BASICS OF MEDICINE

Respiratory Failure

AF713779

BLACKWELL'S BASICS OF MEDICINE

Books in the series:

Acid-Base

Potassium

Salt & Water

Heart Failure

Renal Failure

Respiratory Failure

BLACKWELL'S BASICS OF MEDICINE

Respiratory Failure

Horacio J. Adrogué, MD, FACP
Professor of Medicine
Baylor College of Medicine
Department of Veterans Affairs Medical Center
Houston, Texas

Martin J. Tobin, MD
Professor of Medicine
Chief, Division of Pulmonary and Critical Care Medicine
Loyola University of Chicago, Stritch School of Medicine
and
Edward Hines Veterans Administration Hospital
Chicago, Illinois

Blackwell
Science

Blackwell Science

EDITORIAL OFFICES:
238 Main Street, Cambridge, Massachusetts 02142, USA
Osney Mead, Oxford OX2 0El, England
25 John Street, London WC1N 2BL, England
23 Ainslie Place, Edinburgh EH3 6AJ, Scotland
54 University Street, Carlton, Victoria 3053, Australia
Other Editorial offices:
Arnette Blackwell SA, 224, Boulevard Saint Germain, 75007 Paris, France
Blackwell Wissenschafts-Verlag GmbH Kurfürstendamm 57, 10707 Berlin, Germany Zehetnergasse 6, A-1140 Vienna, Austria

DISTRIBUTORS:
USA
Blackwell Science, Inc.
238 Main Street
Cambridge, Massachusetts 02142
(Telephone orders: 800-215-1000 or 617-876-7000; fax orders: 617-492-5263)

Canada
Copp Clark Professional
200 Adelaide Street, West, 3rd Floor
Toronto, Ontario M5H 1W7
(Telephone orders: 800-815-9417 or 416-597-1616; fax orders: 416-597-1617)

Australia
Blackwell Science Pty, Ltd.
54 University Street
Carlton, Victoria 3053
(Telephone orders: 03-9347-0300;
fax orders 03-9349-3016)

Outside North America and Australia
Blackwell Science, Ltd.
c/o Marston Book Services, Ltd.
P.O. Box 269
Abingdon
Oxon OX14 4YN
England
(Telephone orders: 44-01235-465500;
fax orders 44-01235-465555)

The Blackwell Science logo is a trade mark of Blackwell Science Ltd., registered at the United Kingdom Trade Marks Registry

Acquisitions: Joy Denomme
Development: Kathleen Broderick
Production: Irene Herlihy
Manufacturing: Lisa Flanagan

Typeset by Achorn Graphic Services, Inc.
Printed and bound by Capital City Press

© 1997 by Blackwell Science, Inc.

Printed in the United States of America
96 97 98 99 5 4 3 2 1

All rights reserved. No part of this book may be reproduced in any form or by any electronic or mechanical means, including information storage and retrieval systems, without permission in writing from the publisher, except by a reviewer who may quote brief passages in a review.

Library of Congress Cataloging-in-Publication Data
Adrogué, Horacio J.
Respiratory failure / Horacio J. Adrogué, Martin J. Tobin.
p. cm. — (Blackwell's basics of medicine)
Includes bibliographical references and index.
ISBN 0-86542-478-0 (alk. paper)
1. Respiratory insufficiency. I. Tobin, Martin J. II. Title. III. Series.
[DNLM: 1. Respiratory Insufficiency.
WF 140 A2425r 1997]
RC776.R4A35 1997
616.2—dc20
DNLM/DLC
for Library of Congress 96-9846
CIP

To our families

Sarita
Sofía, Horacio, Soledad,
Matías and Marcos Adrogué

Sareen
Damien, Kate, and Kieran Tobin

Contents

Preface

The practice of medicine is rapidly moving from health care delivered by multiple specialists, each responsible for a single problem, toward comprehensive patient management provided by a single practitioner. A proper response to this trend mandates that health care providers successfully integrate knowledge from multiple disciplines and skillfully apply it to patient care. Yet, past and current education compels students to swallow sizable amounts of information on each of the various basic science disciplines (i.e., anatomy, biochemistry, etc.), and within a short time thereafter, they are force-fed the various components of clinical sciences. Thus, acquisition of clinical knowledge is accomplished with simultaneous loss of fundamental concepts of basic sciences. This undesirable effect is due to our outdated educational curriculum that does not allow proper digestion, incorporation, and integration of knowledge, as well as fails to develop and nurture the skills required to deliver comprehensive health care.

This issue, entitled *Respiratory Failure*, represents the sixth of the Blackwell's Basics of Medicine Series, a book collection that examines relevant topics in medicine using concepts that pertain to the basic sciences as a starting point. The doctrine on which this series has been formulated dictates that two critical elements should be present in order to acquire the skills necessary for optimal patient management. The first element is a thoughtful approach based on solid pathophysiological knowledge. The second element is that this basic medical knowledge needs to be applied using common sense. If properly combined, the presence of these two elements allows the unraveling of difficult and/or obscure clinical situations. This series uses simple questions followed by short answers as well as case presentations to illustrate the various topics presented. The sequential order of the questions chosen provides the reader with layers of knowledge that will steadily increase his/her understanding of each topic. The application of the various concepts mentioned above in the analysis of each case helps to consolidate theoretical principles with practical facts.

Respiratory Failure, like the previous issues of this series, examines a carefully selected topic that is germane to the daily practice of medicine. In it, readers will find the tools for an intelligent interpretation of clinical data based on sound pathophysiological concepts enabling them to provide quality care.

The teaching approach used in this series is at variance with that of the traditional system of medical education that advocates the acquisition of an encyclopedic knowledge as the critical weapon to deal with medical problems. Our belief is, instead, that a larger fraction of time and energy should be spent in integrating theory and practice.

H.J.A.
M.J.T.

Acknowledgments

The authors want to extend their gratitude and indebtedness to Debbie S. Verrett for her patience, secretarial expertise, and dedication in deciphering and typing the manuscript.

Part I: Essentials of Respiration

1. Basic Concepts

INTRODUCTORY CONCEPTS

1 What is respiration? Name the main processes that participate in respiration.

❑ Respiration involves a series of processes that facilitate the exchange of oxygen and carbon dioxide between the atmosphere and body tissues. The starting step of respiration is pulmonary ventilation, which consists of the bulk movement of air toward and from the gas-exchange region of the lung (ie, alveoli). Other processes of respiration include the delivery and distribution of blood through the lungs, the diffusion of oxygen and carbon dioxide across the air-blood barrier, and the transport of these gases between the lungs and the peripheral tissues. Cellular respiration consumes oxygen and produces carbon dioxide, allowing the biosynthesis of ATP, the molecule that powers living processes.

2 What is the principal function of the respiratory system?

❑ The principal function of the respiratory system is to bring ambient air into the pulmonary alveoli, permitting gas exchange with the capillary blood of the pulmonary circulation. This process makes oxygen available and removes carbon dioxide, promoting optimal cellular function of all tissues and organs.

3 What are the components of the respiratory system?

❑ The respiratory system is composed of the airways and the lung alveoli, the pulmonary circulation, the various elements of the chest wall (especially the diaphragm and intercostal muscles), and the corresponding centers of the nervous system (central and peripheral) as well as afferent and efferent pathways. Disorders arising from any component of the respiratory system can lead to respiratory failure.

4 How does the respiratory system achieve its goal of maintaining optimal arterial blood levels of oxygen and carbon dioxide?

❑ The respiratory system maintains optimal arterial blood levels of oxygen and carbon dioxide by modulating the ventilation of the lung alveoli (ie, alveolar ventilation) and the pulmonary capillary blood flow, while preserving a ventilation-perfusion ratio ($\dot{V}/\dot{Q}$) that allows maximal exchange of gases across the alveolocapillary walls (ie, $\dot{V}/\dot{Q}$ ratio of approximately 1.0).

5 What is ventilation? Compare total pulmonary ventilation and alveolar ventilation.

❑ Ventilation is the process whereby the respiratory system provides fresh air to the conducting airways and pulmonary alveoli. Total ventilation ($\dot{V}_E$) represents the total volume of inspired or expired gas in the act of breathing during a time interval, expressed in liters per minute. Alveolar ventilation ($\dot{V}_A$) is the volume of fresh gas that replaces alveolar gas during a time interval, expressed in liters per minute. Total ventilation is larger than alveolar ventilation because it also includes the ventilation of the conducting airway ($\dot{V}_D$), known as dead space (V_D), an area in which no significant gas exchange occurs.

6 Explain inspiration.

❑ Inspiration is the entry of air from the atmosphere to the lungs. For inspiration to occur, a pressure gradient must be created between the nostrils or other airway opening and the alveoli, since air flows only from a high-pressure region to one of low pressure. Contraction of the respiratory muscles (ie, diaphragm, intercostal muscles, scalene muscles) during normal inspiration causes expansion of the thoracic cavity. Accordingly, inspiration is an active phenomenon that consumes energy. The inspiratory enlargement of the chest cavity opposes the normal tendency of the lungs to collapse because of their intrinsic elastic recoil, and creates a normal subatmospheric intrapleural and alveolar pressure that causes air to flow from the atmosphere to the alveoli. The volume of gas entering the lungs is dependent on several factors that include the intrapleural pressure, the magnitude of the opposing forces due to the elastic recoil of the lungs and chest wall, as well as the frictional resistance of the airways and lung tissue. Inspiration also can be achieved artificially by increasing pressure at the airway opening with positive-pressure ventilators.

7 Explain expiration.

❑ Expiration is the exit of air from the lungs to the atmosphere. Expiration is usually a passive phenomenon, accomplished by the energy stored in the expanded elastic structures of the lungs and chest wall during inspiration. Normally, there is fairly equal and synchronous inflation and deflation of the alveoli in different regions of the lungs. However, in patients with pulmonary disease, differences in regional airway resistance or lung distensibility (compliance) can lead to nonhomogeneous filling and emptying, so that expiration may not be completed in some units when inspiration starts again. These units are characterized by a prolonged time constant that is computed as resistance multiplied by compliance of the lungs. Such regional inhomogeneity is likely to occur in patients with a rapid respiratory rate and may lead to progressive gas trapping.

MECHANICS OF BREATHING

8 Explain the physical factors that determine resistance to airflow.

❑ Because air behaves like a fluid of low viscosity, resistance to airflow is determined by the same factors that govern the flow of liquids (eg, circulatory system). Consequently, Poiseuille's law for laminar flow in rigid tubes may be applied, with some limitations, to the airflow in the respiratory system. This law states that the pressure required to produce a given flow varies inversely with the fourth power of the radius. Therefore, the radius of the tube is of great importance in determining the resistance to flow (eg, bronchoconstriction reduces the radius of bronchioles, increasing airway resistance, and to maintain a given airflow will require an increase in the driving pressure).

9 Explain the significance of Poiseuille's law applied to the airways in the presence of bronchial constriction (eg, status asthmaticus).

❑ The significance of Poiseuille's law applied to the airways becomes apparent by recognizing that if the radius of the bronchioles is halved, the pressure must be increased 16-fold to maintain constant flow. Thus, the work of breathing by the respiratory muscles may dramatically increase as a result of severe and generalized bronchospasm.

10 How is airway resistance calculated?

❑ Calculation of airway resistance consists of the ratio of driving pressure and the airflow. Consequently, airway resistance can be calculated as follows:

$$\text{Resistance across the entire airway} = \frac{\text{Mouth pressure} - \text{Alveolar pressure}}{\text{Flow}}$$

11 What is the transpulmonary pressure gradient? What are the pressure levels at the pleural space and at the alveoli during normal breathing?

❑ The transpulmonary pressure gradient is the pressure difference between the pleural space and the alveoli. It is also called *recoil pressure* because it represents a measure of the elastic forces in the lungs that tend to collapse this organ. The pleural pressure is slightly below the atmospheric level during normal respiration (ie, −5 and −7.5 cm H_2O during expiration and inspiration, respectively). The alveolar pressure at the end of expiration is approximately 0 cm H_2O (when the glottis is open and there is no airflow into or out of the respiratory tract, the pressure levels in all the system from the alveoli to the larynx are equal and identical to atmospheric pressure, the reference value that represents 0 cm H_2O). During normal inspiration, the alveolar pressure decreases to approximately −1 cm H_2O. This small negative pressure drives approximately 0.5 L of air into the lungs within 2 seconds of inspiratory effort. Opposite changes in alveolar pressure are observed during expiration in which alveolar pressure rises to approximately +1 cm H_2O and the pressure gradient between the alveoli and the glottis drives 0.5 L of air out of the lungs within 2 to 3 seconds.

12 How can the alveolar ventilation be estimated?

❑ Considering that when breathing room air, inspired carbon dioxide pressure (PCO_2) is practically zero, the effective alveolar ventilation can be estimated as follows:

$$\dot{V}_A = \dot{V}_E \times P_ECO_2/PaCO_2$$

where P_ECO_2 is the partial pressure of carbon dioxide in expired gas. Examination of this equation reveals that if expired and arterial PCO_2 are identical, their ratio will be one, and total ventilation will be identical to the alveolar ventilation. On the contrary, if expired PCO_2 approaches zero, the ratio of expired over arterial PCO_2 will be minuscule, and most of the total ventilation will be wasted in dead space areas, such that carbon dioxide retention will develop.

13 What is the normal level of pulmonary ventilation, also known as *minute volume*?

❑ The normal level of pulmonary ventilation or minute volume is approximately 6.5 L/min. It represents the total amount of fresh air moved into the respiratory tract each minute, and it is equal to the tidal volume (V_T) multiplied by the respiratory rate. Normal V_T is 380 mL, normal respiratory rate is 17 breaths/min, and minute volume is 6.5 L/min. Values reported in the past as normal (eg, V_T of 0.5 L and respiratory rate of 12 breaths/min) were obtained with a spirometer, which induces slow deep breathing. During hyperventilation, V_T as well as respiratory rate generally increase (eg, 2.0 L × 45 breaths/min = 90 L/min). Although V_T can become as large as the vital capacity, only values of V_T that are approximately half the vital capacity can be sustained in response to increased ventilatory demands (exercise).

14 How is pulmonary ventilation measured?

❑ The method used for the direct measurement of pulmonary ventilation differs in patients with and those without a tracheal tube. In the intubated patient, direct measurement of ventilation is easily performed by attaching a spirometer or pneumotachograph to the patient's endotracheal tube. In a nonintubated, critically ill patient, measurement of ventilation with a spirometer or pneumotachograph is difficult because these patients have a low tolerance of devices that require a direct connection to the airway. In addition, use of a mouthpiece and nose clips produces spurious alterations in breathing pattern, causing tidal volume to increase and respiratory frequency to decrease. To overcome these problems, several devices have been developed to measure ventilation indirectly and these are described in the answer to a pertinent question.

2. Oxygen

IMPORTANCE OF OXYGEN

15 What is the role of oxygen in living cells and in the intact organism?

❑ Oxygen is required in chemical reactions that are responsible for more than 95% of the energy spent by living cells and the intact organism. Consequently, oxygen is a critical substrate to sustain life because of its role in the biosynthesis of ATP. The latter molecule is a versatile energy resource used in all forms of life for most cellular functions.

16 What is the fate of most of the absorbed oxygen in the lungs?

❑ Most of the oxygen absorbed in the lungs is transformed by the cells into carbon dioxide as they consume oxygen. Consequently, a close relationship exists between oxygen consumption and carbon dioxide production and is known as the *respiratory exchange ratio* (RE, process that takes place in the lungs) and the *respiratory quotient* (RQ, dependent on chemical reactions that occur in the tissues).

17 How does the oxygen absorbed in the lungs and consumed by the tissues exit from the organism?

❑ The oxygen consumed by cellular metabolism is mostly transformed into either carbon dioxide or water. The carbon atom provided by nutrients (eg, carbohydrates, lipids) combines with oxygen, leading to the generation of carbon dioxide. The metabolic production of water results from the combination of hydrogen derived from the nutrients intake and oxygen absorbed in the lungs (see function of the ''respiratory chain''; answers 18, 20–23).

18 How does oxygen exert its action in living organisms?

❑ Oxygen is used in the dominant pathway for the synthesis of ATP, known as *oxidative phosphorylation* (ie, addition of a "phosphoryl group" to ADP, generating ATP via the oxygen-consuming pathway). The action of oxygen is exerted as follows: (1) The hydrogen generated in chemical reactions in all living cells (ie, metabolism of carbohydrates, lipids, and proteins) is transiently stored in nicotinamide adenine dinucleotide (NAD) and flavin adenine dinucleotide (FAD), two major components of the "respiratory chain"; (2) the "hydrogen carriers" NAD and FAD unload the hydrogen, which combines with molecular oxygen, yielding as the final product H_2O (the so-called metabolic production of water); and (3) the proton or hydrogen ion transport provides the energy needed to phosphorylate ADP to ATP by the chemiosmotic mechanism (Mitchell's hypothesis). Thus, oxygen acts as a hydrogen acceptor that facilitates the oxidation of nutrients and the disposal of hydrogen by the production of water. This role of oxygen allows the generation of ATP, the molecule that powers cell metabolism (ie, chemical reactions within cells).

19 What is the meaning of anaerobic and aerobic energy?

❑ Anaerobic energy refers to processes that obtain energy without the simultaneous consumption of oxygen. Conversely, *aerobic energy* refers to processes that require the simultaneous consumption of oxygen. As indicated elsewhere in this book, most of ATP synthesis occurs as a result of oxygen utilization in the respiratory chain located in the mitochondria of living cells.

20 Explain further the transport of hydrogen toward its final destination through the respiratory chain located in the mitochondria.

❑ The hydrogen molecule consists of a proton (ie, hydrogen ion) and an electron. The hydrogen carriers NAD and FAD receive the hydrogen molecule through chemical reactions in which carbohydrates, lipids, and proteins are decomposed (by processes collectively known as *oxidation of substrates*). Subsequently, the loaded hydrogen carriers NAD and FAD (ie, NADH and $FADH_2$) release the hydrogen, thereby promoting the transport of electrons and protons that flow separately through the respiratory chain. The electrons are transferred through a chain of mobile molecules (eg, ubiquinone, cytochrome *c*) located in the inner mitochondrial membrane. The protons are released into the space separating the inner (juxtaposed to the mitochondrial matrix) from the outer (juxtaposed to the cytosol) membranes of the mitochondrion. The resulting buildup of protons in the intermembrane space creates a concentration gradient that favors the flow of H^+ from this space toward the mitochondrial matrix through proton channels. As the protons flow through the respective channels by passive forces (moving down their concentration gradient), they promote ATP synthesis so that phosphorylation of ADP to ATP occurs (ie, chemiosmotic mechanism of Mitchell's hypothesis). Within the mitochondrial matrix, the electrons and protons interact with oxygen, leading to water formation (eg, $2\ e^- + 2\ H^+ + {}^1\!/_2 O_2 \Rightarrow H_2O$).

21 Name clinically relevant compounds that inhibit the cellular respiratory chain.

❑ Carbon monoxide and cyanide are clinically important toxic substances that inhibit the respiratory chain and might lead to death. These compounds block the last step of the flow of electrons along the respiratory chain that transfers electrons from complex IV to molecular oxygen. Consequently, carbon monoxide and cyanide interrupt the major cellular pathway responsible for the biosynthesis of ATP, the molecule that powers life.

22 What substrates can be used for ATP synthesis in the absence of oxygen? Compare ATP synthesis with and that without oxygen utilization.

❑ Carbohydrates (eg, glucose) can be utilized for ATP synthesis under anaerobic conditions. Degradation of 1 mole of glucose in 2 moles of pyruvic acid produces 3 moles of ATP if the initial carbohydrate is glycogen, and 2 moles of ATP if the initial substrate is glucose itself. The relatively small production of ATP during anaerobic glycolysis contrasts with the 38 moles of ATP per mole of glucose generated in the presence of oxygen (full operation of the Krebs cycle and the respiratory chain).

23 What is the normal intracellular oxygen tension (PO_2) and what is the minimum level required to support metabolic processes?

❑ The mean intracellular PO_2 is approximately 20 mm Hg (the normal range is 5 to 40 mm Hg). Yet, the level required for cellular metabolism is only 1 to 3 mm Hg. Consequently, there is a large margin of safety in the normal state with respect to securing oxygen to vital tissues. It must be recognized that the PaO_2 required to achieve an intracellular PO_2 that allows optimal cellular metabolism is probably at least 55 mm Hg.

OXYGEN CONSUMPTION

24 What is the normal oxygen consumption? Explain the concepts of oxygen extraction ratio and "supply-dependent" and "supply-independent" oxygen consumption.

❑ Oxygen consumption ($\dot{V}O_2$) is normally about 250 mL/min. This can be calculated according to the Fick equation:

$$\dot{V}O_2 = (CaO_2 - CvO_2) \times \dot{Q}t$$
$$= 5 \text{ mL } O_2/\text{dL} \times 10 \text{ dL/L} \times 5 \text{ L/min}$$
$$= 250 \text{ mL } O_2/\text{min}$$

Causes of increased oxygen consumption include fever, adrenergic stimulation, increased muscular activity, and alkalosis. In normal subjects, substantially more oxygen is delivered to the tissue (1000 mL/min) than is used by it (250 mL/min). This relationship ($\dot{V}O_2/DO_2$) is termed the *oxygen extraction ratio* and provides a useful means of evaluating the many factors concerned with tissue oxygenation; normally, the oxygen extraction ratio is 0.25 or 25%. In patients with diseases that impair oxygen delivery, an increase in oxygen extraction initially compensates for the decrease in oxygen delivery, with the result that oxygen consumption remains normal. However, when a critically low oxygen delivery level is reached, this compensatory mechanism breaks down, and a decrease in oxygen delivery causes a proportional decrease in oxygen consumption. This type of delivery-dependent oxygen consumption contrasts with the normal situation in which oxygen uptake is independent of oxygen delivery. In the past, it was believed that patients with acute respiratory distress syndrome (ARDS) and other critical illnesses displayed pathologic supply-dependency of oxygen consumption; that is, oxygen uptake is directly related to oxygen delivery. The studies on which this concept was based were seriously flawed, and the concept of pathologic supply-dependency of oxygen consumption is no longer accepted as valid.

25 What is the major determinant of oxygen consumption?

❑ The major determinant of oxygen consumption is the rate of energy expenditure (ie, rate of ADP formation from the high-energy compound ATP) and not the availability of oxygen (except for conditions of extreme hypoxia). As long as intracellular PO_2

is higher than 1 to 3 mm Hg, the rate of oxygen consumption is independent of oxygen availability. As previously indicated, the PaO_2 required to achieve an intracellular PO_2 that allows optimal cellular metabolism is probably at least 55 mm Hg.

26 How does the oxygen uptake in the pulmonary capillaries increase during strenuous exercise to satisfy the augmented tissue requirements?

❑ The oxygen diffusing capacity of the lung increases threefold during strenuous exercise because of an augmented number of capillaries being perfused and improved ventilation-perfusion matching in the upper pulmonary areas that accompanies the large increase in cardiac output. The reduction in time that the blood remains in the pulmonary capillaries to less than half normal during intense exercise does not reduce the blood oxygenation because this process is achieved within the first one-third of the transit time along the alveolar capillaries. Consequently, blood leaves the pulmonary circulation almost completely saturated with oxygen, and the uptake of oxygen by the pulmonary blood may increase by as much as 20 times the normal level observed at rest (eg, threefold increase in oxygen diffusing capacity multiplied by the sevenfold increase in cardiac output).

27 What is the oxygen debt that follows strenuous muscle exercise?

❑ *Oxygen debt* refers to the larger than resting oxygen consumption (accompanied by hyperventilation) observed after termination of strenuous exercise and lasting for up to 60 minutes. The augmented oxygen consumption allows for (1) elimination of the high lactate levels in muscle and in plasma, by transforming lactate into glucose by the liver and kidney (Cori cycle); (2) replenishment of muscle stores of ATP and phosphocreatine; and (3) return to the original levels the oxygen bound to myoglobin and hemoglobulin (Hb) and that initially present within the respiratory tract.

28 What are the energy sources during strenuous exercise? What is the final product of anaerobic glycolysis in this condition?

❑ The energy sources during strenuous exercise include (1) ATP stored within muscle cells prior to initiation of exercise, (2) new ATP derived from degradation of phosphocreatine (this compound is the most important energy deposit in muscle cells), (3) anaerobic glycolysis from the breakdown of glycogen stores in muscle cells, and (4) oxidative reactions that regenerate ATP. All these processes participate in the provision of energy, yet their relative contributions differ significantly. The first two processes can sustain strenuous exercise for only a few seconds. Similarly, oxidative metabolism is short-lasting because of a rapid decrease in muscle PO_2 during maximal exercise. Consequently, anaerobic glycolysis plays a major role in this condition, producing lactic acid instead of pyruvic acid as the final step of this pathway. The pyruvate is converted to lactate because of an accumulation of the reduced form of nicotinamide adenine dinucleotide (NADH) as a result of the anaerobic condition of exercising muscle.

29 What is the maximum level of oxygen that can be delivered to the peripheral tissues in well-trained marathon runners?

❑ Well-trained marathon runners can increase the oxygen delivery to peripheral tissues by 20-fold the normal resting level. Such increment is accounted for by augmenting the extraction ratio (percentage of the blood that releases oxygen as it travels through the tissue capillaries) from its normal level of 25% to a maximum of 75% to 85% and by increasing the cardiac output. Since the latter can increase up to six or seven times the normal value, the product of the larger extraction ratio and augmented cardiac output (ie, $3 \times 7 = 21$) explains the approximately 20-fold rise in oxygen delivery to the tissues.

30 What is the source of energy in states of respiratory arrest or in acute extreme hypoxia?

❑ The oxygen combined to Hb as well as that contained within the respiratory tract provides aerobic energy for approximately 2 minutes following acute oxygen deprivation. Anaerobic glycolysis utilizing glucose originated from glycogen breakdown provides energy for approximately 1 additional minute. Consequently, beyond 3 minutes from an acute respiratory arrest (or comparable condition of acute hypoxia), all energy sources become depleted so that cellular damage and death become imminent.

ALVEOLAR GAS EQUATION

31 What is the basis for the estimation of alveolar PO_2 and PCO_2 with the alveolar gas equation?

❑ The measurement of alveolar PO_2 and PCO_2 from analysis of a single sample of exhaled alveolar gas is subject to considerable error, but mean alveolar PO_2 can be calculated accurately with the alveolar air equation. The underlying principle is based on the concept that at sea level the total pressure of gases (oxygen, carbon dioxide, nitrogen, and water vapor) in the alveoli equals 760 mm Hg (Patm) and that if the partial pressures of any three of these four are known, the fourth can be obtained by subtraction. Thus,

$$760 \text{ mm Hg} = PO_2 + PCO_2 + PN_2 + PH_2O$$

Consequently,

$$PO_2 = \text{Patm} - PH_2O - PN_2 - PCO_2$$

and

$$PO_2 = 760 \text{ mm Hg} - 47 \text{ mm Hg} - 563 \text{ mm Hg} - 40 \text{ mm Hg} = 110 \text{ mm Hg}$$

considering that PH_2O at 37°C is approximately 47 mm Hg and arterial PCO_2 is used to represent mean alveolar PCO_2, and assuming that PN_2 equals 563 mm Hg. This would be true if the respiratory gas exchange ratio (R) were one (ie, the amount of carbon dioxide added to the alveoli equals the amount of oxygen removed from the alveoli per minute). Actually, more oxygen is removed per minute than carbon dioxide is added (ie, R = 0.8). Consequently, R needs to be incorporated in the alveolar gas equation (see details in answer to pertinent question).

32 What is the precise formula for the alveolar gas equation? What is the formula used for clinical purposes?

❑ The precise formula for the alveolar gas equation (assuming inspired PCO_2 is 0) is

$$\underset{\text{(unknown)}}{P_AO_2} = \underset{\text{(known)}}{PiO_2} - \underset{\text{(measured)}}{P_ACO_2} \quad \underset{\text{(correcting factor)}}{\left[FiO_2 + \frac{1 - FiO_2}{R}\right]}$$

where PiO_2 is inspired oxygen pressure (moist) at sea level; 20.93% of (760 − 47) = 149 mm Hg; P_ACO_2 is alveolar carbon dioxide pressure and is assumed to be equal to arterial PCO_2, which can be measured accurately; and FiO_2 is fractional inspired oxygen. The most commonly used formula for the alveolar gas equation, keeping in mind that most pulmonary patients are receiving supplemental oxygen, is as follows:

$$P_AO_2 = (Patm - PH_2O) \times FiO_2 - \frac{PaCO_2}{0.8}$$

The latter formula must be remembered for the management of patients with respiratory failure.

33 Explain the relationship between PO_2 and PCO_2 in patients breathing room air as defined by the carbon dioxide–oxygen diagram of Rahn and Fenn.

❑ The diagram of Rahn and Fenn shows that a rise in $PaCO_2$ must be accompanied by a fall in PaO_2. The reverse is also true. The slope of this relationship ($\Delta PCO_2/\Delta PO_2$) depends on the respiratory exchange ratio (R), which is assumed to be 0.8. Consequently, an increase in $PaCO_2$ of 10 mm Hg results in a 12.5 mm Hg fall in PaO_2 in a healthy person. In patients in acute respiratory failure with chronic obstructive pulmonary disease (COPD), the lowest PaO_2 level compatible with life is approximately 20 mm Hg while breathing room air. Therefore, the highest tolerable $PaCO_2$ while breathing room air is approximately 80 to 90 mm Hg. In fact, $PaCO_2$ rarely exceeds 80 mm Hg in patients with pulmonary disease breathing room air because of the concomitant presence of an increased alveolar-arterial oxygen gradient.

PRESSURE GRADIENTS AND TRANSPORT OF OXYGEN AND CARBON DIOXIDE

34 Compare the PO_2 levels of the pulmonary alveoli, pulmonary capillary blood, and arterial blood.

❑ The PO_2 in the pulmonary alveoli calculated by the alveolar gas equation is approximately 100 mm Hg. The PO_2 of mixed venous blood reaching the alveolus is approximately 40 mm Hg, and increases up to a value almost identical to that of the alveolar gas (ie, blood PO_2 in the pulmonary capillary is also approximately 100 mm Hg). However, PO_2 of arterial blood is approximately 90 mm Hg, that is, 10 mm Hg lower than that of pulmonary capillary blood. This PO_2 reduction is accounted for by the 2% of blood that is not exposed to the alveolar atmosphere because it belongs to the bronchial circulation that has a venous blood PO_2 of about 40 mm Hg (value similar to that of systemic venous blood). Thus, the bronchial venous blood represents a "shunt" of poorly oxygenated blood which is added to the well-oxygenated blood that exits the alveolar capillaries.

---

35 Compare the PO_2 and PCO_2 and their correspondent pressure gradients (driving force of gas diffusion) between the blood compartment and the peripheral tissues.

❑ The PO_2 of arterial blood is identical to the value found in the arterial end of capillaries (ie, 95 mm Hg), and about fourfold the mean tissue PO_2 (ie, 23 mm Hg). Therefore, there is a large pressure gradient that promotes rapid diffusion of oxygen from the blood into the tissues. Except for the arterial end of the capillaries that have a high PO_2 level, capillary blood PO_2 is approximately 40 mm Hg, a value similar to that found at the venous end of the capillaries and in venous blood. In contrast to the high oxygen gradient that drives oxygen into the tissues, the carbon dioxide gradient that allows exit of this metabolite from the tissues into the blood is very small (ie, only 1 mm Hg). The PCO_2 of arterial blood and that of the arterial end of capillaries are identical (ie, 40 mm Hg). The pressure gradient of carbon dioxide between tissues and capillary blood is only 1 mm Hg because the values of the former and the latter are 46 and 45 mm Hg, respectively. The venous blood PCO_2 is also 45 mm Hg, a value identical to that of capillary blood.

---

36 Compare the amount of oxygen and carbon dioxide transported in the blood and the corresponding values consumed and produced, respectively, by the tissues under normal conditions.

❑ Each deciliter of arterial blood transports 20 mL of oxygen and 48 mL of carbon dioxide toward the peripheral tissues. However, each deciliter of mixed venous blood transports 15 mL of oxygen and 52 mL of carbon dioxide toward the lungs where the capillary blood will gain oxygen and lose carbon dioxide and become, once more, arterial blood. Consequently, 5 mL of oxygen and 4 mL of carbon dioxide per deciliter of blood (mL/dL is also known as *volumes percent*) represent the arteriovenous difference, which is in turn explained by tissue metabolism (at one end) and lung function (at the other end). The ratio of 4 mL of carbon dioxide and 5 mL of oxygen per deciliter of blood (arteriovenous difference) is equal to 0.8, a value that is identical to the respiratory quotient (ie, $\dot{V}CO_2/\dot{V}O_2$) estimated by a different method.

ROLE OF HEMOGLOBIN IN OXYGEN TRANSPORT

37 How much oxygen can be transported by the Hb in the normal state?

❑ Approximately 20 mL of oxygen can be transported by the Hb contained in 100 mL of blood when this molecule is 100% saturated with oxygen (ie, 15 gm of Hb × 1.34 mL of oxygen = 20 mL). Yet, under normal conditions only 5 mL of oxygen (25% of total load, also called *utilization coefficient*) is released to the peripheral tissues. Expressed differently, only 5 volumes percent from the 20 volumes percent is delivered to the tissues, and this expression (ie, volume percent) can be used instead of percent saturation in the oxygen-Hb dissociation curve.

38 Compare the amount of oxygen transported in the dissolved state and that carried by the Hb in the blood in the normal state.

❑ The oxygen content of blood represents the sum of the oxygen dissolved in the fluid phase (ie, solution) and the oxygen bound to Hb. The former is calculated by multiplying the arterial PO_2 times 0.003 (constant factor). Consequently, at the normal arterial PO_2 of 95 mm Hg, the amount of dissolved oxygen is approximately 0.3 mL/dL of blood, whereas at the normal venous PO_2 of 40 mm Hg the amount of dissolved oxygen is about 0.1

mL/dL of blood. Thus, only 0.2 mL of dissolved oxygen per deciliter of blood is released to the tissues as compared to 5 mL of oxygen transported by the Hb in an identical volume of blood that is released to the tissues (dissolved oxygen is only 3% of the total amount released in the tissues).

39 How much oxygen is released under normal conditions from the Hb to the peripheral tissues per deciliter of blood? Compare this value with the oxygen consumption per minute.

❑ Under normal conditions, approximately 5 mL of oxygen per deciliter of blood is released to the tissues (an identical amount is taken up from the pulmonary alveoli replenishing the blood oxygen content). The tissue oxygen consumption can be estimated by subtracting the oxygen content of mixed venous blood (ie, 14.4 mL/dL) from the oxygen content of arterial blood (ie, 19.4 mL/dL). Consequently, the delivery of the 250 mL of oxygen per minute for consumption by the tissues under resting conditions requires a cardiac output of approximately 5 L/min, as follows:

$$\frac{5 \text{ mL } O_2}{0.1 \text{ L blood}} \times 5 \text{ L/min} = 250 \text{ mL/min}$$

40 Elaborate on the clinical importance of the Hb level in the oxygen-carrying capacity of the blood.

❑ The oxygen content of blood represents the sum of oxygen bound to Hb and the oxygen dissolved in the fluid phase (ie, solution), as follows:

$$\begin{aligned}\text{Oxygen content of blood} &= O_2 \text{ combined to Hb} + O_2 \text{ in solution} \\ &= (1.34 \times \text{Hb} \times SO_2) + (PO_2 \times 0.003) \\ &= (1.34 \times 15 \times 0.97) + (95 \times 0.003) \\ &= 19.5 + 0.3\end{aligned}$$

where SO_2 is percent saturation of Hb. Consequently, the Hb level is a critically important determinant of the oxygen-carrying capacity of the blood. It is not possible to effectively increase the oxygen content of blood in patients with substantial anemia (eg, Hb <10 gm/dL) by raising the PO_2 in an attempt to increase the oxygen dissolved in solution. Correction of this defect requires administration of red blood cells (blood transfusion).

41 Is arterial PO_2 a reliable indicator of the oxygen content of blood? Explain the effect of carbon monoxide intoxication on oxygen transport.

❑ No. Arterial PO_2 is not a reliable indicator of the oxygen content of the blood because in the absence of Hb or if Hb is not functional, the oxygen content of blood is extremely small and not compatible with life. Severe carbon monoxide intoxication represents a typical example of this defect as patients affected with this condition frequently have normal arterial PO_2 but life-threatening tissue hypoxia because the oxygen content of blood is greatly reduced as a result of carboxyhemoglobin formation. The Hb bound to carbon monoxide is unable to transport oxygen. In addition, carbon monoxide impairs the ability of the Hb to release oxygen in the tissues because it shifts to the left the dissociation curve of the Hb that remains capable of binding oxygen.

42 Describe conditions in which the fraction of oxygen transported in the dissolved state is either substantially smaller or larger than the value observed in the normal resting state.

❑ The fraction of oxygen transported in the dissolved state decreases (although the absolute value increases) during strenuous exercise because the amount of oxygen released from the Hb to the tissues might increase threefold; consequently, as little as 1.5% of the total oxygen delivered to the tissues originates from that transported as dissolved oxygen during exercise. On the contrary, a substantially larger fraction of oxygen transported in the dissolved state is observed in patients breathing an oxygen-rich mixture. In the latter condition, the high PaO_2 can lead to the development of a syndrome of oxygen toxicity.

43 Does Hb participate in the transport of gases other than oxygen and carbon dioxide?

❑ Besides transporting oxygen from lungs to tissues and carting back carbon dioxide, Hb distributes a third gas, nitric oxide. Consequently, Hb seems to be able to make the blood vessels expand or contract by regulating the amount of nitric oxide to which they are exposed. The iron of Hb is known to have a strong affinity for nitric oxide after it has released its oxygen in the tissues, where it picks up carbon dioxide and nitric oxide. Another part of the Hb, a segment of its protein chain known as a *cysteine residue,* can hold and release super nitric oxide (one electron added to nitric oxide), a chemical form that is not mopped up by the iron atoms of Hb. When a red blood cell enters the lung, its Hb molecules release carbon dioxide and pick up both oxygen and super nitric oxide (produced in the lungs and transferred to the cysteine residues in Hb). The red blood cell travels through the arteries and into the capillary blood vessels of peripheral tissues where oxygen is released. Free of oxygen, the iron atoms of Hb can then trap any local excess of ordinary nitric oxide, making blood vessels contract. But the Hb changes shape as the oxygen leaves and can also release super nitric oxide, making blood vessels relax. When the red blood cell returns to the lungs, it releases carbon dioxide and the ordinary kind of nitric oxide bound to the iron atoms. The Hb then picks up more oxygen and super nitric oxide and the cycle continues.

OXYHEMOGLOBIN DISSOCIATION CURVE

44 What is the oxyhemoglobin dissociation curve?

❑ The oxyhemoglobin dissociation curve represents the relationship between the percent saturation of Hb with oxygen (depicted in the standard diagram on the vertical or "y" axis since SaO_2 is the dependent variable) and the ambient PO_2 (depicted on the horizontal or "x" axis since PO_2 is the independent variable). As the PO_2 increases, there is a progressive increase in the percentage of the Hb that is bound with oxygen. The shape of the curve has a major impact on the uptake of oxygen by Hb in the lungs and its release in peripheral tissues. In addition, physiologic conditions as well as diseases can shift the oxyhemoglobin dissociation curve to the left (ie, increased affinity of Hb for oxygen) or to the right (ie, decreased affinity of Hb for oxygen).

45 What are the PO_2 levels associated with a Hb SO_2 of 10, 30, 50, 70, and 90% (at normal temperature of 37°C and pH 7.40). Explain the concept of P_{50}.

❑ Examination of the normal oxyhemoglobin dissociation curve reveals that the PO_2 values corresponding to 10, 30, 50, 70, and 90% SO_2 are approximately 10, 19, 26.6, 37, and 58 mm Hg, respectively. The PaO_2 that results in 50% SO_2, known as *P_{50}*, is commonly used as a measure of the affinity of Hb for oxygen (normal value is 26.6 mm Hg). A higher P_{50} is observed when the oxyhemoglobin curve shifts to the right, decreasing the affinity of Hb for oxygen (salutary effect). Conversely, a lower P_{50} is observed when the oxyhemoglobin curve shifts to the left, increasing the affinity of Hb for oxygen (nonsalutary effect).

46 What are the major influences on the oxyhemoglobin dissociation curve? When does this curve shift to the right or to the left? What are the effects of these shifts on the release of oxygen to the tissues?

❑ Major factors that modify the oxyhemoglobin dissociation curve include the type of Hb (eg, fetal, adult, and other types), blood temperature, PCO_2, blood pH, level of 2,3-diphosphoglycerate (2,3-DPG) in the red blood cells, and concentration of carboxyhemoglobin. A shift of the curve to the right indicates a decreased oxygen affinity, therefore facilitating the release of oxygen to the tissues; this effect is observed in the presence of abnormal Hbs (eg, E, Seattle, Kansas), hyperthermia, hypercapnia, acidosis, and increased 2,3-DPG levels. Conversely, a shift of the curve to the left indicates increased oxygen affinity, therefore decreasing the release of oxygen to the tissues; this effect is observed in the presence of large quantities of fetal Hb (and other types including Hb Yakenia, Chesapeake, Ranier), hypothermia, hypocapnia, alkalosis, decreased 2,3-DPG levels, and high concentration of carboxyhemoglobin.

47 Explain further the shape of the oxyhemoglobin dissociation curve and its physiologic importance.

❑ The oxygen dissociation curve of a solution of pure Hb is hyperbolic whereas it has a sigmoid shape when red blood cells are intact due to interaction of Hb with 2,3-DPG and other factors that participate in its physiologic control. The initial part of the curve is steep, having large changes in Hb saturation with modest changes in PO_2 (ie, SO_2 increases from 10% to 70% when PO_2 increases from 10 to 37 mm Hg). Conversely, the final part of the curve is flat, having small changes in Hb saturation with large changes in PO_2 (ie, SO_2 increases from 70.0% to 97.5% when PO_2 augments from 37 to 100 mm Hg). The steep portion of the curve facilitates the unloading of oxygen from the Hb in peripheral tissues in the presence of a mild decrease in PO_2. On the other hand, the flat portion of the oxyhemoglobin curve facilitates adequate loading with oxygen in the lungs, even in the presence of a large decrease of PO_2 in the pulmonary alveoli that can occur because of a low PiO_2 or pulmonary disease. The behavior of the Hb favors a nearly maximum uptake of oxygen in the lungs and the release of this gas in the tissues.

48 Explain the role of Hb in the maintenance of a relatively constant PO_2 in peripheral tissues in the presence of large changes of alveolar PO_2 (ie, caused changes in PiO_2 and pulmonary diseases).

❑ The relatively flat upper portion of the oxygen-hemoglobin dissociation curve accounts for the small change in the percent oxygen saturation of arterial blood when the alveolar PO_2 decreases to 60 mm Hg (ie, 89% SO_2) or increases to 500 mm Hg (ie, 99% SO_2); these values represent a decrease of only 8% and an increase of only 2% with respect to the normal saturation of 97%, respectively. Because the tissues will remove about 5 mL of oxygen per deciliter of blood, the corresponding values for SO_2 in mixed venous blood will be 77% (43 mm Hg PO_2) and 67% (35 mm Hg PO_2). Consequently, the PO_2 in the tissues does not change more than a few millimeters of mercury in spite of a large change in alveolar PO_2.

49 Compare the amount of oxygen released by the Hb under normal conditions and that observed with shifts in either direction of the oxyhemoglobin dissociation curve.

❑ A shift in either direction of the oxyhemoglobin dissociation curve may substantially change the oxygen released to the tissues. For example, at a blood pH of 7.20 the oxygen released by Hb is approximately 30% larger than that released at a blood pH of 7.60 (these pH values correspond to curves shifted to the right and to the left, respectively, as compared to the normal oxyhemoglobin curve at pH 7.40).

50 How does the oxyhemoglobin dissociation curve shift during exercise? What are the determinants of the shift?

❑ A shift to the right of the oxyhemoglobin dissociation curve of the capillary blood that perfuses muscle is observed during exercise. The main factors responsible for this effect include (1) increased muscle temperature of up to 3°C, (2) higher tissue PCO_2 levels caused by augmented carbon dioxide production, (3) acidemia caused by the higher PCO_2 and lower plasma bicarbonate concentration ($[HCO_3^-]_p$) (secondary to lactic acidosis), and (4) release of phosphate compounds from muscle. Consequently, 75% to 85% of the oxygen transported by the Hb can be released to the tissues, in contrast to only 25% observed in the normal resting state.

51 What are the levels of PO_2 and the percent saturation of the Hb with oxygen in arterial and mixed venous blood in healthy humans?

❑ The oxygen saturation of arterial blood is approximately 97% because PaO_2 is approximately 95 mm Hg in healthy humans. The values for SO_2 and PO_2 in mixed venous blood (collected from the pulmonary artery and representing a sample of normal venous blood returning from peripheral tissues) are 75% and 40 mm Hg, respectively.

52 What is the Bohr effect? What is its importance?

❑ The Bohr effect refers to the shift of the oxygen-Hb dissociation curve caused by changes in blood PCO_2. This process has important physiologic significance because it facilitates oxygen loading of the Hb in the lungs as well as its unloading in the tissues. The loss of carbon dioxide from the blood to the pulmonary alveoli reduces the blood carbonic acid level and its $[H^+]$. Consequently, an upward displacement of the curve that also shifts to the left is observed with the carbon dioxide loss, thereby augmenting the oxygen uptake by the Hb as blood passes through the lungs. The opposite phenomenon occurs in peripheral tissues as carbon dioxide gain by the blood shifts the curve to the right. This rightward displacement of the oxyhemoglobin dissociation curve promotes larger unloading of oxygen in the tissues.

53 How does the Hb help to maintain a relatively constant PO_2 in peripheral tissues in states of augmented tissue oxygen demands (eg, heavy exercise)?

❑ The steep lower portion of the oxygen-Hb dissociation curve is characterized by a large change in the percent saturation of Hb with oxygen in association with a relatively small decrease in PO_2.

This portion of the dissociation curve facilitates the release of oxygen in the tissues, especially during exercise. In the normal state SvO_2 is 75% and PO_2 is 40 mm Hg, but during heavy muscular exercise SvO_2 is 30% and PO_2 is 20 mm Hg. Thus, SvO_2 decreases by 45% (ie, from 75% to 30%) during exercise. The relatively small decrease in tissue PO_2 from 40 to 20 mm Hg is accompanied by the release of an additional 9 mL of oxygen per deciliter of blood (eg, 15 gm of Hb $\times$ 1.34 mL of O_2 $\times$ 0.45 = 9 mL). Thus, the Hb helps to maintain a relatively constant PO_2 in the tissues when PaO_2 decreases markedly and when tissue oxygen demands augment substantially; this property is often referred to as the effect of Hb to "buffer" the tissue oxygen tension.

3. Carbon Dioxide

SOURCES OF CARBON DIOXIDE

54 What are the sources of carbon dioxide and how large are the whole-body stores of this gas? Compare the daily production of volatile and fixed acids by normal adults.

❑ In humans consuming an acid ash diet, intermediary metabolism results in the production of both volatile (carbonic acid) and fixed acids; the former are excreted as carbon dioxide by the lungs, whereas the latter are eliminated by the kidneys. The daily rate of carbon dioxide production by cellular metabolism in normal adults under basal conditions is approximately 15,000 mmol. During maximal exercise carbon dioxide production increases by as much as 20-fold, but as noted, the associated hyperpnea maintains the PCO_2 in body fluids relatively constant. The daily rate of nonvolatile (fixed) acids requiring excretion amounts to 70 to 100 mmol in normal adults and is therefore orders of magnitude smaller than that of volatile acids. Consequently, the values for the daily production of volatile and fixed acids presented above indicate that the level of the former is about 200-fold that of the latter. This marked difference between the rates of production and excretion of carbon dioxide and those of the metabolic acids affords insight into the almost immediate derangement in acid-base balance that follows severe pulmonary hypoventilation; on the other hand, it takes days to alter plasma acidity to a similar degree after cessation of renal function. In normal individuals maintaining a relatively uniform level of activity and diet, the daily rate of carbon dioxide production is remarkably constant. Diets very rich in carbohydrates yield greater amounts of carbon dioxide and this effect might have clinical implications in patients with respiratory failure and those with limited ventilatory reserve. The whole-body stores of carbon dioxide are large even at normal PCO_2, amounting to approximately 1.8 L/kg of body weight. Most of these extractable carbon dioxide stores are present as bone carbonates, followed by carbon dioxide retained in the form of bicarbonate ions that are distributed throughout the body fluids.

55 How is the daily production of volatile acid measured?

❑ The daily production of volatile acid (ie, carbonic acid) is assessed by measuring pulmonary carbon dioxide excretion because the lungs are the exclusive organs involved in the final disposal of volatile acids. As was the case for production and excretion of fixed acids, in a steady state, production and excretion of volatile acids are identical. Thus, measurement of pulmonary carbon dioxide excretion permits quantification of carbon dioxide production.

CARBON DIOXIDE TRANSPORT

56 Outline the transport of carbon dioxide from the cells to the external environment.

❑ The uninterrupted flow of blood continuously transports the carbon dioxide produced by the tissues to the lungs for final excretion to the atmosphere. Most of the carbon dioxide entering the circulation is converted to nongaseous forms for transport by mechanisms that depend largely on certain properties of Hb. Yet, the process of diffusion is the fundamental driving force responsible for the steady flow of carbon dioxide from the tissues to the blood and from the blood to the alveolar spaces of the lungs. Accordingly, a progressive pressure gradient for carbon dioxide is required to transfer carbon dioxide across the several membranes between its sites of production and the alveolar spaces. However, because of the efficiency with which gaseous carbon dioxide is converted to other molecular forms in the bloodstream, the transport of carbon dioxide from tissues to lungs is accomplished with a remarkably small gradient for PCO_2; thus, the impact of carbon dioxide production per se on the level of acidity is greatly minimized. The PCO_2 gradient between tissues and pulmonary alveoli is only 6 mm Hg, as mean tissue PCO_2 and alveolar PCO_2 are approximately 46 and 40 mm Hg, respectively. If the transport of carbon dioxide were to occur exclusively as physically dissolved gaseous carbon dioxide in the plasma, a partial pressure gradient of carbon dioxide between tissues and lungs greater than 10 times the normal value would be required to secure excretion of the daily carbon dioxide load.

57 Explain further the transport of carbon dioxide in the blood.

❑ The content of carbon dioxide in the blood increases as a function of PCO_2. Such relationship, known as the *carbon dioxide dissociation curve,* is relatively linear, as opposed to the oxyhemoglobin dissociation curve (sigmoid shape). The higher carbon dioxide content in blood as PCO_2 increases is caused by a larger amount of carbon dioxide in all different forms of this gas within blood (ie, free carbon dioxide, carbon dioxide chemically combined with water, Hb, and plasma proteins). At the normal arterial PCO_2 of 40 mm Hg, the carbon dioxide content of blood is 48 mL/dL whereas at the normal mixed venous PCO_2 of 45 mm Hg, the carbon dioxide content is 52 mL/dL. Only 5% of the carbon dioxide content of mixed venous blood is transported in the dissolved state (eg, 2.7 mL/dL represents 5% of 52 mL/dL).

58 Compare the diffusion of oxygen and carbon dioxide in body tissues.

❑ Carbon dioxide diffuses approximately 20 times as rapidly as oxygen. This property explains the much smaller pressure gradient of carbon dioxide as compared to oxygen in the tissues and the lungs. The PO_2 in the pulmonary alveoli is approximately 100 mm Hg and the PO_2 of mixed venous blood is about 40 mm Hg, resulting in a PO_2 gradient of 60 mm Hg between the alveolar gas and capillary blood. As PCO_2 in mixed venous blood is 45 mm Hg and alveolar PCO_2 is 40 mm Hg (identical to blood PCO_2 in the last two-thirds of the pulmonary capillaries and to arterial PCO_2), this gradient is about one-tenth of the PO_2 gradient (ie, 5 and 60 mm Hg are the PCO_2 and PO_2 gradients between alveolar gas and capillary blood, respectively).

59 How does carbon dioxide elimination occur from the capillary blood to the pulmonary alveoli?

❑ The entire sequence of events that results in the transfer of carbon dioxide from the tissues to the bloodstream is reversed in the pulmonary capillaries. Considering that the PCO_2 in the alveoli is lower than that in the blood compartment, the carbon dioxide pressure gradient allows for the unloading of carbon dioxide. The reduction in PCO_2 of the blood perfusing the pulmonary alveoli results in local alkalemia that challenges the Hb and other nonbicarbonate buffers of the blood; thus, these compounds release hydrogen ions that titrate bicarbonate ions inside and outside the red blood cells producing carbonic acid. Since oxygenation of the Hb transforms this compound into a stronger acid by decreasing the pK′ value of the imidazole group of histidine, the release of hydrogen ions by the Hb is further enhanced. The newly generated carbonic acid is rapidly dehydrated by red cell carbonic anhydrase as well as carbonic anhydrase residing on the endothelial surface of the alveolar capillaries. Carbamino carbon dioxide is also released for excretion. The very high permeability of the alveolar capillary membrane to carbon dioxide, about 20 times greater than that to oxygen, allows for the rapid equilibration of the blood and alveolar compartments, which occurs in a fraction of the transit time of the red cells along the pulmonary capillaries.

60 Explain the importance of the circulatory system in carbon dioxide excretion.

❑ The elimination of carbon dioxide requires adequate function of the circulatory system, in addition to the previously considered carbon dioxide transporting properties of the blood and the pulmonary ventilation. According to the Fick principle, the total carbon dioxide excretion is a function of the cardiac output ($\dot{Q}$, in

L/min) and the difference in the concentrations of carbon dioxide in venous and arterial blood, expressed as (Cv − Ca) CO_2:

$$\dot{V}CO_2 = \dot{Q} \times (Cv - Ca)\ CO_2$$

As can be seen from this equation, in the presence of a constant difference in the venoarterial carbon dioxide content, an increase in the cardiac output results in an increase in carbon dioxide excretion, and the converse is true if cardiac output decreases. This consideration has critical implications for the proper interpretation of arterial and venous blood gases in patients with abnormal circulatory status.

61 Elaborate further on the carbon dioxide transport in the blood. What is the Haldane effect?

❑ The initial step in this process is the entry of carbon dioxide from the tissues to the plasma in the form of carbon dioxide dissolved in water. A very small portion of metabolically produced carbon dioxide is transported as physically dissolved carbon dioxide; this amount is equal to the physical solubility coefficient for carbon dioxide (equal to 0.0301 mmol/L/mm Hg), times the partial pressure of carbon dioxide. Thus, at the normal value of mixed venous PCO_2 level of 45 mm Hg, the concentration of dissolved carbon dioxide in plasma is 1.35 mmol/L. The largest fraction of the carbon dioxide entering the plasma diffuses into the erythrocytes where conversion to nongaseous forms take place. The hydration of carbon dioxide in the red blood cell forms carbonic acid under the catalytic influences of erythrocytic carbonic anhydrase; carbonic acid then ionizes, with consequent production of bicarbonate ions and hydrogen ions. The buffer properties of Hb, which are enhanced in the tissue capillaries because of Hb's deoxygenation, neutralize the newly generated hydrogen ions; most of the bicarbonate ions formed diffuse from the erythrocyte into the plasma. At any given PCO_2, poorly oxygenated blood displays an enhanced capacity for transporting carbon dioxide as compared with oxygenated blood, a phenomenon known as the *Haldane effect.* The amount of carbon dioxide carried by whole blood in vitro increases as PCO_2 rises, approximating a straight line over the physiologic range of PCO_2, and no saturation point for carbon dioxide is reached. This pattern contrasts sharply with the sigmoid shape of the curve relating the oxygen content of whole blood to the prevailing PO_2, in which blood becomes fully saturated with oxygen at the upper range of physiologic PO_2 level.

62 How important is the Haldane effect in the transport and elimination of carbon dioxide from the tissues to the atmosphere?

❑ The increased capacity of the blood to transport carbon dioxide when exposed at low PO_2 and vice versa at high PO_2, known as the Haldane effect, is very important in the elimination of carbon dioxide. The Haldane effect doubles the amount of carbon dioxide taken by the blood in the tissues as well as doubles the amount of carbon dioxide released from the blood in the lungs. In other words, if there were no shift in the carbon dioxide dissociation curve with the change in PO_2 (absence of the Haldane effect), only 2 mL of carbon dioxide per deciliter of blood (as opposed to the normal value of 4 mL of carbon dioxide per deciliter of blood) would be loaded in the tissues and unloaded in the lungs in response to the change in PCO_2 of approximately 5 mm Hg (ie, $PaCO_2$ and $PvCO_2$ are 40 and 45 mm Hg, respectively). The Haldane effect is quantitatively far more important in facilitating carbon dioxide transport than is the Bohr effect in facilitating oxygen transport.

63 How important for the transport of carbon dioxide is the presence of carbonic anhydrase in red blood cells and in the pulmonary capillaries?

❑ Carbonic anhydrase accelerates the formation and decomposition of carbonic acid ($H_2CO_3 \Leftrightarrow CO_2 + H_2O$) by about 5000-fold. Consequently, the blood loading and unloading of carbon dioxide in the peripheral times and lungs, respectively, are achieved within a fraction of a second, instead of requiring many seconds or minutes to occur. Approximately 70% of the carbon dioxide transported between the tissues and the lungs is under the influence of the carbonic anhydrase.

64 What is the "chloride shift" in red blood cells? Explain the relative importance of each of the three mechanisms of carbon dioxide transport in the overall process of carbon dioxide excretion.

❑ The exit of bicarbonate from the red blood cells to the plasma would alter the electrical neutrality of the erythrocytes, which is restored by diffusion of chloride ions into the cells, a phenomenon known as the *chloride shift.* The rapid transport of anions is a distinct function of the red cell membrane that allows the "exchange diffusion" of chloride at a rate 2.5 million times faster than that of cations, such as potassium. This process is mediated by an anion exchanger protein of the erythrocytic membrane, known as *band 3 protein.* In the absence of the chloride shift, the buildup of cellular bicarbonate would limit the capacity of the erythrocytes to transport carbon dioxide. A substantial but smaller portion of the carbon dioxide entering the red cells combines directly and reversibly with certain amino groups of the Hb molecule forming carbamino compounds. The contributions of the three carbon dioxide transport processes of the blood, namely, dissolved carbon dioxide, carbamino compounds, and bicarbonate ions, to the total transport of carbon dioxide between tissues and lungs are approximately 8%, 10%, and 82%, respectively.

65 Compare the effects of differences in the carbon dioxide and the oxygen dissociation curves in the blood.

❑ The alteration in arterial blood gases (ABGs) that accompanies the various diseases of the lung is, to a significant extent, a reflection of differences in the carbon dioxide and oxygen dissociation curves in the blood. The nearly linear shape of the dissociation curve of carbon dioxide over the physiologic range allows greater than normal carbon dioxide excretion (due to hypoxemia-induced enhanced ventilation) from areas of the lungs with relatively undisturbed gas exchange. This phenomenon offsets the effects of simultaneous carbon dioxide retention occurring in areas of the lung that are consolidated or underventilated. On the other hand, the shape of the oxyhemoglobin dissociation curve explains the fact that hyperventilation of lung areas in which Hb is already saturated to the maximum with oxygen will not offset the right-to-left shunting of hypoxic blood perfusing capillaries in underventilated areas. As a consequence, arterial hypoxemia in association with hypocapnia, eucapnia, or hypercapnia is observed in "hypoxemic respiratory failure."

RESPIRATORY EXCHANGE RATIO

66 What is the respiratory exchange ratio?

❑ The respiratory exchange ratio (RE) is the quotient of carbon dioxide output to oxygen uptake in the lungs. The value of this ratio measured over a period of 60 minutes or longer is identical to the respiratory quotient of the chemical reactions occurring in the tissues. The average value of RE is 0.825, but it changes according to the substrate being metabolized (eg, carbohydrates and fats have RE values of 1.0 and 0.7, respectively).

67 Is the value of the respiratory quotient constant in the normal state?

❑ No. Since the respiratory quotient (RQ) is the ratio of carbon dioxide production and oxygen consumption, its value is dependent on the substrate providing energy to the tissues. Carbohydrate consumption raises the RQ to 1.0 whereas oxidation of fatty acids decreases its value to 0.7. In addition, physical exercise increases RQ toward 1.0. Considering that a mixture of energy substrates is generally utilized in body tissues, the RQ is approximately 0.8, a value that is applied in the alveolar gas equation (see pertinent questions).

4. Pulmonary Circulation

PULMONARY HEMODYNAMICS

68 What is cardiac output and how is it measured? Report the normal value of cardiac output (ie, pulmonary blood flow and systemic blood flow).

❑ Cardiac output is the volume of blood pumped per unit of time (usually expressed as L/min) by the heart into the systemic or pulmonary circulation, and is the product of stroke volume and heart rate. The two pumps in series, right and left ventricles, propel equal amounts of blood per minute and are responsible for the blood flow in the entire system. Consequently, the same volume of blood flows through each segment of the circulation each minute (cardiac output), and the velocity of blood in the arteries, capillaries, and veins is inversely proportional to their respective cross-sectional area. Thus, cardiac output is identical to both pulmonary blood flow and systemic blood flow. Cardiac output can be measured in patients by the Fick method (based on the Fick principle which states that blood flow through an organ or the whole body is equal to the amount of a substance taken up per unit of time such as oxygen, divided by the arterial minus the venous level of the substance, known as the arteriovenous [A-V] difference) and the indicator dilution method. In the latter technique, a known amount of an indicator (eg, dye such as indocyanine green, or radioactive isotope) is injected into an arm vein, and the concentration of the indicator in serial samples of arterial blood is measured (ie, cardiac output is equal to the amount of indicator injected divided by its average concentration in arterial blood after a single circulation through the heart). The indicator dilution technique most commonly used is based on thermodilution and the indicator injected is cold saline solution (ie, injected into the right atrium via a double-lumen catheter and the temperature change of blood is measured by a thermistor probe located in the pulmonary artery). Cardiac output is best expressed per unit of body surface area (usually in square meters), known as *cardiac index* (normal range, 2.3 to 3.9 L/min/m^2). A cardiac index of less than 2.0 L/min/m^2 produces severe tissue hypoperfusion.

69 Is the blood flow produced by the left ventricle identical to that of the right ventricle? Are the functions of the right and left ventricles of equal importance in maintaining the circulation under normal conditions?

❑ The left ventricular output is theoretically slightly higher than that of the right ventricle due to the small blood flow in the bronchial arteries that drains into the pulmonary veins, and the coronary blood flow that drains into the left atrium and ventricle through the thebesian veins. In addition, changes in body position, respiratory cycle (inspiration and expiration), and physiologic adjustments might cause transient and very short-lasting periods (seconds) in which a substantial differential in left and right ventricular outputs develops. However, the mean cardiac output of the left and right ventricles is, for practical purposes, identical. In experimental settings, the right ventricle is not required for maintenance of pulmonary blood flow and arterial pressure at rest. When this chamber is excluded from the circulation (ie, experimentally bypassed), the left ventricle maintains the entire circulation although fluid retention and a mild increase in venous pressure develop. By contrast, right ventricular function is important in maintaining adequate circulation during exercise, in states of increased pulmonary vascular resistance, and during hypovolemia.

70 What are the general determinants of arterial blood pressure in both pulmonary and systemic circulations?

❑ The determinants of arterial blood pressure are conveniently grouped as physical and physiologic. The physical determinants of arterial pressure are (1) the blood volume within the arterial system (arterial blood volume) and (2) the elastic characteristics (pressure-volume relationship or compliance) of the arterial compartment. The physiologic determinants modify the physical ones, that is, the arterial blood volume and compliance, through changes in total circulating blood volume, arterial "inflow" or cardiac output, arterial "outflow" or peripheral runoff, and properties of the vascular wall (structural and functional changes). Thus, physiologic factors operate on the physical determinants of arterial blood pressure in the pulmonary circulation as well as on the systemic circulation.

71 What are the specific determinants of arterial blood pressure in both pulmonary and systemic circulations?

❑ Mean arterial pressure is determined by cardiac output and vascular resistance (impediment to blood flow through the vessels) according to Ohm's law (electric circuit theory) and Poiseuille's law (flow of fluids theory). Ohm's law applied to the circulation establishes that

$$\dot{Q} \text{ (fluid flow)} = \frac{\Delta P \text{ (pressure difference)}}{R \text{ (resistance)}}$$

in which $\dot{Q}$ is blood flow or cardiac output, ΔP is the pressure difference between the beginning and end of the circulation (eg, since the systemic circulation ends in the right atrium, which has a pressure of about 0 mm Hg, ΔP is identical to mean arterial pressure), and R is vascular resistance. Poiseuille's law specifically applies to straight and rigid tubes filled with homogeneous fluid and having steady laminar flow. Although these conditions do not strictly apply to blood vessels in vivo, the law is often used to describe blood flow in vivo. Poiseuille's law establishes that

$$\text{Fluid flow} = \frac{\pi \times \text{Pressure difference} \times \text{Radius}^4}{8 \times \text{Vessel length} \times \text{Fluid viscosity}}$$

where π and 8 are constants of proportionality. The hydraulic resistance according to this law is

$$R = \frac{\text{Pressure difference}}{\text{Fluid flow}}$$

$$= \frac{8 \times \text{Vessel length} \times \text{Fluid viscosity}}{\pi \times \text{Radius}^4}$$

Consequently, Poiseuille's law allows for further dissection of the various components responsible for vascular resistance in the circulation (pulmonary and systemic).

72 What principles governing the pulmonary and systemic circulations derive from Ohm's and Poiseuille's laws?

❑ These laws and corresponding equations establish that (1) blood flow is directly proportional to the pressure difference but inversely proportional to the vascular resistance; (2) vascular resistance is dramatically and inversely influenced by vessel radius because the latter is raised to the fourth power; (3) blood vessels connected in parallel (an advantageous arrangement found in most capillary beds) have less resistance to flow than if they were connected in series, and in addition, parallel arrangement of blood vessels provides a greater total cross-sectional area with the same resistance as a single wide tube (ie, the total resistance of 16 small tubes with four times the total cross-sectional area is the same as that of a single wide tube); and (4) blood viscosity, which might be altered by changes in hematocrit, serum proteins, and temperature, might have a significant effect on flow and circulatory pressure when acting on small vessels of the pulmonary and systemic circulations.

73 How is the resistance to blood flow in the pulmonary and systemic circulations, known as *vascular resistance*, measured and expressed?

❑ The impediment to blood flow through vessels (simply called *vascular resistance*) cannot be measured directly but must be calculated from measurements of blood flow and pressure differences along the circulation. Vascular resistance is calculated by dividing mean pressure difference between two points in the vascular system by the blood flow between them (ie, mean amount of blood passing from one point to the other per unit of time). Vascular resistance might be expressed in various units, including the following:

1. Peripheral resistance units (PRUs), in which the pressure gradient is expressed in millimeters of mercury and blood flow in milliliters per second. Because in normal adults at rest the pressure difference between the systemic arteries and veins is about 100 mm Hg, and the simultaneously measured cardiac output is about 100 mL/sec (ie, 6 L/min amounts to 6000 mL flowing through the circulatory system in 60 seconds), the total peripheral resistance is about 1 PRU (100/100 = 1).
2. CGS (cm-gm-sec) units, which are obtained by multiplying PRUs by a conversion factor of 1332 and allows for expression of vascular resistance in $dyn \cdot sec \cdot cm^{-5}$ which is the conventional unit employed in both fluid mechanics and hemodynamic monitoring.
3. R units in which the pressure gradient is expressed in millimeters of mercury and blood flow in liters per minute. This unit may be converted to CGS units by multiplying its value times 80. Calculation of vascular resistance in R units and subsequent multiplication by 80 is the standard method utilized in clinical settings including intensive care units and hemodynamics laboratories.

74 What are the major factors that control the caliber or lumen diameter of blood vessels of the pulmonary and systemic circulations?

❑ The caliber of blood vessels is controlled by vascular smooth muscle that contracts and relaxes in response to various stimuli, a process known as *vasomotion.* The major factors that influence vasomotion include (1) the autonomic nervous system, whose fibers innervate the blood vessels and locally release norepinephrine or acetylcholine, which has a major role in the control of the caliber of vessels in the systemic circulation but only a modest role in the pulmonary circulation; (2) metabolic, chemical, and hormonal substances locally produced or carried in the bloodstream; and (3) the vascular endothelium, which produces vasodilatory (eg, nitric oxide, also known as *endothelium-derived relaxing factor* or EDRF) and vasoconstrictor (eg, endothelin-1) substances that are involved in the local modulation of vascular smooth-muscle contraction. The relative importance of these mechanisms varies markedly from one vascular bed to another. In most organs the autonomic nervous system works synergistically with nonneural influences (eg, PO_2, PCO_2, K^+, prostaglandins, nitric oxide) to regulate regional blood flow.

75 Compare the normal levels of systemic and pulmonary vascular resistance.

❑ The mean normal systemic vascular resistance (SVR) expressed in CGS units in an adult is about 1200 units (ie, [90 mm Hg ÷ 6 L/min] × 80 = 1200 units) and the range is 770 to 1500 dyn · sec · cm^{-5}. SVR can be transiently as high as four times the mean normal value (about 5000 units) in the presence of generalized vasoconstriction. Conversely, SVR can be transiently as low as one-fourth of the mean normal value (about 300 units) in the presence of generalized vasodilation. SVR is calculated from hemodynamic monitoring data as follows:

$$\text{SVR} = \frac{\text{MAP (mm Hg)} - \text{CVP (mm Hg)}}{\text{Cardiac output (L/min)}} \times 80$$

where MAP (mean arterial pressure) might be calculated as follows:

$$\text{MAP} = (\text{systolic BP} - \text{diastolic BP})\ \tfrac{1}{3} + \text{diastolic BP}$$

and CVP (central venous pressure) is either measured or estimated. The mean normal pulmonary vascular resistance (PVR) expressed in CGS units in an adult is about 70 units (ie, [5 mm Hg ÷ 6 L/min] × 80 = 67 units). The conventional normal range of PVR is 20 to 120 dyn · sec · cm^{-5}. PVR is calculated from hemodynamic monitoring data as follows:

$$\text{PVR} = \frac{\text{MPAP (mm Hg)} - \text{PAOP (mm Hg)}}{\text{Cardiac output (L/min)}}.$$

where MPAP is mean pulmonary artery pressure (eg, 13 mm Hg), and PAOP is pulmonary artery occlusion pressure that measures mean pulmonary wedge pressure, which is approximately equal to the left atrial pressure (eg, 8 mm Hg; range, 2 to 12 mm Hg).

76 Should increased and decreased vascular resistance in the pulmonary and systemic circulation be equated with arteriolar constriction and dilation, respectively?

❑ No. The interpretation of increases and decreases in vascular resistance as indicative of vasoconstriction and vasodilation, respectively, is a gross oversimplification. Other factors including vascular occlusion (which increases vascular resistance), active bleeding (which decreases vascular resistance), and changes in blood viscosity modify calculated levels of vascular resistance.

77 Explain the determinants of cardiac pumping toward the pulmonary and systemic circulations. What are cardiac preload and afterload, two major determinants of stroke volume and of performance of the intact ventricle (left or right)?

❑ *Preload* is the cardiac filling at the end of diastole (ie, end-diastolic filling pressure) which, according to Starling's law of the heart, helps determine the force of ventricular contraction during systole. *Afterload* is the resistance to ejection of blood at the initiation of ventricular contraction during systole (eg, aortic blood pressure for left ventricle, pulmonary artery pressure for right ventricle). The concepts of preload and afterload arise from in vitro studies of papillary muscle or atrial myocardium in which one end of the muscle is attached to a tension transducer and the other end is attached to a lever that is free to move. A small weight, termed *preload,* is placed on the lever to stretch the muscle, and a "stop" is applied so that any weight added on the lever will neither stretch the muscle nor be sensed by this tissue until it starts contraction in response to electrical stimulation. Loads added once the "stop" has been applied represent the *afterload.* Total load imposed on the preparation equals the sum of preload and afterload.

78 How do changes in total blood volume and fraction of blood volume held in the thorax modify cardiac preload? What is the effect of increased intrathoracic pressure on cardiac preload?

❑ A decreased and increased total blood volume will decrease and increase preload, respectively, in the absence of compensatory mechanisms. However, activation of the adrenergic nervous system allows maintenance of a constant preload if reductions of blood volume are small (<15% of total volume) or gradual. At any given total blood volume, preload increases when a greater fraction of blood is held in the thorax (eg, recumbent posture, deep inspiration, head-out water immersion, inflation of a lower-body positive-pressure suit, absence of gravitational force during space flight). Conversely, preload decreases when a greater fraction of blood is held outside the thorax (eg, increased intrathoracic pressure due to pneumothorax or application of positive-pressure ventilation, upright posture, suction applied to the lower extremities and trunk). Increased pericardial pressure due to effusion within this cavity and constrictive pericarditis also reduce preload.

79 How reliable is measurement of ejection fraction (ratio of stroke volume and end-diastolic volume) in the evaluation of myocardial contractility of patients with cardiorespiratory failure? What is its normal value?

❑ Ejection fraction is a commonly used and reliable index of cardiac performance that can be estimated by different techniques including radionuclide or radiocontrast angiography, two-dimensional echocardiography, and cinemagnetic resonance imaging. However, ejection fraction is significantly altered by changes in ventricular loading conditions, both preload and afterload, thereby precluding its use as a reliable index of myocardial contractility. Thus, a decreased ejection fraction and cardiac output may be observed with reduced preload (eg, hypovolemia) or increased afterload (eg, pulmonary or systemic hypertension) despite normal myocardial contractility. The ejection fraction (normal range, 0.55 to 0.78; mean value, 0.67; significant depression is <0.50) remains a useful clinical index of ventricular contractility despite the limitations.

80 What is the pressure gradient along the pulmonary and systemic circulations?

❑ Since the left and right ventricles pump blood directly into the aorta and pulmonary artery, respectively, these vessels have the highest pressure within each circuit. The systolic and diastolic pressures in the aorta and systemic arteries are about 120 and about 75 mm Hg, respectively, and the mean value is about 90 mm Hg. The systolic and diastolic pressures in the pulmonary artery are about 25 and about 10 mm Hg, with a mean pressure of about 15 mm Hg. The mean arterial pressure in each circuit can be estimated as the sum of systolic pressure, plus diastolic pressure multiplied by two, and the value obtained is divided by three. The large resistance to blood flow through the arterioles is responsible for the major decrease in pressure that occurs when blood flows from arteries to capillaries (about 17 and 7 mm Hg in the systemic and pulmonary capillaries, respectively). The lowest blood pressure in the circulation occurs at the termination of the venae cavae in the right atrium (about 0 mm Hg) and at the entrance of pulmonary veins in the left atrium (about 2 mm Hg).

STARLING'S LAW APPLIED TO THE PULMONARY CAPILLARIES

81 Describe Starling's law of fluid exchange across capillary walls of the pulmonary circulation and other vascular beds.

❑ Osmotic forces contribute to the distribution of water across capillary walls, yet the high permeability of these membranes to sodium salts and glucose makes these solutes ineffective determinants of intravascular volume. By contrast, plasma proteins are effective osmoles in the vascular space as these large molecules do not significantly cross the capillary walls. The transfer of fluid by convection across the capillary walls is determined by the difference between forces that favor filtration and forces that favor reabsorption. Starling's law can be generally expressed as follows:

$$\text{Net fluid transfer} = \text{Permeability of the capillaries} \times (\text{Filtration forces} - \text{Reabsorption forces})$$

82 Provide a more detailed explanation of the various components of Starling's law of capillary-interstitial fluid exchange.

❑ Starling's law can be described as follows, using the general formula of fluid transfer by convection, described earlier:

$$J_V = (\Delta P + \Delta\pi) \times A \times L_P$$

where J_V is net fluid transfer or net volume flux, ΔP is hydrostatic pressure gradient, $\Delta\pi$ is osmotic pressure gradient, A is membrane area for volume flow, and L_P is hydraulic permeability of the membrane. The ΔP is calculated as follows:

$$\Delta P = P_{cap} - P_{ISF}$$

where P_{cap} is capillary hydrostatic pressure and P_{ISF} is interstitial fluid hydrostatic pressure. The $\Delta\pi$ is calculated as follows:

$$\Delta\pi = \pi_p - \pi_{ISF}$$

where π_p is plasma oncotic pressure and π_{ISF} is interstitial oncotic pressure (due to filtered plasma proteins and interstitial mucopolysaccharides). The term K_f (filtration coefficient, or net permeability of capillary membrane) is most frequently used in Starling's equation to replace the terms $A \times L_P$ (surface area available for fluid transfer multiplied by hydraulic permeability of the capillary wall) because the composite value expressed as K_f can be quantified precisely, whereas the individual components cannot be measured with accuracy.

83 What are the values of Starling's forces in the capillaries of the pulmonary circulation?

❑ The ΔP is approximately 16 mm Hg since P_{cap} is about 14 mm Hg and P_{ISF} is -2 mm Hg. The $\Delta\pi$ is approximately 16 mm Hg since π_p is about 25 mm Hg and π_{ISF} is 9 mm Hg. Thus, forces favoring fluid reabsorption (volume flux entering the capillaries) are identical to forces favoring filtration (volume flux leaving the capillaries). Consequently, the pulmonary alveoli remain "dry," allowing optimal gas exchange. These values of Starling's forces in the pulmonary capillaries represent composite levels of all pulmonary zones. Zone 1 (comprising the apical areas) has a vascular pressure lower than the alveolar one, while in zone 3 (comprising the basal areas), the vascular pressure is higher than the alveolar.

84 Describe other major mechanisms that alter net fluid transfer across the capillaries in the lung and other tissues (eg, increased capillary permeability).

❑ Since hydrostatic and oncotic pressures are the major physiologic determinants of net fluid transfer across the capillaries, changes in any of these variables can significantly alter fluid exchange in body tissues. Consequently, an increased capillary hydrostatic pressure due to increased venous pressure (eg, congestive heart failure) or a decreased colloid osmotic pressure (eg, low serum albumin concentration due to protein malnutrition, liver cirrhosis, or nephrotic syndrome) favors fluid accumulation in peripheral tissues. Increased capillary permeability is the third major mechanism (the first and second mechanisms are increased filtration pressure and decreased colloid osmotic pressure gradient) that enhances fluid exit from the intravascular compartment. Histamine, kinins, and substance P are some of the humoral factors known to increase capillary permeability.

85 Is the interstitial fluid pressure approximately equal in the lung and other tissues?

❑ No. Interstitial fluid pressure differs among the various tissues, with the lowest value found in the lung (approximately −2 mm Hg) and the highest one in the brain (approximately +6 mm Hg). Intermediate levels are present in subcutaneous tissue, liver, and kidney; a subatmospheric level, approximately −1 mm Hg, is found in the first of these tissues, and supra-atmospheric levels in the last two organs (approximately +2 to 4 mm Hg).

86 Describe the three pulmonary zones that result from the gravity-dependent, apex-to-base distribution of pulmonary blood flow in upright lungs (eg, standing or sitting position).

❑ The three pulmonary zones, known as 1, 2, and 3, comprise approximately the upper, middle, and lower third of the lungs, respectively. In zone 1 or the upper area, the pulmonary capillaries are almost bloodless because their internal pressure is less (or about the same) than the external or alveolar pressure, making blood flow either very low or absent. In theory, zone 1 should not have any capillary perfusion because the relationship among pressures is as follows: $P_A > P_a > P_v$ (alveolar, arterial, and venous pressures, respectively). In zone 2 or the middle area, the pulmonary blood flow is intermediate between the very low one observed in zone 1 and the larger capillary flow found in zone 3. Capillary pressure at the arterial side in zone 2 exceeds alveolar pressure; the latter in turn exceeds capillary pressure at the venous side (thus, $P_a > P_A > P_v$). In zone 3 or the lower area, the capillary vessels are constantly distended (as opposed to the collapse of capillaries at their venous end in zone 2) and have the highest blood flow because the internal pressure in the capillaries at the arterial and venous ends are higher than the alveolar pressure (thus, $P_a > P_v > P_A$). To reliably measure pulmonary capillary wedge pressure (PCWP) with a pulmonary artery catheter, the tip of the catheter must be placed in zone 3. It should be recognized that the use of positive end-expiratory pressure (PEEP) can modify a lung area that belongs to zone 3 to one with the characteristics of zone 1 or 2 because of alveolar distention with vascular collapse caused by increased intrathoracic pressure.

5. Respiratory Control

CONTROL OF VENTILATION

87 How is alveolar ventilation regulated by the respiratory control system?

❑ The neurons of the respiratory centers located in the brain stem receive information from the chemoreceptors, the peripheral sensory receptors, and the cerebral cortex. This information is integrated, and the resulting neural output to the chest bellows (respiratory muscles) and lungs determines PaO_2 and $PaCO_2$. The cerebral cortex can also transmit signals to the chest bellows through a neural pathway that bypasses the brain stem respiratory neurons.

88 Briefly describe the main components of the respiratory control system responsible for the stability of PaO_2 and $PaCO_2$. Explain the role of the control centers, sensors, and effectors of the ventilatory system.

❑ The main components of the mechanism that regulates pulmonary ventilation are the control centers, sensors, and effectors. The control centers contain the neurons that regulate ventilation and are located at several levels of the brain stem, with the most important network residing in the medulla oblongata where the respiratory rhythm is generated. These brain stem centers are responsible for the automatic control of breathing, but they can be overridden by the cerebral cortex, as occurs during speech and other actions requiring the voluntary control of ventilation. The respiratory sensors consist of the chemoreceptors (central and peripheral) and other sensory receptors. The central chemoreceptors respond primarily to $PaCO_2$ and the peripheral chemoreceptors respond primarily to PaO_2. Other groups of receptors include the peripheral sensory receptors that are located in the chest wall, airways, and lungs. Among the chest wall receptors are the mechanoreceptors in the respiratory muscles that respond to stretch.

The receptors of airways and lungs consist of (1) irritant (rapidly adapting) receptors, which respond to physical or chemical stimulation; (2) pulmonary stretch (slowly adapting) receptors, which respond to marked increases in lung volume; and (3) C-fiber receptors that are located deep within the lung parenchyma (J receptors) and in the bronchi, which respond to vascular engorgement and congestion, to chemical stimulation, and less so to mechanical stimulation. The effectors of respiratory center output are the respiratory muscles, which move air in and out of the thoracic cavity, and facilitate the pulmonary gas exchange. The changes in thoracic configuration, PaO_2, and $PaCO_2$ are fed back to the central nervous system by afferent nerves arising in the lungs, chest wall, and chemoreceptors, informing the control centers about the adequacy of pulmonary ventilation.

89 What are the functions of the respiratory muscles?

❑ The major function of the respiratory muscles is expansion of the thoracic cavity aimed at developing a subatmospheric intrathoracic pressure and thus facilitate airflow toward the lung. The respiratory muscles also fulfill other functions that include expulsive efforts (such as coughing, vomiting, and defecation) and stabilization of the rib cage and abdomen for posture and physical tasks. The respiratory muscles are the only skeletal muscles essential for life because their repetitive contraction is responsible for breathing, a vital function.

90 What are the main anatomic and physiologic features of the diaphragm? Explain the effects of contraction of costal and crural fibers.

❑ The diaphragm is composed of costal fibers that arise from the lowest six ribs and crural fibers that arise from the first three lumbar vertebrae. Both the costal and crural portions of the diaphragm are inserted into a central tendon. The costal and crural portions of the diaphragm differ in embryologic origin, segmental innervation, fiber composition, and mechanical action. Diaphragmatic contraction causes the dome of the diaphragm to move downward without changing its shape; the effect is similar to that of a piston. The result is an increase in abdominal pressure with consequent abdominal expansion. At the same time, the lower rib cage expands because of two forces: (1) contraction of costal diaphragmatic fibers at their point of insertion (''bucket-handle'' action) and (2) the increase in abdominal pressure, which acts directly through the area of apposition between the diaphragm and rib cage. The crural component of the diaphragm also causes an increase in abdominal pressure. However, the crural fibers do not expand the rib cage; in fact, they produce inward motion of the rib cage.

91 Compare the change in blood flow to the diaphragm with that of other skeletal muscles in the course of muscle contraction.

❑ Contrary to the change in blood flow in other skeletal muscles, diaphragmatic blood flow increases in parallel with the intensity of muscle contraction. This differential response is believed to occur because the diaphragm is not influenced by compressive forces as it lies between the thoracic and abdominal cavities. In addition, unlike other skeletal muscles, the diaphragm lacks fascial planes that can slide and crimp the supplying vessels. However, as the work of breathing rises to a level likely to induce muscle fatigue, diaphragmatic blood flow decreases. Furthermore, experimental reduction of cardiac output has resulted in diaphragmatic fatigue presumably caused by a reduction in blood flow to this muscle.

92 What are the main anatomic and physiologic features of the intercostal and accessory muscles? Do the internal intercostal muscles have an expiratory action? Are the scalene muscles accessory respiratory muscles?

❑ The intercostal muscles consist of the external and internal intercostals. The latter are subdivided into a parasternal (intercartilaginous) component and an interosseous component. Traditionally, the external intercostals were thought to have an inspiratory action and the internal intercostals to have an expiratory action. It is now recognized that both muscle groups have an expiratory action at high lung volumes and an inspiratory action at low lung volumes. The sternomastoid muscles and the scalene muscles have conventionally been considered accessory muscles of respiration. However, the scalene muscles are active during normal breathing, and thus should not be classified as accessory muscles. Vigorous respiratory efforts, such as when minute ventilation reaches 50 to 100 L/min, or after 75% of the vital capacity has been inhaled, will normally recruit the sternomastoids.

93 What fiber types are present in the respiratory muscles?

❑ Three kinds of fibers known as types 1, 2A, and 2B are present in the respiratory muscles. Type 1 fibers (slow twitch type with high oxidative and low glycolytic capacity) make up about 55% of the diaphragm, 65% of the intercostal muscles, and 30% to 60% of the abdominal muscles. Type 1 fibers have the highest resistance to fatigue and they are best suited for sustained tonic activity. Conversely, type 2 fibers (2A and 2B) are of a fast twitch type and best prepared for either a sustained phasic activity (ie, type 2A) or short-term activity (ie, type 2B). Fiber types 2A and 2B account for about 20% and 25%, respectively, of the diaphragm muscle.

94 Do the abdominal muscles have any role in the process of inspiration?

❑ Yes. In addition to being the primary muscles of expiration, the abdominal muscles may facilitate inspiration by three mechanisms:

1. *Contraction*: During expiration, abdominal muscle contraction causes lung volume to decrease below its passively de-

termined end-expiratory level. This action pushes the diaphragm upward toward the rib cage and lengthens its fibers, allowing them to function over a more favorable portion of the length-tension curve.

2. *Upward motion of the diaphragm*: This action causes the diaphragm to become more curved and the resulting decrease in the radius of curvature may improve its mechanical efficiency on the basis of Laplace's law.
3. *Elastic energy*: During expiration, elastic energy is stored in the abdominal muscles and release of this energy during inspiration can enhance inspiratory flow.

---

95 Which are the motor and sensory nerves of the respiratory muscles? What spinal cord segments participate in the innervation of these muscles?

❑ The phenic nerves, the only motor nerves of the diaphragm, arise from the third, fourth, and fifth cervical segments of the spinal cord. In addition to their motor function, the phrenic nerves are the main source of diaphragmatic sensory innervation. Likewise, the intercostal nerves provide both motor and sensory innervation of the intercostal muscles. They arise from the first to the twelfth thoracic segments (T1–T12) of the spinal cord. The scalene muscles are now considered necessary rather than accessory muscles of respiration, and they are innervated by the lower five cervical nerves (C4–C8). The abdominal muscles are innervated by the lower six intercostal nerves (T7–T12) and the first lumbar nerve. The major accessory muscles of respiration are the sternomastoid muscles, and in some patients, the trapezius muscles also play a role. The sternomastoid muscles are innervated by the spinal accessory nerve and the second and third cervical segments (C2–C3), and the trapezius muscles are innervated by the accessory nerve and the third and fourth cervical segments (C3–C4).

96 What spinal cord areas participate in the motor innervation of the major respiratory muscle groups? What is the importance of this information with respect to the risk of respiratory failure after a cord injury?

❑ The major respiratory muscles and their corresponding motor innervation are as follows: diaphragm—phrenic nerve, cervical spinal cord C3–C5; intercostal muscles—intercostal nerves, thoracic spinal cord T1–T12; and abdominal muscles—T7 and T12 and lumbar L1. Other groups of respiratory muscles include sternomastoid (accessory [XI] nerve, C2–C3), trapezius (accessory [XI] nerve, C3–C4), and scalene (C4–C8) muscles. Knowledge of the motor innervation of the respiratory muscles helps to understand the risk of respiratory failure observed with spinal cord injury and with neuromuscular diseases predominantly affecting some body areas. Thus, lesions at or above C5 result in serious respiratory compromise because the major muscle of respiration, the diaphragm, is impaired.

97 What sensory receptors are present in the respiratory muscles? How does their information reach the brain? Explain the role of muscle spindles in the genesis of dyspnea.

❑ Two main types of sensory receptors are present in the respiratory muscles: muscle spindles and tendon organs. The muscle spindles, which are abundant in the intercostal muscles, are relatively scarce in the diaphragm. Muscle spindles are found within the special intrafusal fibers that are arranged in parallel with the main, extrafusal muscle fibers. The contractile extrafusal fibers of a muscle receive the integrated output of the respiratory centers through alpha motoneurons, whereas the axons of gamma motoneurons, also present in peripheral nerves, innervate the intrafusal fibers within the muscle spindles (fusiform system). A disturbance in the equilibrium between the two fiber systems may be important in the generation of the dyspnea sensation in some patients.

Tendon organs are found in both the intercostal muscles and the diaphragm. The diaphragm is richly innervated with tendon organs, in contrast to the low density of muscle spindles. Tendon organs are arranged in series within the muscle fibers and provide a restricted but accurate estimate of the forces generated by muscle contraction. Despite the presence of alpha- and beta-adrenergic receptors in the smooth muscle of airways, adrenergic nerves do not appear to have a physiologic role in the control of airway resistance. Practically all of the afferent information collected by the sensory receptors in the airways and lungs travels in the vagus (parasympathetic) nerve. Afferent information originating in the sensory chemoreceptor cells of the carotid body travels in a branch of the carotid sinus nerve and reaches the brain stem via the glossopharyngeal (ninth cranial) nerve.

98 Explain further the determinants of the rate of carbon dioxide excretion and how the brain centers are informed to adjust pulmonary ventilation in accordance with changes in carbon dioxide production.

❑ The rate of carbon dioxide elimination by the lungs is determined by the partial pressure of carbon dioxide in the alveolar space (P_ACO_2) and the level of alveolar ventilation ($\dot{V}_A$). Under steady-state conditions, the rate of carbon dioxide elimination by the lungs is equal to the rate of carbon dioxide production ($\dot{V}CO_2$) by the tissues. Assuming that no limitation to gas diffusion exists and that ventilation and perfusion of pulmonary units are homogeneous, P_ACO_2 and $PaCO_2$ (alveolar and arterial PCO_2, respectively) can be taken as identical. Thus,

$$PaCO_2 = K \times \dot{V}CO_2 / \dot{V}_A$$

Accordingly, the value of $PaCO_2$ is determined at all times by the interaction of two factors, the rate of carbon dioxide production and the rate of alveolar ventilation. If the rate of carbon dioxide production is constant, $PaCO_2$ varies inversely with alveolar ventilation. Alternatively, an increase in carbon dioxide production in the presence of a constant alveolar ventilation will increase PCO_2 and decrease pH in arterial blood. These changes are recognized by central chemoreceptors located on the ventral surface of the medulla oblongata in the brain stem, and by peripheral chemoreceptors located in the carotid and aortic bodies. The increased rate of impulses, predominantly from the central chemoreceptors and less importantly from the peripheral chemoreceptors, stimulate the respiratory centers in the brain stem. The enhanced activity of the respiratory centers will in turn stimulate the motor neurons of the respiratory muscles, resulting in pulmonary hyperventilation mediated by increased respiratory rate and tidal volume. The increased alveolar ventilation corrects the initial deviation in PCO_2 and pH such that this negative feedback loop allows stabilization of ABGs.

99 Explain the changes in airway resistance and control of breathing during sleep.

❑ During normal sleep, reduced respiratory center output to the upper-airway muscles that normally dilate the oropharynx and larynx on inspiration produces an increase in upper-airway resistance, providing a basis for progression to complete obstruction in patients at such risk (ie, episode of obstructive apnea). In addition, during nonrapid eye movement (NREM) sleep, activation of the intercostal, laryngeal, and pharyngeal muscles diminishes slightly while activation of the diaphragm remains basically unaltered. During rapid eye movement (REM) sleep, there can be wide fluctuations of systemic blood pressure, heart rate, respiratory frequency, and metabolic rate accompanying a decrease in skeletal muscle tone. The ventilatory response to hypoxia and hypercapnia is decreased during sleep as well as the hypoxic arousal response.

6. Pulmonary Function Laboratory

SPIROMETRIC EVALUATION

100 What is the purpose of pulmonary function testing?

❑ Pulmonary function tests are used (1) to quantitate functional impairment of the respiratory system, (2) to establish pattern of disease (ie, obstructive, restrictive), and (3) to determine surgical risk. Knowledge of pattern of disease may help to establish a specific diagnosis. Evaluation of surgical risk is of importance especially when lung resection is being considered for a particular patient.

101 Name the lung volumes that can be measured with a spirometer and those that require other techniques for their evaluation.

❑ The spirometer is a commonly used device that allows measurement of expired or inspired gas volume and plots the values obtained as a function of time. The lung volumes that can be quantitated and recorded in a spirographic tracing include the tidal volume (V_T, volume of gas inspired or expired with each breath), vital capacity (VC, maximal volume of gas that can be voluntarily expired following a maximal inspiration), inspiratory capacity (IC, maximal volume of gas that can be voluntarily inspired following a normal expiration), expiratory reserve volume (ERV, maximal volume of gas that can be voluntarily expired following a normal expiration), and inspiratory reserve volume (IRV, maximal volume of gas that can be voluntarily inspired following a normal inspiration). The lung volumes that cannot be measured with a spirometer include the residual volume (RV, volume of gas remaining in the lungs following maximal expiration), the functional residual capacity (FRC, volume of gas that remains in the lungs after a normal expiration), and total lung capacity (TLC, volume of gas retained within the lungs at maximal inspiration). Measurement of residual volume, functional residual capacity, and total lung capacity is obtained with body plethysmography or helium dilution techniques.

102 Explain further the relationship among the previously mentioned lung volumes.

❑ Vital capacity includes the inspiratory capacity and the expiratory reserve volume (ie, VC = IC + ERV). Alternatively, vital capacity can be viewed as the sum of inspiratory reserve volume, tidal volume, and expiratory reserve volume (ie, VC = IRV + V_T + ERV) or as the difference between total lung capacity and residual volume (ie, VC = TLC − RV). Inspiratory capacity includes the inspiratory reserve volume and tidal volume (ie, IC = IRV + V_T). Alternatively, inspiratory capacity can be viewed as the difference between vital capacity and expiratory reserve volume (ie, IC = VC − ERV) or as the difference between total lung capacity and functional residual capacity (ie, IC = TLC − FRC). Functional residual capacity includes residual volume and expiratory reserve volume (FRC = RV + ERV); functional residual capacity can also be viewed as the difference between total lung capacity and inspiratory capacity (ie, FRC = TLC − IC). Proper understanding of the relationship among the various pulmonary volumes facilitates recognition of the patterns of abnormal lung function.

103 Name the lung volumes measured in the pulmonary laboratory. What are their normal values for men and women?

❑ Lung volumes measured in the pulmonary laboratory include vital capacity, inspiratory capacity, functional residual capacity, total lung capacity, residual volume, and expiratory reserve volume. The approximate values for average-size normal men and women, respectively, are as follows: total lung capacity of 6 to 7 L and 5 to 6 L and vital capacity of 4 to 5 L and 3 to 4 L. Other lung volumes for average-size normal individuals of either sex are inspiratory capacity of 2 to 4 L, functional reserve capacity of 2 to 3 L, residual volume of 1 to 2 L, and expiratory reserve volume of 1 to 2 L.

104 What spirometric parameters derived from volume-time curves are commonly obtained for the assessment of patients? What are their approximate values for normal men and women?

❑ Commonly used spirometric parameters obtained from volume-time curves include forced vital capacity (FVC), forced expiratory volume in 1 second (FEV_1), and FEV_1/FVC. The approximate values for average-size normal men and women, respectively, are as follows: FVC equal or higher than 4.0 and 3.0 L, and FEV_1 higher than 3.0 and 2.0 L. FEV_1/FVC, referred to as FEV_1%, is higher than 70% in normal men and women.

105 What clinically relevant measurements of ventilatory function can be performed?

❑ Clinically relevant measurements of ventilatory function include determination of lung volumes under static conditions and evaluation of expiratory and inspiratory flow rates under dynamic conditions. Because flow rates are closely linked to lung volumes, it is common practice to plot flow rates during expiration and inspiration (vertical axis) against lung volume (horizontal axis), thereby obtaining flow-volume curves.

106 How are the values for lung volumes and inspiratory and expiratory flow rates interpreted?

❑ A comparison of the values measured with those expected according to age, height, gender, and race of the patient is the basis of interpretation of the data collected. The results of a given patient are expressed as percent of the predicted normal values, the latter being available in the form of regression equations. Because there is substantial variability among normal individuals, values between 80% and 120% of predicted are generally considered normal. The ratio FEV_1/FVC is approximately 0.75 to 0.80 (ie, 70 to 80%) in normal subjects, although this value decreases slightly with advancing age.

107 What dynamic measurements of ventilatory function are commonly performed?

❑ Clinically useful measurements of airflow are generally obtained by requesting the patient to take a maximal inspiration and then perform a forceful maximal expiration, while a tracing is obtained with the spirometer. Thus, a volume-time recording, known as a *spirogram,* is obtained, allowing measurement of the following three parameters: (1) FEV_1, which represents the volume of gas exhaled during the first second of expiration; (2) FVC or forced vital capacity, which represents the total volume expired; and (3) $FEF_{25\%-75\%}$ or forced expiratory flow from 25% to 75% of the vital capacity, also known as *MMFR* or maximal midexpiratory flow rate, which represents the average expiratory flow rate during the middle 50% of the vital capacity.

108 What other dynamic measurements of ventilatory function can be performed?

❑ An additional dynamic measurement of ventilatory function includes maximum voluntary ventilation (MVV), which represents the maximum volume of air that can be inspired or expired per minute by a patient breathing as fast and as deep as possible. Other derived values can be obtained for the dynamic measurement of ventilatory function.

109 Describe the test that evaluates muscle endurance known as *maximum sustained ventilation* (MSV) and compare with MVV.

❑ The volume of air that can be inhaled and exhaled with maximum effort over 1 minute is called the *maximum voluntary ventilation* (MVV). Typically, the measurement is made over 15 seconds, and the value is multiplied by 4. Normal values range from 50 to 250 L/min. Only about 60% of MVV can be sustained for 15 minutes or longer. This level of ventilation, known as *maximum sustained ventilation* (MSV), is a measure of respiratory muscle endurance. MSV is measured as the maximal level of ventilation that can be sustained for 15 minutes under normocapnic conditions. Unfortunately, because MSV depends on a patient's motivation and cooperation, its application is limited to research use.

110 What is the relationship between the patient's level of effort and measured expiratory flow rates?

❑ A low level of effort by the patient during a forced expiration that has been preceded by maximal inspiration may result in abnormally low flow rates. If several forced expiratory maneuvers are performed using increasing muscular effort, expiratory flow rates will increase until a certain level of effort is reached. Beyond this level, forced expiratory flow rates become constant and therefore they are effort independent. The main determinants of the effort-independent forced expiratory flow include (1) the elastic recoil of the lung (eg, decreased in pulmonary emphysema), (2) the airflow resistance between the alveoli and the site of flow limitation (eg, augmented in acute attack of asthma), and (3) the airway wall compliance at the site of flow limitation (variable depending on the specific defect). At any given lung volume, the expiratory flow rate decreases with diminished elastic recoil, augmented airflow resistance, or increased airway wall compliance.

111 What are the main features and causes of an obstructive pattern on pulmonary function tests? How is the presence of an acute reversible obstruction established?

❑ An obstructive pattern of pulmonary function tests is characterized by a decreased FEV_1 and FEV_1/FVC, and it occurs primarily with asthma and COPD. The airflow obstruction is considered to be acutely reversible by inhaled bronchodilator administration if immediately after use of this medication FEV_1 or FVC increases by 15% or more.

112 What are the main features and causes of a restrictive pattern on pulmonary function tests? How does evaluation of diffusing capacity for carbon monoxide (DLCO) help in the differential diagnosis of conditions with a restrictive pattern?

❑ Main features of a restrictive pattern include a decreased total lung capacity that is often associated with a decreased FVC and a normal or increased FEV_1/FVC ratio. A restrictive pattern is observed with diffuse infiltrative lung diseases, chest wall disorders, and neuromuscular diseases. Evaluation of DLCO helps in the differential diagnosis of disorders with a restrictive pattern. A reduction in DLCO corrected for lung volume, known as *DLCO/VA,* is observed with diffuse infiltrative lung diseases, but this value is normal with chest wall disorders and neuromuscular diseases.

113 Are airflow rates measured by FEV_1 and FVC abnormally low in patients with a restrictive defect in the absence of an obstructive defect?

❑ Yes. Airflow rates measured by FEV_1 and FVC are often abnormally low in patients with a pure restrictive defect (ie, absence of airway obstruction) because of the reduced lung volumes of these patients. Yet, the FEV_1/FVC ratio is normal or increased in patients with restrictive defects but it decreases if an obstructive defect is also present.

114 How do pulmonary function tests assist in the diagnosis of a restrictive ventilatory defect?

❑ Patients exhibiting a restrictive ventilatory defect have a decreased vital capacity associated with a normal FEV_1/FVC ratio.

Additional data that can support this diagnosis include the presence of decreased values of total lung capacity, lung compliance, and DLCO normalized for lung volume (ie, DLCO/VA). As previously indicated, DLCO/VA decreases in diffuse infiltrative lung diseases, but remains normal in chest wall disorders and neuromuscular diseases.

115 What parameters that assess resistance to airflow are measured in the pulmonary function laboratory? What are their approximate normal values?

❑ Parameters that assess resistance to airflow include airway resistance (Raw) and specific conductance (SGaw). The normal values for average-size men are as follows: Raw lower than 2.5 cm H_2O/sec/L and SGaw higher than 0.13 cm H_2O/sec.

116 What pulmonary function tests might help to evaluate extrathoracic airway obstruction?

❑ Screening spirometric tests measuring FEV_1 and FVC determine exclusively expiratory flow, and therefore could fail to detect an extrathoracic obstruction that limits predominantly the inspiratory flow (this defect is typically observed with nonfixed extrathoracic obstruction). Therefore, spirometric tests that evaluate inspiratory flow are required to identify all forms of extrathoracic obstructions. Typical features of a variable extrathoracic obstruction located above the thoracic inlet include flattening of the inspiratory portion of the flow-volume loop and a reduction of the ratio of inspiratory to expiratory flow (ie, <1.0, measured at the middle portion of vital capacity). The presence and type of upper-airway obstruction is further established by examination of the shape of the flow-volume loop, which as well as other tests (eg, computerized tomography of the neck) may reveal a distinct deformation.

117 How does preoperative spirometry (ie, FEV_1) help predict surgical risk in patients scheduled for either lung resection or nonpulmonary surgery?

❑ Preoperative spirometry is commonly used in the evaluation of surgical risk for both pulmonary and nonpulmonary surgery. However, spirometry does not reliably predict surgical outcome or mortality for patients undergoing extrathoracic surgery. A predicted postoperative FEV_1 that exceeds 0.8 L is considered sufficient pulmonary reserve to permit resection of lung tissue. Quantification of predicted postoperative FEV_1 after lung resection requires a preoperative evaluation of FEV_1 and a perfusion lung scan. The percent of perfusion of the anticipated residual lung multiplied by the preoperative FEV_1 provides the expected postoperative FEV_1. This calculation is relevant only in patients having a preoperative FEV_1 lower than 2.0 L.

118 How might pulmonary function tests help in the differentiation of respiratory symptoms (eg, dyspnea) caused by heart failure from those due to lung diseases?

❑ Pulmonary function testing in patients with dyspnea and other respiratory symptoms caused by heart failure might reveal (1) reduction in arterial PCO_2 and PO_2; (2) diminished vital capacity, total lung capacity, pulmonary compliance, and pulmonary diffusion capacity during exercise and frequently at rest; (3) normal residual volume and functional residual volume; and (4) moderately augmented resistance to airflow with evidence of air trapping and increased dead space. None of the abnormalities in the pulmonary function tests is specific for heart failure or constant in this disease. Thus, the results of pulmonary function tests must be interpreted considering all the clinical and laboratory information obtained from the patient.

PRESSURE-VOLUME CURVES AND COMPLIANCE

119 Explain the pressure-volume curve of the lungs isolated from the chest wall and that of the chest wall isolated from the lungs.

❑ The lungs and the chest wall are elastic structures with variable volume that is dependent on the applied pressure that either expands or contracts them, and these effects are graphically depicted by means of the pressure-volume curves (ie, pressure is plotted on the horizontal axis or abscissa and volume is plotted on the vertical access or ordinate). In the absence of a distending pressure (ie, 0 cm H_2O), the elastic properties of the lung isolated from the chest wall result in complete collapse of this structure. Consequently, either a negative (this is a commonly used expression but represents a misnomer because external pressure is not strictly negative) or subatmospheric external pressure (eg, pleural pressure) or a positive internal pressure (eg, supra-atmospheric level applied within the airway by a positive-pressure ventilator) is required to expand the lung. The distending pressure also known as *transpulmonary pressure* or P_{TP} is equal to the difference between the internal pressure (ie, at the alveoli) and external pressure (ie, at the pleural surface). Inspection of the pressure-volume curve of the normal lung isolated from the chest wall demonstrates that the P_{TP} values required to achieve the residual volume, FRC, and total lung capacity are approximately 2, 8, and 40 cm H_2O, respectively. Inspection of the pressure-volume curve of the chest wall (in the absence of the lungs) demonstrates that the resting volume of the thorax (observed in the absence of applied pressure, or in other words, when the transthoracic pressure is zero) is approximately 75% of total lung capacity and is positioned at equal distance from FRC and total lung capacity (ie, larger than the FRC and smaller than total lung capacity). Expansion of the chest wall to reach a volume identical to total lung capacity requires a pressure of approximately 6 cm H_2O; conversely, contraction of the chest wall (ie, its volume becomes smaller than the resting volume) to reach FRC and residual volume requires an opposite pressure equal to 8 and 40 cm H_2O, respectively.

120 Let us examine the combined effects of the pressure-volume curve of the lung with that of the chest wall, which determine the pressure-volume curve of the intact respiratory system (observed when the lungs are held within the thorax).

❑ At FRC, which represents the end of a normal expiration, the tendency of the lungs to contract is counteracted by an equal tendency of the chest wall to expand. Thus, at FRC identical absolute pressures of about 6 cm H_2O but opposite in sign are present so that the pressure of the combined system (ie, lungs in situ) equals 0 cm H_2O. During inspiration to volumes above FRC (eg, tidal volume, inspiratory capacity), the tendency of the lungs to decrease their volume, and thereby return to FRC, requires work by the inspiratory muscles to overcome the passive retraction of the lungs resulting from their elastic nature. Maximal inspiration reaching total lung capacity produces the highest force, due to inward recoil of the lungs, that is balanced by the outward expansion of the chest wall caused by active work of inspiratory muscles. Consequently, the principal determinants of total lung capacity are the stiffness of the lungs (stiffer or less compliant lungs reduce total lung capacity and more compliant or less stiff lungs increase total lung capacity) and the strength of the inspiratory muscles (major weakness of these muscles reduces total lung capacity). Expiration below FRC requires active work of the expiratory muscles to overcome the tendency of the respiratory system (ie, sum of effects of lungs and chest wall) to increase volume to its resting condition (ie, FRC). The volume of gas contained within the lungs at residual volume increases with weakness of the expiratory muscles (since it requires active work of these muscles) and intrinsic airway disease (closure of airways decreases the volume of expired gas).

121 What are the pressure-volume and the pressure-flow curves measured in the pulmonary function laboratory? How are a decrease in lung compliance and increase in airway resistance detected with these measurements?

❑ The pressure-volume curve refers to the effect of changes in the intrapleural pressure (in cm H_2O), graphically depicted on the horizontal axis (x axis), on lung volume (L), depicted on the vertical axis (y axis). In patients with decreased lung compliance, a considerably greater change in intrapleural pressure is required to achieve a given change in lung volume, resulting in a flatter (more horizontal) pressure-volume curve as compared to that of normal subjects. The pressure-flow curve refers to the effect of changes in the intrapleural pressure (in cm H_2O), graphically depicted on the horizontal axis (x axis), and on airflow (in L/min), depicted on the vertical axis (y axis). In patients with increased airway resistance, a considerable greater change in intrapleural pressure is required to achieve a given change in airflow, resulting in a flatter (more horizontal) pressure-flow curve as compared to that of normal subjects.

122 What are the flat and the steep portions of the pressure-volume curve? How do normal breathing and PEEP (positive end-expiratory pressure) correlate with each portion of the curve?

❑ The pressure-volume curve has two flat portions, located at the initiation and at completion, and a steep portion (intermediate area of the curve). The flat portions indicate that large changes in pressure produce small changes in volume (depicted in the vertical or y axis). Conversely, the steep portion indicates that small changes in pressure produce large changes in volume. During normal respiration a tidal breath begins at FRC, which is on the intermediate or steep portion of the pressure-volume curve of the lung. A collapsed airway or alveolus results in a low FRC, which corresponds to the low flat portion of the curve, where a large change in pleural pressure is required for even a small volume change.

PEEP shifts the FRC to the steep portion of the curve, but it may also cause a normal alveolus to move to the upper flat portion of the curve with consequent overdistention and risk of barotrauma.

123 Explain the concept of static compliance of the respiratory system. What is its normal value?

❑ The static compliance (Cst) of the thorax (lungs and chest wall) is calculated as the ratio of the change in its volume (ie, tidal volume) to the change in inspiratory pressure (ie, distending pressure at end-inspiration, known as *static pressure, alveolar pressure,* or *plateau pressure*). The normal range for static compliance is 50 to 100 mL/cm H_2O.

124 Explain the concept of effective dynamic compliance. Is this parameter a reliable index of thoracic compliance? Enumerate conditions that can decrease effective dynamic compliance.

❑ Effective dynamic compliance (Cdyn) is calculated by dividing the ventilator-delivered volume per respiratory cycle by the peak airway pressure minus PEEP. This index is not a measure of true thoracic compliance, because the peak airway pressure also includes the resistive pressure component of the applied pressure. The Cdyn may be decreased by disorders of the airways, lung parenchyma, or chest wall; Cdyn falling to a greater extent than the total thoracic compliance suggests an increase in airway resistance (eg, bronchospasm, mucus plugging, kinking of the endotracheal tube, or an excessive flow rate). The Cdyn is normally about 50 to 80 mL/cm H_2O.

125 Compare the static and dynamic pressure-volume relationships of the intact respiratory system (ie, lungs and chest wall) during positive-pressure ventilation. How are static compliance and dynamic compliance measured?

❑ At the completion of inspiration the pressure gradient between the proximal airways and the alveolar sacs that is responsible for airflow into the lungs has dissipated, resulting in a single pressure level (known as *static* or *plateau pressure*). However, proximal-airway pressure exceeds alveolar pressure during inspiration because it provides the pressure gradient for airflow into the lungs. Measurement of the peak proximal airway pressure (Ppeak) during inspiration provides an index of the dynamic pressure-volume relationship. Dynamic compliance of the thorax (lungs and chest wall) is calculated as the ratio of the change in its volume (ie, tidal volume) to the peak pressure measured during inspiration. Conversely, the "plateau level" of pressure (Pplateau) at the end of inspiration, as opposed to the peak pressure (Ppeak) observed during inspiration, is utilized in the evaluation of static compliance.

126 How is thoracic compliance measured in patients receiving ventilator support? What conditions might alter static compliance and dynamic compliance?

❑ The physician can obtain a rough measure of combined lung and chest-wall static compliance by occluding the expiratory tubing and determining the ratio between the tidal volume delivered by the ventilator and the plateau in airway pressure (minus PEEP) displayed on the ventilator manometer (normal value of static compliance is 60 to 100 mL/cm H_2O). Similarly, dynamic compliance can be estimated by dividing the delivered tidal volume (V_T) by the peak airway pressure minus PEEP (normal range for dynamic compliance is 50 to 80 mL/cm H_2O). The development of a pneumothorax and main-stem bronchial intubation represent the most common causes of a decrease in static compliance in patients receiving ventilator support. Dynamic compliance falling to a greater extent than static compliance suggests an increase in airway resistance, such as that caused by bronchospasm or kinking of the endotracheal tube.

127 What is the importance of subtracting PEEP (extrinsic and intrinsic) in the evaluation of thoracic compliance? How can the level of auto-PEEP be measured?

❑ Failure to take into account the presence of extrinsic/intrinsic PEEP (its value must be subtracted from the plateau pressure to calculate compliance) may lead to a large underestimation of thoracic compliance (eg, 50% reduction). Patient-generated PEEP, known as *auto-PEEP* or *intrinsic PEEP,* has also been termed *occult PEEP,* because it is not registered on the ventilator manometer, as the latter is open to the atmosphere. If, however, the expiratory port of the ventilator circuit is occluded immediately before the onset of the next breath, the pressure in the lungs and ventilator circuit will equilibrate, and the level of auto-PEEP will be displayed on the manometer.

128 What parameters that assess pulmonary compliance can be measured in the laboratory for pulmonary studies? What are their normal values?

❑ Parameters that assess pulmonary compliance measured in the laboratory include the static recoil pressure at total lung capacity (Pst TLC), static compliance of lungs (CL), and compliance of lungs and thorax, abbreviated as C(L+T). The values for average-size normal men are as follows: the static recoil pressure at total lung capacity, 25 ± 5 cm H_2O; static compliance of lungs, 0.2 L/cm H_2O; and compliance of lungs and thorax, 0.1 L/cm H_2O.

129 How can thoracic compliance be measured? What are the causes of a reduced level?

❑ In patients receiving mechanical ventilation and making no respiratory effort, respiratory system compliance can be estimated by dividing the tidal volume (V_T) by the distending transthoracic pressure. Conditions of zero gas flow are necessary and can be achieved by employing the "inspiratory hold" option on the ventilator; at zero gas flow the airway pressure falls to a plateau. Alternatively, the inspiratory plateau in the pressure tracing is achieved by temporary occlusion of the expiratory tubing. If the patient is receiving PEEP or has auto-PEEP, its value must be first subtracted from the plateau pressure before calculating the total thoracic compliance, that is, compliance = volume delivered/(plateau pressure − PEEP). The normal range for thoracic compliance is 60 to 100 mL/cm H_2O. A decrease in thoracic compliance is observed with disorders of the thoracic cage or a reduction in the number of functioning lung units (eg, resection, bronchial intubation, pneumothorax, pneumonia, atelectasis, pulmonary edema).

EVALUATION OF RESPIRATORY MUSCLES

130 What is meant by the terms *strength, endurance,* and *fatigue* of respiratory muscles? How is strength measured?

❑ Respiratory muscle function can be described in terms of strength and endurance. Strength is usually measured as the maximal respiratory pressure that can be generated during a static effort against an occluded airway. Strength is dependent on the number of contractile elements or myofibrils. Endurance is the capacity of a muscle to sustain a contractile force and is dependent on the density of muscle capillaries and mitochondria, and on overall oxidative enzyme capacity. The converse of endurance is fatigue, which can be defined as a loss in the capacity for developing force and velocity of a muscle, and is reversible by rest. Generally, fatigue is considered a relatively acute loss of contractile force, from which a muscle usually recovers spontaneously. Fatigue impairs proper contraction as well as relaxation (slows down this process) of the respiratory muscles.

131 What noninvasive test can be used to assess the strength of respiratory muscles? How is it performed?

❑ Measurements of maximum airway pressures are used to assess respiratory muscle strength. Such measurements are usually made while the patient makes a maximum effort against an occluded airway. The mouthpiece is connected to a manometer and should contain a small leak to ensure that the glottis remains open.

Like other skeletal muscles, the respiratory muscles generate a maximum force that is related to their length; consequently, it is important to control the lung volume at which the pressure measurements are made. Maximum inspiratory airway pressure (PImax) is usually measured after expiration to residual volume. Maximum expiratory airway pressure (PEmax) should be measured after an inspiration to total lung capacity because the expiratory muscles are maximally stretched in this position. Proper performance of these tests depends on excellent cooperation from the patient.

132 What are the normal values of maximum airway pressures? How does measurement of this parameter help to predict the development of hypercapnia (ie, acute respiratory failure)?

❑ In general, healthy men have a mean PImax of about 115 ± 27 cm H_2O and a PEmax of approximately 180 ± 40 cm H_2O; values in women are approximately 25% lower. In both sexes, the values decline linearly with age by about 20% between ages 20 and 70 years. A reduction in maximum airway pressure can be caused by neuromuscular disease, pulmonary disease, or poor cooperation by the patient. In patients with neuromuscular disease but who are free of lung disease, hypercapnia is likely to develop when PImax decreases to one-third of its normal predicted value. Hypercapnia can be observed with less severe reductions (PImax of less than one-half normal) in patients who have COPD because of the associated abnormalities in gas exchange and increased work of breathing.

133 What methods work best for assessing respiratory muscle dysfunction at the bedside? What other methods might be used for the evaluation of respiratory muscle strength?

❑ Detailed evaluation of the patient's pattern of breathing provides the most useful bedside information regarding respiratory muscle performance. In addition, respiratory muscle strength can be determined at the bedside by measuring maximal airway pressures; subnormal pressures may result from neuromuscular disease, pulmonary disease, or poor cooperation. A number of techniques have been used to study respiratory muscle fatigue in the research setting, but all of them have limitations that prevent their easy application at the patient's bedside. Evaluation of maximum transdiaphragmatic pressure can assist in diagnosing diaphragmatic paralysis. Respiratory muscle fatigue can be assessed with serial measurements of maximum sustained ventilation, transdiaphragmatic pressure response to phrenic stimulation, or electromyographic power spectral analysis; however, problems associated with each of these techniques limit their clinical utility.

134 How can the pleural pressure swings characteristic of breathing abnormalities be evaluated?

❑ Early studies of the sleep apnea syndrome measured intrapleural pressure with an intraesophageal balloon catheter. This evaluation distinguished obstructive from central apnea, as wide swings in intrapleural pressure occurred in the former and were absent in the latter. The discomfort associated with swallowing an esophageal balloon catheter has limited the application of this method. In mixed apnea (having a central plus an obstructive component), there is absence of intrapleural pressure swings indicative of a central apnea component followed by swings of intrapleural pressure during the obstructive phase of the apnea.

7. Blood Gases

PO_2, $P_A\text{-}aO_2$, PaO_2/P_AO_2, PaO_2/FiO_2

135 How can the pulmonary gas exchange be assessed?

❑ ABG analysis is universally employed in the assessment of pulmonary function. In addition, a number of indices have been derived from ABG values to assist with assessing the efficiency of pulmonary gas exchange, including (1) alveolar-arterial oxygen tension difference ($P_A\text{-}aO_2$); (2) arterial-alveolar oxygen tension ratio (PaO_2/P_AO_2); (3) arterial-inspired oxygen ratio (PaO_2/FiO_2); and (4) physiologic dead space or wasted ventilation (V_D/V_T). These indices are explained in the answers to pertinent questions.

136 What are the normal values for ABGs and alveolar-arterial difference for oxygen at sea level?

❑ The normal values for ABGs at sea level are PaO_2 of 95 ± 5 mm Hg, $PaCO_2$ of 40 ± 5 mm Hg, SaO_2 of 97 ± 2%, pH 7.40 ± 0.02, $[HCO_3^-]$ of 24 ± 2 mmol/L, and base excess (BE) of 0 ± 2 mmol/L. Because PaO_2 is dependent on the inspired fraction of oxygen (FiO_2), it is important to estimate $P_A\text{-}aO_2$, which has a normal value of up to 20 mm Hg. The $P_A\text{-}aO_2$ needs to be assessed at a constant FiO_2 in order to obtain useful information.

137 What are the effects of body temperature on the blood gases measured in vitro at 37°C?

❑ In patients with hyperthermia, application of a correction factor to convert the PO_2 and PCO_2 measured in vitro at 37°C to the in vivo levels at the patient's body temperature produces an increase in PO_2 and PCO_2 and a fall in pH; hypothermia has the opposite effects. A number of nomograms and equations have been published to correct ABG values measured at 37°C in vitro to the values expected at the patient's body temperature. However, it is generally recommended that clinical decisions should be based on ABG measurements made at 37°C without correcting for extremes of body temperature.

138 How can the effect of age on PaO_2 values be predicted?

❑ The effect of age on PaO_2 can be calculated as follows:

$$PaO_2 = 104.2 - 0.27 \times \text{age (years)}$$

The value obtained is the predicted PaO_2 in normal seated adults.

139 What factors modify mixed venous oxygen tension? What is the effect of changes in mixed venous oxygen tension on PaO_2?

❑ The factors affecting PvO_2 can be seen by rearranging the Fick equation from

$$\dot{V}O_2 = \dot{Q}t \times (CaO_2 - CvO_2)$$

to

$$\begin{aligned} CvO_2 &= CaO_2 - (\dot{V}O_2/\dot{Q}t) \\ &= 1.34 \times Hb \times SaO_2 - (\dot{V}O_2/\dot{Q}t) \end{aligned}$$

Thus, PvO_2 is low when the cardiac output ($\dot{Q}t$) is low, when the Hb level is low (anemia), when oxygen consumption ($\dot{V}O_2$) is increased, and of course, with a decrease in oxygen saturation. For any lung unit, the end-capillary PO_2 (and for both lungs, the PaO_2) is influenced by the mixed venous PO_2 (PvO_2). The magnitude of this effect depends on the ventilation-perfusion ratio

($\dot{V}_A/\dot{Q}$) of that lung unit and is greatest with low $\dot{V}_A/\dot{Q}$ ratios or a shunt.

140 How can the clinician establish the underlying mechanism of a patient's hypoxemia?

❑ Clinically significant hypoxemia might occur as a result of one or more of the following mechanisms: (1) decreased partial pressure of oxygen in the inspired gas (PiO_2), (2) alveolar hypoventilation, (3) ventilation-perfusion defect, and (4) right-to-left blood shunting. Measurement of PaO_2 and evaluation of the alveolar-arterial oxygen gradient (P_A-aO_2), as well as the response in PaO_2 to breathing 100% oxygen, represent the basic elements for the differential diagnosis of hypoxemia. The results of these tests in each of the previously mentioned conditions are examined in the answers to subsequent questions.

141 Explain the possible role of abnormal diffusion as a determinant of a disturbance of pulmonary gas exchange.

❑ Normally, blood takes 0.75 second to travel through the pulmonary capillary bed. As only one-third of this time is required for equilibration between blood and alveolar gas, there is a wide margin of safety before abnormal pathology causes nonequilibration, that is, a diffusion impairment. From a clinical standpoint, diffusing capacity is assessed by measuring the transfer of carbon monoxide (DLCO). It is estimated that the DLCO must fall to less than 10% of normal before it affects PaO_2 at rest. For diffusing capacity to play an important role in the hypoxemia of disease, at least two of the following three conditions need to be met: thickening of the alveolar capillary membrane, which increases the distance for diffusion; a marked decrease in FiO_2 (eg, high altitude); and a shortened residence time for blood in the capillaries (increased cardiac output or capillary bed destruction). Even when these conditions are met, diffusion impairment plays only a minor role in the resulting hypoxemia.

142 Explain the use of ABG measurements in the diagnosis of abnormalities of pulmonary gas exchange.

❑ Measurement of ABGs while breathing room air and 100% oxygen can be helpful in diagnosing the mechanism of abnormal gas exchange. If the hypoxemia is due to pure $\dot{V}A/\dot{Q}$ inequality, inhaling 100% oxygen will cause the PaO_2 to increase to almost 600 mm Hg. If the hypoxemia is due to a shunt, a much smaller increase in PaO_2 will be noted, depending on the level of the shunt.

143 How can the partial pressure of oxygen in the alveolar space (P_AO_2) be calculated from the alveolar gas equation?

❑ The P_AO_2 can be estimated from the simplified alveolar gas equation as follows:

$$P_AO_2 = PiO_2 - (PaCO_2/RQ)$$

where RQ is the respiratory quotient (ie, ratio of carbon dioxide production and oxygen consumption, usually about 0.8), respectively.

The PiO_2 can be obtained as follows:

$$PiO_2 = FiO_2 \times (Patm - PH_2O)$$

where FiO_2 is the fraction of the inspired gas that is oxygen (eg, 21% in room air), the Patm is the atmospheric pressure (eg, 760 mm Hg at sea level), and PH_2O is the vapor pressure of water (ie, 47 mm Hg).

144 What is the alveolar-arterial oxygen gradient (P_A-aO_2)?

❑ The P_A-aO_2 is the difference between the estimated partial pressure of oxygen in the alveolar space (determined from the alveolar gas equation) and the measured PO_2 in arterial blood, where P_AO_2 and PaO_2 represent the alveolar and arterial oxygen pressure, respectively. The normal P_A-aO_2 is 10 to 15 mm Hg in young subjects breathing room air. P_A-aO_2 increases with the patient's age, the PO_2 in inspired air, and conditions that interfere with oxygen exchange between the alveoli and pulmonary capillaries.

145 How can the change in P_A-aO_2 that accompanies increasing age be estimated?

❑ The patient's age expressed in years multiplied by 0.4 (constant factor) allows estimation of the expected P_A-aO_2. Consequently, the expected P_A-aO_2 level in a healthy 75-year-old man is approximately 30 mm Hg (ie, $0.4 \times 75 = 30$).

146 Estimate the P_AO_2 and the P_A-aO_2 in a patient breathing room air whose PaO_2 and $PaCO_2$ are 90 and 40 mm Hg, respectively.

❑ The simplified alveolar gas equation indicates that

$$P_AO_2 = FiO_2\ (Patm - PH_2O) - (PaCO_2/RQ)$$

and substituting we obtain

$$\begin{aligned} P_AO_2 &= 0.21\ (760 - 47) - (40 \div 0.8) \\ &= 150 - 50 \\ &= 100 \text{ mm Hg} \end{aligned}$$

Thus, P_AO_2 is 100 mm Hg and P_A-aO_2 is 10 mm Hg (ie, $100 - 90 = 10$ mm Hg); this value is within normal limits.

147 What elements might help to determine the physiologic mechanism of hypoxemia and the FiO_2 required for the treatment of patients in acute respiratory failure?

❑ The patient's clinical presentation and $P_{A}\text{-}aO_2$ might help to determine the physiologic mechanism responsible for the hypoxemia. Hypoventilation is likely in the presence of a normal $P_{A}\text{-}aO_2$ and the absence of pulmonary infiltrates on chest x-ray films, and usually responds to a small increase in the inspired oxygen concentration (eg, FiO_2 of 24% or 28%). A ventilation-perfusion ($\dot{V}/\dot{Q}$) mismatch is likely in the presence of an increased $P_{A}\text{-}aO_2$, clinical features of pneumonia, or infiltrates on the chest film, and indicates the need for a higher concentration of inspired oxygen (eg, FiO_2 of 50%).

148 Describe the distribution of the pulmonary ventilation among the various lung areas. Does the $\dot{V}/\dot{Q}$ ratio alter gas exchange?

❑ Since a fraction of the pulmonary ventilation remains in areas distant to the alveoli where gas-exchange processes occur, the relationships among total pulmonary ventilation, alveolar ventilation, carbon dioxide output, and $PaCO_2$ must be recognized and understood. The pulmonary ventilation that effectively reaches the alveolar spaces is called the *alveolar ventilation* ($\dot{V}_A$). The complementary portion of the total ventilation ($\dot{V}_E$) that serves to flush the conducting, non-gas-exchanging portion of the airways and does not reach the alveoli is the *dead space ventilation* ($\dot{V}_D$). Thus,

$$\dot{V}_A = \dot{V}_E - \dot{V}_D$$

The efficiency of alveolar gas exchange is modified if an unequal distribution of alveolar ventilation with respect of pulmonary perfusion ($\dot{V}_A/\dot{Q}$) is present.

149 What are the effects on the alveolar gas exchange of a high and a low $\dot{V}_A/\dot{Q}$ ratio?

❑ The composition of gas leaving alveoli without blood flow is equal to that of inspired air and represents a component of dead space ventilation. Similarly, areas of the lungs with ratios of ventilation to perfusion higher than normal exhibit a waste of ventilation, which further increases the dead space ventilation. The unequal distribution of alveolar ventilation to pulmonary perfusion ($\dot{V}_A/\dot{Q}$) may produce the opposite effect, that is, a decrease in this ratio; in one extreme situation, areas of the lung may lack ventilation but maintain normal blood perfusion. Under these circumstances, there is no alveolar gas exchange and a shunt effect will occur. The overall impact of qualitative inhomogeneities of alveolar ventilation to pulmonary perfusion, independent of the direction of the change, is a reduction in the efficiency of the pulmonary gas exchange.

150 Explain the development of hypoxemia due to ventilation-perfusion ($\dot{V}/\dot{Q}$) abnormalities and provide examples of this condition.

❑ Mismatching of pulmonary ventilation and perfusion wherein the former process is relatively low with respect to the latter (ie, low $\dot{V}/\dot{Q}$ ratio) causes hypoxemia. Most pulmonary diseases including pneumonias, ARDS, and many other conditions are associated with some degree of $\dot{V}/\dot{Q}$ mismatching that causes a reduced PaO_2 level.

151 Explain the development of hypoxemia due to a right-to-left shunt in patients with pulmonary diseases.

❑ A right-to-left shunt is said to be present when venous blood returning from the tissues passes to the systemic arterial circulation without coming into contact with gas-containing alveoli. Shunt is the major mechanism of abnormal gas exchange in patients with pulmonary edema, ARDS, pneumonia, and atelectasis. In these instances, the shunt results from the perfusion of alveoli that are unventilated due to being filled with fluid or atelectatic. While a shunt may appear to represent one extreme of $\dot{V}_A/\dot{Q}$ inequality (perfusion but absent ventilation), its effect on gas exchange and response to therapy is different. A shunt typically produces more severe hypoxemia than does $\dot{V}_A/\dot{Q}$ mismatching, and the fall in PaO_2 induces hyperventilation, which causes hypocapnia.

152 What specific conditions are associated with hypoxemia caused by right-to-left blood shunting through abnormal anatomic pathways?

❑ A right-to-left blood shunting process can result from the presence of abnormal anatomic pathways including atrial or ventricular septal defects, patent ductus arteriosus, and pulmonary arteriovenous fistulae.

153 What is venous admixture? How is it calculated?

❑ Venous admixture ($\dot{Q}\bar{v}a/\dot{Q}t$) is a measure of the true shunt ($\dot{Q}\bar{v}a/\dot{Q} = 0$) plus the functional shunt from low $\dot{V}_A/\dot{Q}$ (shuntlike) regions. It is calculated according to the equation

$$\dot{Q}\bar{v}a/\dot{Q}t = (Cc'O_2 - CaO_2)/(CcO_2 - C\bar{v}O_2)$$

where $\dot{Q}\bar{v}a/\dot{Q}t$ is the venous admixture, $\dot{Q}t$ is the cardiac output, and $Cc'O_2$, CaO_2, and $C\bar{v}O_2$ are the oxygen contents of "ideal" end-capillary, arterial, and mixed venous blood, respectively. The oxygen content of ideal end-capillary blood ($Cc'O_2$) is derived from P_AO_2 as calculated from the alveolar gas equation, assuming that PaO_2 equals P_AO_2. An increased $\dot{Q}\bar{v}a/\dot{Q}t$ is caused by a ventilation-perfusion mismatch or shunt. By breathing 100% oxygen ($FiO_2 = 1.0$), the contribution of the ventilation-perfusion mismatch is abolished, and calculation of $\dot{Q}\bar{v}a/\dot{Q}t$ quantitates the amount of shunt. However, administration of 100% oxygen washes out the nitrogen that may be keeping alveoli open and converts some areas of $\dot{V}_A/\dot{Q}$ inequality into a shunt. Although an accurate and informative parameter, $\dot{Q}\bar{v}a/\dot{Q}t$ is not commonly measured because a pulmonary artery catheter is necessary to obtain a mixed venous blood sample and the calculations are cumbersome. Modifications of the venous admixture equation have been proposed with the intention of simplifying the calculations. However, the assumptions on which these modifications are based (eg, an arteriovenous oxygen content difference [$CaO_2 - C\bar{v}O_2$] of 4 to 5 mL/dL) are frequently inaccurate, and such modifications should be avoided.

154 Enumerate the conditions that have an abnormal (enlarged) $P_A\text{-}aO_2$.

❑ An enlarged $P_A\text{-}aO_2$ is characteristically present with ventilation-perfusion ($\dot{V}/\dot{Q}$) defects and right-to-left blood shunting processes. As previously indicated, $P_A\text{-}aO_2$ is within normal limits in patients with hypoxemia caused by decreased PiO_2 as well as in the hypoventilation-induced mechanism.

155 How might the evaluation of $P_A\text{-}aO_2$ help differentiation of the causes of hypoxemia? Name the mechanisms of hypoxemia associated with a normal and abnormal $P_A\text{-}aO_2$.

❑ Hypoxemia caused by decreased PiO_2 and hypoventilation is characterized by the presence of a normal $P_A\text{-}aO_2$. Conversely, an abnormally elevated $P_A\text{-}aO_2$ is observed in association with a ventilation-perfusion defect and right-to-left blood shunting. Further characterization of each mechanism requires additional tests (eg, evaluation of PaO_2 while breathing 100% oxygen).

156 Explain the use of the alveolar-arterial oxygen difference in the evaluation of pulmonary gas exchange. What is its major limitation?

❑ Alveolar-arterial oxygen tension difference ($P_A\text{-}aO_2$) is commonly employed as a measure of gas-exchange efficiency. It is little affected by changes in overall minute ventilation, and thus, it remains normal when hypoxemia is solely due to hypoventilation. Any other factor making gas exchange less efficient will widen the P_A-aO_2. A major limitation of this index is that it changes unpredictably (depending on the $\dot{V}_A/\dot{Q}$ distribution) with changes in FiO_2, which limits its clinical applicability in the management of critically ill patients.

157 Explain the use of the PaO_2/P_AO_2 and PaO_2/FiO_2 ratios in the evaluation of pulmonary gas exchange. What are the advantages of these ratios?

❑ The PaO_2/P_AO_2 ratio remains more stable than the alveolar-arterial oxygen difference with changing levels of FiO_2. Thus, it is a preferable index of gas exchange, and it can be used to predict the expected PaO_2 when FiO_2 is altered. The PaO_2/FiO_2 has been advocated because it is the easiest index to calculate as it does not require solving the alveolar gas equation. Unlike the PaO_2/P_AO_2 ratio, it fails to adjust for fluctuations in $PaCO_2$, although this has little influence on calculations at high levels of FiO_2.

158 Explain further the differentiation of hypoxemia caused by decreased PiO_2 from the hypoventilation-induced mechanism.

❑ ABG measurements help this task because PCO_2 is either low or normal (ie, hypocapnia or eucapnia, respectively) when hypoxemia is caused by decreased PiO_2, but high (ie, hypercapnia) in patients with alveolar hypoventilation. The P_A-aO_2 is normal in the two conditions, and therefore is not helpful for their differential diagnosis. The response to breathing 100% oxygen is also noncontributory for the differential diagnosis, yet if performed, it will demonstrate a normal response.

159 How does the response to breathing 100% oxygen allow differentiation of the three mechanisms of hypoxemia (ie, diffusion abnormality, $\dot{V}/\dot{Q}$ mismatch, right-to-left shunt) characterized by an abnormal (enlarged) alveolar-arterial oxygen gradient?

❑ Patients having hypoxemia caused by a right-to-left shunt characteristically exhibit an abnormal response to breathing 100%

oxygen (ie, this maneuver fails to raise PaO_2 to the levels observed in normal individuals). Conversely, the response to breathing 100% oxygen is normal in patients with hypoxemia caused by a diffusion abnormality as well as in those having ventilation-perfusion mismatch.

PCO_2, P_ECO_2, V_D/V_T

160 What body fluid can be sampled to assess acid-base status and lung function? How do PCO_2 levels compare in arterial and venous blood?

❑ Arterial or venous blood or both can be sampled to evaluate acid-base status. However, evaluation of lung function on acid-base composition requires arterial blood sampling; in addition, a sample of arterial blood allows one to assess the level of oxygenation. Venous blood has higher PCO_2 levels than does arterial blood.

161 Why is arterial blood commonly chosen to assess blood PCO_2? Is arterial PCO_2 a good indicator of tissue PCO_2 levels?

❑ An arterial blood sample is commonly chosen to assess blood PCO_2 because it provides an excellent indication of the lung's ability to excrete carbon dioxide and also provides information about the PCO_2 levels of the blood that reaches all body tissues. Venous PCO_2 is a good indicator of the PCO_2 levels within peripheral tissues whereas arterial PCO_2 is not because venous PCO_2 is dependent on the metabolism in each individual tissue/organ while arterial PCO_2 is identical for all tissues.

162 Elaborate on the daily production and excretion of volatile acids. Provide comparable information with respect to the net daily production of fixed acids.

❑ The daily production of volatile acid (ie, carbonic acid or H_2CO_3) is approximately 15,000 mEq/day and is excreted by the lungs. The net daily production of fixed acids is only 70 to 100 mEq/day and is excreted by the kidney. It becomes apparent that the production of volatile acid is approximately 200 times that of fixed acid. Such discrepancy helps to explain the severe acidemia observed within minutes of severe hypoventilation whereas it takes days to reach a similar decrease in blood pH in patients with severe renal failure.

163 How does the approximately 2 mEq/L of arteriovenous difference of $[HCO_3^-]_p$ (ie, plasma bicarbonate level in mixed venous blood minus its value in arterial blood) relate to the 15,000 mEq/day of volatile acid production?

❑ The product of the arteriovenous difference of $[HCO_3^-]$ per liter of blood and the cardiac output (in L/min) yields the carbon dioxide production (in mmol/min). This value multiplied by 1440 minutes provides the daily carbon dioxide production (in mmol or mEq). Thus, 2 mEq/L × 5 L/min of cardiac output × 1440 min/day = 14,400 mEq/day (approximately 15,000 mEq/day).

164 What determines the level of PCO_2 and bicarbonate in body fluids?

❑ The level of PCO_2 in body fluids is determined by the relationship between carbon dioxide production by the tissues and its excretion by the lungs. The $[HCO_3^-]$ in body fluids results from ongoing processes that decompose bicarbonate, counterbalanced by other processes that regenerate it. The major component of bicarbonate decomposition is the release of fixed acids derived from cellular metabolism; regeneration of bicarbonate stores is accomplished by excretion of acid by the kidneys.

165 Elaborate on the determinants of PCO_2 in body fluids.

❑ The level of carbon dioxide in body fluids is ultimately the result of the relationship between carbon dioxide production by cellular metabolism and carbon dioxide excretion by the lungs. The large increase in carbon dioxide production that accompanies maximal exercise is attended by a prompt and effective enhancement in its excretion due to pulmonary hyperpnea, such that a substantial increase in PCO_2 in body fluids is prevented. On the other hand, primary changes in carbon dioxide production that are not associated with parallel alterations in carbon dioxide excretion will result in abnormal levels of PCO_2. Similarly, primary alterations of carbon dioxide excretion that are not accompanied by parallel changes in carbon dioxide production will lead to deviations in the steady-state levels of carbon dioxide.

166 What are the determinants of $PaCO_2$? Explain the effects of changes in minute ventilation ($\dot{V}E$), dead-space ventilation ($\dot{V}D$), and tidal volume (VT) on $PaCO_2$. What are the possible causes of an increased $PaCO_2$?

- ❑ $PaCO_2$ is determined by the following relationship:

$$PaCO_2 = k \frac{\dot{V}CO_2}{\dot{V}A}$$

where $\dot{V}CO_2$ is carbon dioxide production, $\dot{V}A$ is alveolar ventilation, and k is constant of proportionality. Since an increase in $\dot{V}CO_2$ is never solely responsible for an increase in $PaCO_2$, the development of hypercapnia indicates a reduction in alveolar ventilation. Substituting the term alveolar ventilation from the previous equation, we obtain

$$PaCO_2 = k \frac{\dot{V}CO_2}{\dot{V}E\ (1 - VD/VT)}$$

where $\dot{V}E$ is minute ventilation, VD is dead space, and VT is tidal volume. From the last equation it is apparent that an increase in $PaCO_2$ may result from (1) an increase in the dead space to tidal volume ratio (VD/VT), if $\dot{V}CO_2$ and $\dot{V}E$ remain unchanged, (2) a decrease in $\dot{V}E$, if $\dot{V}CO_2$ and VD/VT remain unchanged, (3) an increase in $\dot{V}CO_2$ (although this is never solely responsible for hypercapnia), or (4) a combination of all these factors.

167 What is the normal range of $PaCO_2$ and arterial $[HCO_3^-]_p$ at sea level? Is $[HCO_3^-]_p$ equal in arterial and venous blood?

❑ The normal range of $PaCO_2$ at sea level is 35 to 45 mm Hg and that of $[HCO_3^-]_p$ in arterial blood is 24 ± 2 mmol/L (22 to 26 mmol/L). The $[HCO_3^-]_p$ is higher in venous blood than in arterial blood because the bulk of the carbon dioxide added to the blood for its ultimate excretion into the atmosphere is carried in the form of bicarbonate in the plasma of venous blood. The value of venous $[HCO_3^-]_p$ is about 2 mEq/L (mmol/L) higher than the arterial one.

168 What are hypocapnia and hypercapnia? Compare these terms with the normal level of PCO_2 in arterial blood.

❑ Under normal conditions, the level of $PaCO_2$ is maintained relatively constant, between 35 and 45 mm Hg. The terms *hypocapnia* and *hypercapnia* denote decreases and increases in $PaCO_2$ levels below and above the normal value, respectively. Because the hydrogen ion concentration of body fluids is determined by the ratio of the PCO_2 and $[HCO_3^-]$, changes in PCO_2 are accompanied by alterations in $[H^+]$ to the same direction. Thus, hypocapnia will result in alkalemia, and hypercapnia in acidemia. Abnormalities in PCO_2 elicit secondary responses in both renal as well as extrarenal tissues that culminate in changes in $[HCO_3^-]$ to the same direction. These adaptive changes in $[HCO_3^-]$ are considered an integral part of the respiratory acid-base disorder rather than independent metabolic abnormalities.

169 Why is venous PCO_2 higher than arterial PCO_2? Is it possible to have identical PCO_2 in arterial and venous blood?

❑ Venous PCO_2 is higher than arterial PCO_2 due to the interposition of peripheral tissues (which add carbon dioxide to the blood) between the arterial and venous compartments, and also to the presence of the lungs (which release the carbon dioxide from the blood to the atmosphere) between the venous and the arterial compartments. Arterial and venous PCO_2 may be transiently identical during respiratory arrest because of the absence of carbon dioxide excretion (eg, respiratory arrest with preserved function of the circulatory system).

170 What is the normal mean arteriovenous difference for PCO_2? What is the most likely explanation for the presence of an enlarged arteriovenous difference of PCO_2 levels in a patient?

❑ The normal mean arteriovenous difference for PCO_2 is 4 to 6 mm Hg. For this calculation, mixed venous blood (obtained from the pulmonary artery or "central" venous blood collected from the right atrium or vena cava) is used for the evaluation of venous PCO_2. The most common explanation for an enlarged arteriovenous PCO_2 difference is the presence of a reduced cardiac output.

171 How would a reduced cardiac output enhance the arteriovenous difference of PCO_2?

❑ A reduced cardiac output prolongs the transit time of blood, leading to greater carbon dioxide accumulation per liter of blood flowing through the tissues (leading to venous hypercapnia) as well as greater carbon dioxide excretion per liter of blood perfusing the lungs (leading to arterial hypocapnia). Therefore, arterial hypocapnia and venous hypercapnia are the characteristic features observed in patients with decreased cardiac output. This unique situation is a form of respiratory acidosis accompanied by arterial hypocapnia (ie, "pseudorespiratory alkalosis") that is observed in patients with profound depression of cardiac function and relative preservation of respiratory function.

172 What is the highest possible $PaCO_2$ in patients breathing room air according to the alveolar gas equation?

❑ The constraints of the alveolar gas equation establish that patients breathing room air cannot reach $PaCO_2$ levels much higher than 80 mm Hg, because the degree of hypoxemia that would develop at higher values is incompatible with life. Thus, extreme hypercapnia occurs only during oxygen therapy, and indeed severe carbon dioxide retention is often the result of uncontrolled oxygen administration.

173 How does the PCO_2 level measured with the capnometer relate to the arterial PCO_2? Is this relationship similar in health and disease?

❑ In healthy subjects, the end-tidal carbon dioxide tension ($P_{ET}CO_2$), measured as the plateau value of an exhaled sample, is 1 to 5 mm Hg lower than the $PaCO_2$. Patients with pulmonary disease who have an uneven distribution of ventilation display a steadily rising expired carbon dioxide signal that does not achieve a plateau. In these patients, the $PaCO_2$-$P_{ET}CO_2$ gradient increases unpredictably by 10 to 20 mm Hg or more (reflecting inefficient alveolar gas exchange), with the result that $P_{ET}CO_2$ is no longer a reliable reflection of $PaCO_2$.

174 How does capnography help the evaluation of physiologic dead space (V_D)? What conditions can lead to an increased V_D?

❑ Measurement of expired carbon dioxide tension (P_ECO_2) permits calculation of the V_D according to the Bohr alveolar equation: $V_D/V_T = (PaCO_2 - P_ECO_2)/PaCO_2$. In healthy subjects, the V_D/V_T ratio is between 0.33 and 0.45. The V_D/V_T ratio is increased in a number of disease states associated with regions of the lung possessing high ventilation-perfusion ratios, such as pulmonary embolism, venous air embolism, hypovolemia, ARDS, and emphysema, and with the employment of positive-pressure ventilation with high V_T or PEEP.

175 How can physiologic dead space or wasted ventilation be measured?

❑ Physiologic dead space or wasted ventilation (V_D/V_T) can be estimated from simultaneous samples of arterial blood (to measure $PaCO_2$) and expired gas (to measure mixed expired carbon dioxide tension, $P_{E}CO_2$). Expired gas is collected in a mixing chamber over a 2- to 3-minute period, and the V_D/V_T ratio is calculated according to the Bohr equation:

$$V_D/V_T = (PaCO_2 - P_ECO_2)/PaCO_2$$

In healthy subjects the V_D/V_T ratio is between 0.33 and 0.45. V_D/V_T is increased in a number of disease states associated with regions of lung possessing high $\dot{V}/\dot{Q}$ ratios such as pulmonary embolism, ARDS, and emphysema and with the employment of positive-pressure ventilation. Increases in V_D/V_T require an increase in minute ventilation if hypercapnia is to be prevented. In patients being evaluated for a trial of weaning from mechanical ventilation, an increase in V_D/V_T to 0.6 or above is generally considered to predict an unsuccessful outcome because the necessary increase in minute ventilation for satisfactory gas exchange causes marked encroachment on ventilatory reserve.

176 What are the normal values of V_D, the ratio of dead space volume to tidal volume (V_D/V_T) known as physiologic dead space, and the diffusing capacity for carbon monoxide (single-breath test)?

❑ The normal value of V_D is 50 ± 25 mL. The physiologic dead space (V_D/V_T) is as much as 35% V_T at rest and decreases to 20% V_T during exercise. The normal value of the diffusing capacity for carbon monoxide (single-breath test), known as DLCO, is 25 mL of CO/min/mm Hg.

177 What clinical conditions are associated with sudden or gradual increases in end-tidal carbon dioxide tension ($P_{ET}CO_2$)?

❑ Conditions leading to a sudden increase in $P_{ET}CO_2$ include a bolus intravenous injection of sodium bicarbonate, a sudden increase in cardiac output, as well as an abrupt sudden release of a tourniquet (applied to a limb to reduce peripheral venous return). A gradual increase in $P_{ET}CO_2$ is observed in the presence of hypoventilation and with increased carbon dioxide production.

RESPIRATORY AND METABOLIC COMPONENTS OF ACID-BASE STATUS

178 Is the pH of body fluids modulated by direct physiologic control of $[H^+]$? What organs regulate the level of PCO_2 and $[HCO_3^-]_p$? How do the PCO_2 and $[HCO_3^-]_p$ interact to determine blood pH?

❑ The pH of body fluids is not modulated by direct physiologic control of $[H^+]$. Acidity is modulated by altering the levels of the components that determine $[H^+]$, namely, PCO_2 and $[HCO_3^-]$. The PCO_2 is regulated by the lungs and the plasma $[HCO_3^-]$ ($[HCO_3^-]_p$) is regulated by the kidneys. The PCO_2 and $[HCO_3^-]_p$ interact to determine blood pH, as follows:

$$H^+ + HCO_3^- \Leftrightarrow H_2CO_3 \Leftrightarrow H_2O + CO_2$$

When $[H^+]$ is expressed as nanomoles per liter, $[HCO_3^-]$ in millimoles per liter, and the dissolved carbon dioxide as PCO_2 in millimeters of mercury, the following relationship is obtained:

$$[H^+] = 24 \frac{PCO_2}{[HCO_3^-]}$$

The above relationship is known as the Henderson equation (the logarithmic form is known as the *Henderson-Hasselbalch equation*) and needs to be used in the evaluation of accuracy of blood acid-base data collected from patients (see answer to pertinent question).

179 What are the initial elements necessary to assess the acid-base status of a patient? What is specifically measured to assess the acid-base status?

❑ The initial elements necessary to assess the acid-base status of a patient include the measurement of the acidity of body fluids and its respiratory and metabolic components. To accomplish this goal, the pH of a blood sample is measured with a glass electrode and the PCO_2 determined with an ad hoc electrode (PCO_2 can be obtained also with an indirect method such as the ''interpolation'' technique of Siggaard Andersen). $[HCO_3^-]_p$ is calculated from the measured pH and PCO_2 using the Henderson-Hasselbalch equation.

180 Why is the metabolic component often assessed by a parameter that is different from the actual $[HCO_3^-]_p$ (eg, base excess)?

❑ The Henderson equation establishes that the $[H^+]$ is dependent on the ratio of a so-called respiratory component (ie, PCO_2) and a metabolic component (ie, $[HCO_3^-]_p$). While the former is regulated by the lungs, the latter is regulated by the kidneys. It is assumed that these components are basically independent of each other. Yet, a major interdependency exists between PCO_2 (the respiratory component) and HCO_3^- (the metabolic component). The need to obtain an estimate of the metabolic component that was truly independent of the respiratory component led to the creation of other parameters including standard HCO_3^-, buffer base, and base excess. These metabolic parameters of acid-base status are commonly reported when ABG determinations are requested; therefore, it is important to understand the precise meaning of each of them.

181 Why does $[HCO_3^-]_p$ increase with hypercapnia?

❑ It is frequently but erroneously concluded that the increment in $[HCO_3^-]_p$ during hypercapnia is exclusively the result of the renal response to a primary increment in PCO_2. However, humans or animals without any kidney function, or simply a blood sample in vitro, will develop hyperbicarbonatemia during acute hypercapnia. This reaction is explained as follows: Hydration of carbon dioxide results in the formation of H_2CO_3, which subsequently dissociates into a H^+ and a HCO_3^-. The H^+ is, to some extent, bound by the non-HCO_3^- buffers; thus, the reaction is further sustained, resulting in an increment in $[HCO_3^-]$. This reaction,

$$CO_2 + H_2O \Leftrightarrow H_2CO_3 \Leftrightarrow HCO_3^- + H^+$$

$$HCO_3^- + H^+ + Buf^- \Leftrightarrow Buf\ H^+ + HCO_3^-$$

is best known as the *interaction reaction* of body buffers and is responsible for the rise in $[HCO_3^-]_p$ during acute hypercapnia.

182 What is standard bicarbonate, or more precisely, what is the plasma standard bicarbonate concentration (standard $[HCO_3^-]_p$)? What is the buffer base or buffer value of plasma?

❑ Standard $[HCO_3^-]_p$ is the plasma bicarbonate concentration from a blood sample fully saturated with oxygen and equilibrated in vitro at 38°C with PCO_2 equal to 40 mm Hg. The mean normal value is 24 mmol/L, which is identical to the actual $[HCO_3^-]_p$ in a patient with a normal PCO_2 of 40 mm Hg. Singer and Hastings defined the plasma buffer base concentration ($[BB]_p$) as the sum of the concentration of the buffer anions in the plasma; this includes bicarbonate and proteins. The mean normal value is 41.7 mEq/L, as follows:

$$\begin{aligned}[BB]_p &= HCO_3^- \text{ buffers} + \text{non-}HCO_3^- \text{ buffers}\\ &= [HCO_3^-] + [\text{Proteins}]\\ &= 24 + 17.7\\ &= 41.7 \text{ mEq/L}\end{aligned}$$

183 Is the buffer base of blood different from that of plasma?

❑ Yes. The buffer value or buffer base of blood ($[BB]_b$) is the sum of the buffer value of plasma and the buffer value of Hb. Thus, $[BB]_b = 41.7 + 0.42\ [Hb]$, where 41.7 is the [BB] of plasma; 0.42 is a constant that allows calculation of [BB] of Hb, which is equal to 0.42 mEq/L for each gram of Hb per 100 mL of blood; [Hb] is the Hb concentration (in gm/dL). Thus, for a normal [Hb] of 15 gm/dL,

$$[BB]_b = 41.7 + (0.42 \times 15)$$
$$= 41.7 + 6.3$$
$$= 48 \text{ mEq/L}$$

184 How does the level of oxygenation influence the $[BB]_b$?

❑ When oxygenated Hb releases oxygen, it becomes less acid and can more easily accept protons. Therefore, the $[BB]_b$ is increased when the Hb releases its oxygen content. The increased [BB] of deoxygenated Hb allows removal of the bulk of H^+ resulting from production of H_2CO_3 by the tissues. Consequently, tissue production of H^+ results in only a very small reduction in blood pH (ie, venous blood pH is approximately 0.03 unit lower than arterial blood pH).

185 What is blood base excess, or more precisely, what is blood base excess concentration ($[BE]_b$)? Compare blood base excess and blood buffer base.

❑ The $[BE]_b$ is the amount of acid or alkali that must be added to a liter of fully oxygenated blood exposed in vitro to a PCO_2 of 40 mm Hg at 38°C to achieve a normal pH (7.40). When the initial blood pH is lower (more acid) than normal, alkali must be added to titrate the blood; thus, the blood sample under evaluation has a "negative base excess," which is also called a *base deficit.* On the other hand, if the initial blood pH is higher (more alkaline) than normal, acid must be added to titrate the blood; thus, the blood sample under evaluation has a "positive base excess" or simply *base excess.* The $[BE]_b$ is expressed in milliequivalents of acid or alkali per liter of blood. Its normal value is theoretically zero as no correction of the metabolic component is required to normalize pH in the presence of a normal respiratory component. The ranges of normal values for men and women are −2.4 to +2.2 and −3.3 to +1.3 mEq/L, respectively. The $[BE]_b$ is also equal to the difference between the measured level of the buffer base in a blood sample and its normal value.

186 Does evaluation of the metabolic component with standard $[HCO_3^-]_p$, buffer base ($[BB]_p$), and base excess ($[BE]_p$) provide an assessment of the metabolic component in vivo that is truly independent of the respiratory component?

❑ No. The above-mentioned parameters are truly independent of the respiratory component within the closed in vitro system where they are analyzed. In vivo, however, the blood sample might have been equilibrated with an abnormal respiratory component within the blood/nonblood compartments of the body fluids, interfering with the independence of the respiratory and metabolic components. In vitro, the carbon dioxide–induced increase in $[HCO_3^-]$ is identical to the decrease in the concentration of non-HCO_3^- buffers that bind the H^+ released from the H_2CO_3; in vivo, however, a more complex situation develops and is explained in the answers to the next six questions.

187 What is the pseudometabolic acidosis associated with acute hypercapnia?

❑ A decrease in the metabolic component of the acid-base equilibrium (eg, blood base deficit) observed in response to acute hypercapnia in vivo is called a *pseudometabolic acidosis.* Combined respiratory acidosis and metabolic acidosis has been repeatedly described in patients undergoing general anesthesia associated with inadequate ventilation. The observed base deficit had been attributed to the production of fixed acids secondary to hypoventilation. A striking feature of the acid-base disturbance was the disappearance of the metabolic acidosis without alkali therapy as soon as proper ventilation was secured. The nature of this obscure acid-base disorder was properly clarified as being actually a pseudometabolic acidosis associated with acute hypercapnia.

188 Explain why, when assessed in vivo, standard $[HCO_3^-]_p$, $[BB]_b$, and $[BE]_b$ decrease in response to acute hypercapnia.

❑ Standard $[HCO_3^-]_p$, $[BB]_b$, and $[BE]_b$ all decrease in response to acute hypercapnia because the in vivo effects of this maneuver are quite different from the in vitro effects: Acute hypercapnia acting in vivo on the intravascular and cellular compartments, rich in non-HCO_3^- buffers, results in the production of significant quantities of new HCO_3^-, increasing the concentration of HCO_3^- in these compartments. Carbon dioxide, a rapidly diffusible gas, increases its tension to a similar degree in the interstitial fluid, which, contrary to what happens in the intravascular and intracellular fluid, is practically devoid of non-HCO_3^- buffers. There is no generation of HCO_3^- in the interstitial compartment during acute hypercapnia; therefore, the concentration of this ion initially remains unchanged. The concentration gradient for HCO_3^- created thereby among the body fluid compartments leads to the migration of HCO_3^- from the intravascular, and possibly from the intracellular compartment, to the interstitial compartment. Thus, the smaller rise in $[HCO_3^-]_p$ during acute hypercapnia in vivo, compared to the one in vitro, as well as the base deficit observed in vivo, are the result of the previously described transitory loss of bicarbonate from the blood to the interstitial fluid. When acute hypercapnia subsides, the opposite sequence of events takes place, and bicarbonate ions move back from the interstitial to the intravascular compartment, with subsequent disappearance of the base deficit. The phenomenon of pseudometabolic acidosis that accompanies acute hypercapnia is, therefore, the result of compartmental redistribution of bicarbonate.

---

189 What is the magnitude of the pseudometabolic acidosis associated with acute hypercapnia?

❑ Whereas in the adult an acute rise in PCO_2 to 100 mm Hg results in a base deficit of about 6 to 7 mEq/L, in the newborn the effect is even greater, the base deficit reaching approximately 10 mEq/L. The greater effect in the newborn is due to a stronger buffering capacity within the intravascular compartment (blood volume of 100 mL/kg, compared to 70 mL/kg in the adult; Hb of 18 gm/dL, compared to 15 gm/dL in the adult) as well as the bigger extracellular fluid volume (400 to 450 mL/kg, compared to 230 to 270 mL/kg in the adult). If, for example, a newborn develops severe respiratory depression, with PCO_2 up to 100 mm Hg, resulting from the administration of narcotics to the mother during labor, it is expected that the newborn will have a base deficit of 10 mEq/L, which does not represent a true metabolic acidosis and will disappear with correction of the hypoventilation.

---

190 How might the non-HCO_3^- buffer system be assessed separately from the HCO_3^- buffer system in vitro and in vivo?

❑ The non-HCO_3^- buffer system can be assessed in vitro and in vivo by titration with carbon dioxide gas. From the Henderson equation,

$$CO_2 + H_2O \Leftrightarrow H_2CO_3 \Leftrightarrow H^+ + HCO_3^-$$

the newly generated H^+ resulting from the dissociation of H_2CO_3 is picked up by non-HCO_3^- buffers. The amount of HCO_3^- that is generated during the carbon dioxide titration is identical to the amount of H^+ removed from the solution by the non-HCO_3^- buffers. Therefore, the change in $[HCO_3^-]_p$ per unit change in PCO_2

or per unit change in blood pH quantifies the buffering response of non-HCO_3^- buffers. The increase in $[HCO_3^-]_p$ observed in a patient with acute hypercapnia reflects the action of the nonbicarbonate body buffers that generate bicarbonate in response to carbon dioxide retention.

191 What parameters should be chosen to assess the respiratory and metabolic components that determine the acid-base status?

❑ The respiratory component is usually assessed by the blood PCO_2. The metabolic component is usually assessed by measurement of actual $[HCO_3^-]_p$, standard $[HCO_3^-]_p$, or $[BE]_b$. These three metabolic parameters are closely interrelated, and change in parallel in metabolic acid-base disturbances. The relationship between changes in standard $[HCO_3^-]_p$ and in $[BE]_b$ is not entirely linear and varies with the [Hb]; if the [Hb] is abnormally low, a change in $[BE]_b$ is approximately equal to the change in standard $[HCO_3^-]_p$, whereas for a normal [Hb] the relationship can be expressed as $\Delta[BE]_b = 1.3 \times \Delta$standard $[HCO_3^-]_p$. None of the various parameters is truly superior as compared with the others. We recommend that for patient management the physician use the parameter that is reported by the laboratory to evaluate the acid-base status, and learn the advantages and limitations that characterize the specific parameter measured.

192 What are the expected changes in actual $[HCO_3^-]_p$, standard $[HCO_3^-]_p$, and $[BE]_b$ when PCO_2 changes rapidly (within minutes) from 40 to 80 mm Hg?

❑ Actual $[HCO_3^-]_p$ increases by approximately 4 mEq/L, while standard $[HCO_3^-]_p$ decreases by about 3 mEq/L, and $[BE]_b$ decreases by approximately 5 mEq/L when PCO_2 rises from 40 to 80 mm Hg. These values represent experimental data collected during acute hypercapnia. The reasons for the disruption of the expected parallel alteration in the three metabolic parameters relate to the redistribution of buffers among body compartments that occurs with acute hypercapnia, as discussed in the answers to pertinent questions.

193 Why is the word *primary* generally included in the definition of acidosis and alkalosis? Explain a manner of establishing the primary process in an acid-base disorder.

❑ The term *primary* indicates the initial event, the original insult, or the first alteration in the acid-base composition of the patient. The production of a given acid-base disorder in an experimental animal is the result of imposing a primary insult (eg, the addition of carbon dioxide to the inspired air of an experimental animal) onto a previously normal acid-base equilibrium. The response to this newly created primary acid-base disturbance provides information on the secondary physiologic response. In an experimental model, the investigator starts with a normal animal on which he or she imposes a specific abnormality such as an increase in PCO_2. The resulting acid-base disorder is called *respiratory acidosis* or *primary hypercapnia* because the original insult was an increase in PCO_2. In a manner comparable to that described in the experimental models, the identification of the primary process or insult responsible for an acid-base disorder in a patient should be made by means of the clinical history.

194 Describe a thoughtful approach to obtain the correct acid-base diagnosis in a patient. How should this systematic approach to the analysis of acid-base disorders begin?

❑ Reaching the correct acid-base diagnosis requires a systematic approach that includes the evaluation of a number of components, each of which is critical. The absence of even one of these components might lead to an erroneous diagnosis. The first step would be to assess the accuracy of the acid-base parameters using the Henderson equation:

$$[H^+] = 24\,\frac{PCO_2}{[HCO_3^-]}$$

pH values must be converted to $[H^+]$ in nanoequivalents per liter in order to apply this equation. There are three commonly used methods to make this conversion (see below).

195 What is the importance of assessing the accuracy of the acid-base parameters using the Henderson equation (ie, first step in acid-base diagnosis)?

❑ Verification of the accuracy of the acid-base data by ensuring that the available values for pH, $PaCO_2$, and $[HCO_3^-]_p$ satisfy the mathematical constraints of the Henderson equation is a critically important first step in the analysis of acid-base results. Not rarely, acid-base values that appear to pose major diagnostic challenge and lead interpreters to propose the most complex mixed acid-base disorders are merely sets of parameters that lack internal consistency (ie, incorrect data).

196 Describe the most precise method of converting pH values to $[H^+]$ in nanoequivalents per liter and vice versa.

❑ The pH value under study must be first subtracted from 9.00 and its antilog subsequently obtained, in order to convert pH values to $[H^+]$ in nanomoles per liter (nEq/L). The reverse, to convert $[H^+]$ in nanoequivalents per liter to pH, is accomplished by obtaining first the log of the nanoequivalent-per-liter value under study and then subtracting it from 9.00. This method is the most precise for converting pH values to $[H^+]$ in nanoequivalents per liter and vice versa.

197 Describe other methods of converting pH values to $[H^+]$ in nanoequivalents per liter.

❑ A second method is to apply the rule whereby for each 0.01 pH unit below or above its normal value, 1 nEq/L is respectively added or subtracted. Since a pH of 7.40 is equal to 40 nEq/L of $[H^+]$, pH values of 7.50 and 7.30 correspond to $[H^+]$ of 30 and

50 nEq/L, respectively. This rule is relatively accurate for a limited range of pH of about 0.2 pH unit below and above the normal value (7.20 to 7.60). It must be recognized, however, that this rule is inaccurate for extreme deviations of pH, and therefore should not be used in those circumstances. A third approach is the 80% method (or 0.8 method), which is useful for any blood pH value and does not require a calculator with a logarithmic capability. This method requires remembering that a pH of 7.40 and one of 7.00 correspond to $[H^+]$ of 40 and 100 nEq/L, respectively. For an increase in pH of 0.10 unit, starting from any pH value, one must multiply the $[H^+]$ that corresponds to the starting pH by 0.8, in order to obtain the $[H^+]$ that corresponds to the higher pH. For example, the $[H^+]$ values for pHs of 7.10 and 7.20 are 80 and 64 nEq/L, respectively. The $[H^+]$ for a pH of 7.10 (ie, 80 nEq/L) is obtained by multiplying 0.8×100 nEq/L, the $[H^+]$ for a pH of 7.00. The $[H^+]$ for a pH of 7.20 (ie, 64 nEq/L) is obtained by multiplying $0.8 \times 0.8 \times 100$ nEq/L (ie, it is necessary to multiply twice by 0.8 because pH 7.20 is 0.20 pH unit higher than pH 7.00).

198 Determine the $[H^+]$ for a pH of 7.50 (ie, increase of 0.10 pH unit from the normal blood value) using the three methods. Apply the 80% method for a decrease of 0.10 pH unit.

❑ The $[H^+]$ values for a pH of 7.50 determined from the three methods are as follows: (1) the log method yields pH 7.50 = 31.6 nEq/L; (2) the 0.01 rule yields pH 7.50 = 30 nEq/L; and (3) the 80% (0.8) method yields pH 7.50 = 32 nEq/L. It should be noted that the value derived from the 80% method is closer to that of the log method (gold standard) than is the one from the 0.01 method. To estimate the $[H^+]$ of a sample that has a ΔpH of 0.10 starting from any pH value, by applying the 80% rule, the $[H^+]$ that corresponds to the starting pH is multiplied by either 0.8 (for a pH increase) or 1.25 (for a pH decrease). For example, the $[H^+]$ for a pH of 6.90 is 125 nEq/L since a pH of 7.00 represents a $[H^+]$ of 100 nEq/L (ie, $100 \times 1.25 = 125$ nEq/L).

199 What is the second major step in the systematic approach to the analysis of acid-base disorders?

❑ The second major step, frequently overlooked, is to obtain a good clinical history and perform a complete physical examination, searching for clues to a particular acid-base disturbance. For example: Does the patient have a history of COPD or chronic carbon dioxide retention? Has he or she been vomiting or had diarrhea? Has he or she been taking diuretics or toxic substances? Is the patient diabetic? Has the patient been drinking large amounts of alcohol? The clinical history and physical examination may provide fundamental information that allows one to formulate the correct acid-base diagnosis by determining the primary derangement of acid-base status.

200 What is the third major step in the analysis of acid-base disorders?

❑ The third major step is the estimation of the plasma anion gap. According to the principle of electroneutrality, in any solution, including the plasma, the sum of cations is identical to the sum of anions. The plasma contains one major measured cation (Na^+) and two major measured anions (Cl^- and HCO_3^-). Although other cations are also routinely measured (K^+, Ca^{++}, Mg^{++}), their contribution to overall cation equivalency is small in health and disease. The remaining anions are not routinely measured. Because measured cations exceed measured anions, the difference is called the *plasma anion gap.* Alterations in plasma anion gap allow detection of abnormal levels of organic and inorganic acids. Thus, estimation of the plasma anion gap represents a critical element in acid-base diagnosis. Changes in the anionic equivalency of plasma proteins might also substantially alter the level of the plasma anion gap.

201 How is the plasma anion gap calculated and what is the normal value? Explain the so-called normalization of the plasma anion gap.

❑ The plasma anion gap and its normal value are calculated in the following way: (1) Computation: $[Na^+]_p$ – $([Cl^-]_p$ +

$[HCO_3^-]_p$); and (2) normal value equals 12 ± 4 mEq/L (mean ± 2 standard deviations). In order to make a sound interpretation of the plasma anion gap in the assessment of acid-base disorders, it is mandatory to correct the anion gap of the patient, taking into consideration the prevailing levels of plasma proteins and pH; this process is called *normalization of the plasma anion gap.* Plasma proteins are polyanions and account for the largest fraction of the plasma unmeasured anions. Accordingly, substantial abnormalities in protein concentration are associated with appreciable (parallel) changes in the plasma anion gap. In addition, there are considerable pH-mediated effects on the plasma anion gap arising from changes in protein electrical charge and as a result of changes in the plasma levels of organic acids. The computation of these changes or normalization of the plasma anion gap is made as follows: (1) Concentration of plasma proteins: for each gram of plasma protein per deciliter below or above the normal range (4.0 gm/dL for albumin or 6.5 gm/dL for total proteins), the amount of 2 mEq/L must be subtracted from or added to the normal anion gap (12 mEq/L), respectively. (2) The pH-mediated effects (changes in electrical charge of plasma proteins and in the plasma levels of organic acids) are as follows: (a) In acidemic states anion gap decreases by 1 to 3 mEq/L (eg, about −1 mEq/L for pH of 7.20 to 7.30, about −2 mEq/L for a pH of 7.10 to 7.20, and about −3 mEq/L for a pH of 7.10 or less), and (b) in alkalemic states anion gap increases by 3 to 5 mEq/L (eg, about +3 mEq/L for a pH of 7.50, +4 mEq/L for a pH of 7.60, and about +5 mEq/L for a pH of 7.70). The pH-mediated effects must be subtracted (acidemia) or added (alkalemia) to the normal anion gap (12 mEq/L). The assessment of the anion gap in a patient is made by comparing the anion gap estimated from the patient's electrolytes to a "normalized" plasma anion gap.

---

202 How does the presence of an increased plasma anion gap help in interpreting the correct acid-base diagnosis in a patient with respiratory acidosis?

❑ The increased plasma anion gap leads to a reduction in the initial $[HCO_3^-]_p$ independent of the secondary response to respiratory acidosis (ie, increase in $[HCO_3^-]_p$ caused by a primary increase in PCO_2). Estimation of the initial $[HCO_3^-]_p$ (assuming that the high anion gap acidosis has disappeared) allows one to assess with precision the magnitude of the observed metabolic response to hypercapnia (eg, acute, chronic) and evaluate the possible presence of additional acid-base disorders (eg, mixed acid-base condition with more than two components such as respiratory acidosis, plus high anion gap acidosis, plus vomiting-induced metabolic alkalosis).

---

203 What are the next steps in the systematic approach to reach the correct acid-base diagnosis?

❑ The fourth step is to identify the primary acid-base disturbance and assess whether a simple or a mixed acid-base disturbance is present. Thus, the initial formulation of a presumptive acid-base diagnosis requires the completion of the three previous steps, namely, (1) checking for internal consistency of acid-base parameters, (2) obtaining a complete history and performing a physical examination, and (3) evaluating the plasma anion gap. The fourth step is the formulation of a presumptive acid-base diagnosis. The final step in the systematic approach to the analysis of acid-base disorders consists of examining the plasma electrolytes and other ancillary data, including, in some instances, the electrolytes and the acid-base composition of the urine, which permits the formulation of a definite diagnosis, instead of merely a presumptive one.

8. Dyspnea

204 What is the neuroanatomic basis of dyspnea? Explain the theory of "length-tension inappropriateness" of the respiratory muscles.

❑ Significant controversy still remains with respect to the mechanisms responsible for the development of dyspnea (ie, disturbance of chemosensitivity, pulmonary receptors, respiratory muscle receptors, outgoing respiratory motor command). Yet, there is a considerable body of evidence implicating the respiratory muscles as a major source of dyspnea. At the breaking point of a breath-hold, performing a rebreathing maneuver can decrease the discomfort and prolong the breath-holding time, even though PCO_2 increases and PO_2 falls. This effect suggests that movement of the chest wall and lungs may alleviate the distressing sensation of breath holding. The previous information and other studies led to the formulation of a general hypothesis for the mechanism of dyspnea, known as the *length-tension inappropriateness theory.* During normal breathing, it is believed that there is an appropriate relationship between the tension developed by the respiratory muscles and the resulting change in muscle length. Breath holding is the ultimate form of length-tension inappropriateness and the relief achieved by a rebreathing maneuver at the break point of a breath-hold is attributed to shortening of the respiratory muscles, leading to a correction of length-tension inappropriateness. This theory has formed the framework for much of the experimental work that has been conducted into determining the mechanisms responsible for the sensation of dyspnea.

205 What is the difference between the sensation of breathlessness (dyspnea) brought on by physical exercise or emotional stress in respiratory diseases compared to that elicited in normal individuals?

❑ The main difference between the dyspnea observed in patients with pulmonary diseases compared to that of normal individuals is the intensity of the physical exercise or emotional stress required to trigger this symptom. While normal individuals, especially those engaging in regular exercise, require relatively intense physical or emotional stress to trigger dyspnea, those with pulmonary diseases experience this symptom in response to a milder stress. Thus, the main distinction between dyspnea in normal conditions and that in patients with disease may be quantitative (a less intense stress initiates dyspnea in pulmonary disease as well as other illness), although there may also be some qualitative differences. Because exertional dyspnea occurs in normal individuals, it is important to determine whether there has been a change in the level of exertion causing it. Patients with exertional dyspnea will usually report that a level of activity that previously did not cause breathlessness (eg, walking to a particular location from their homes at a given pace) now does so. As respiratory disease worsens, the level of exercise that causes dyspnea decreases. It must be recognized that denial of dyspnea by some patients with overt pulmonary disease might be due to their sedentary life (bedridden patients or those confined indoors) such that they do not perform even low-level physical activities.

206 What is orthopnea?

❑ *Orthopnea* is dyspnea that develops in the supine (recumbent) position and improves or disappears when the thorax is elevated toward the upright position. Most patients relieve their orthopnea by adding one or more extra pillows under their head and upper body while in the recumbent position. Consequently, questions as to the number of pillows used by the patients to rest comfortably should be asked by the treating physician. Because some normal individuals prefer to lay with their head elevated by pillows (for comfort reasons rather than relief of breathlessness), it is important to determine whether a change in the degree of head elevation necessary to provide comfort (eg, increase in number of pillows) has occurred to establish whether orthopnea is present or not. One of the major reasons for the development of orthopnea is an increase in venous return from body regions below the heart (abdomen and all extremities) in the recumbent as compared to the upright position; this imposes a load on a failing heart that is beyond its pumping capability so that pulmonary venous congestion develops. By contrast, the normal heart can accept and eject the increased venous return under these circumstances. Sometimes, patients while in the supine position experience a nonproductive cough instead of dyspnea (manifestation of orthopnea), and this symptom is often called a *dyspnea equivalent.* Some patients with COPD develop orthopnea, as a result of poorly understood alterations in the efficiency of respiratory muscle contraction.

207 What is paroxysmal nocturnal dyspnea?

❑ *Paroxysmal nocturnal dyspnea* (commonly called *PND*) is an important manifestation of congestive heart failure wherein intermittent attacks of dyspnea interrupt or disturb rest or sleep; this symptom develops while the patient is in the supine position for 1 hour or longer. Once PND occurs, the patient sits up in bed to relieve dyspnea and frequently moves to a sofa in an attempt to resume rest in a semirecumbent position. Although the term *PND* denotes a nighttime occurrence of the symptom, it might also occur during the day in patients who rest or sleep at this time. The 1-hour or longer delay for the start of dyspnea in PND, a feature that distinguishes it from other forms of orthopnea (eg, an acute asthma attack), is due to a summation of factors, including (1) slow reabsorption of extracellular fluid accumulation (edema) from dependent areas (eg, lower extremities), causing increased venous return to the heart and thereby pulmonary venous congestion associated with expansion of intrathoracic blood volume; (2) increased work of breathing due to the gravity effects of abdominal viscera that displace the diaphragm and compress the lung bases; and (3) decreased sympathetic tone to the heart during sleep that further impairs myocardial contractility. Pulmonary venous congestion in PND produces fluid accumulation in the pulmonary interstitium and bronchial mucosa, compressing the small bronchi. The wheezing sounds evident on lung auscultation are due to edema of the bronchial walls and associated bronchospasm and account for the term *cardiac asthma* frequently used instead of PND. When associated with chest pain or "heaviness," PND might represent a symptom of myocardial ischemia or so-called angina equivalent.

---

208 What elements help differentiate between pulmonary dyspnea and nonpulmonary dyspnea due to either anxiety, neurosis, or malingering intentions?

❑ Careful examination of patients with shortness of breath based on malingering (eg, false claim of disease in an effort to obtain monetary compensation) and that due to anxiety neurosis might disclose the following distinct features that allow differentiation from dyspnea of pulmonary origin: (1) Dyspnea is present at rest and its intensity is not increased with exercise, (2) patient complains of being unable to take a deep breath, (3) a sighing pattern of breathing is commonly observed, (4) respiration is irregular or effortless during exercise testing, and (5) patient does not have other objective evidence of pulmonary disease that explains the shortness of breath.

---

209 Describe the major clinical features of pulmonary dyspnea that help to differentiate it from cardiac dyspnea.

❑ Pulmonary dyspnea is often associated with a history of smoking, noxious inhalants, bronchial asthma, or chronic lung disease. Sputum production is frequently present and coughing up bronchial secretions alleviates pulmonary dyspnea. The chest x-ray film often shows evidence of lung disease and pulmonary function tests reveal a ventilatory defect that is obstructive (ie, chronic bronchitis, emphysema) or restrictive (ie, pulmonary fibrosis). A restrictive ventilatory defect is also present in patients with congestive heart failure. Cardiac dyspnea generally develops without a history of smoking or pulmonary disease. In addition, sputum production is absent, chest-x-ray films may show features of heart disease and lung congestion, and pulmonary function tests may reveal a restrictive ventilatory defect (eg, congestive heart failure).

210 How can the cause of dyspnea be determined (eg, lung disease, cardiac disease, anxiety)?

❑ A thorough clinical evaluation can establish the cause of dyspnea in most patients without requesting expensive or complicated laboratory determinations. Yet, the cause of dyspnea (eg, anxiety, lung disease, cardiac disease, superimposition of heart and lung disease in a single patient) might remain undiagnosed after clinical examination so that further studies are mandatory. Differentiation between pulmonary and cardiac dyspnea in clinical practice often requires additional evaluation including the response to Valsalva's maneuver, exercise studies, pulmonary function testing, or measurement of the circulation time.

211 What is Valsalva's maneuver? What is its role in the differential diagnosis of dyspnea?

❑ *Valsalva's maneuver* is a forced expiration against a resistance (eg, closed glottis, column of water, manometer) so that intrathoracic pressure rises, producing characteristic hemodynamic effects. A typical Valsalva maneuver is performed during defecation. This test has been standardized (as explained in the answer to another question) and is useful in the diagnosis of heart failure. Consequently, evaluation of the hemodynamic response to Valsalva's maneuver might help differentiation of cardiac dyspnea from lung dyspnea.

212 How is the standardized Valsalva maneuver performed and what are its hemodynamic effects in normal individuals? What phases of Valsalva's maneuver allow evaluation of cardiovascular function?

❑ The patient is asked to forcefully expire (blow) against a resistance of 40 mm Hg (aneroid manometer) for 30 seconds. Intrathoracic pressure rises during Valsalva's maneuver, decreasing systemic venous return to the heart and leading to reduced stroke volume and increased systemic venous pressure. The following changes in blood pressure and heart rate occur: (1) Arterial pressure immediately rises with initiation of the expiration effort due to transmission of the increased intrathoracic pressure. (2) Thereafter, arterial pressure decreases (systolic, diastolic, and pulse pressure levels) due to diminished systemic venous return during sustained expiration; the arterial hypotension characteristic of this phase produces reflex tachycardia mediated by depressed activity of arterial baroreceptors. (3) Subsequently, blood pressure decreases further on release of expiration effort due to transmission of the fall in intrathoracic pressure. (4) Finally, arterial pressure and pulse pressure abruptly increase, accompanied by reflex bradycardia on discontinuation of the expiratory effort; the increase in systemic venous return observed during this phase produces the rise in blood pressure that in turn acts on arterial baroreceptors (stimulation) to produce reflex bradycardia. Thus, changes in blood pressure during phases 1 and 3 (initiation and interruption of expiratory effort) of Valsalva's maneuver result from transmission of changes in intrathoracic pressure and thereby, are independent of hemodynamic responses. Consequently, only phases 2 and 4 of Valsalva's maneuver evaluate cardiovascular function.

---

213 What are the hemodynamic effects of Valsalva's maneuver in patients with heart failure? What information can be obtained with careful evaluation of the arterial pulse during this maneuver?

❑ Patients with heart failure exhibit neither the decreased arterial pressure with tachycardia of phase 2 (sustained expiration) nor the increased arterial pressure with bradycardia of phase 4 (recovery phase after expiration) that are characteristic of normal individuals. The lack of changes in arterial pressure during phases 2 and 4 of patients with heart failure is due to the constancy of their stroke volume throughout the course of this maneuver. The absences of reflex tachycardia and bradycardia of phases 2 and 4, respectively, are due to the lack of inhibition and stimulation, respectively, of arterial baroreceptors, leading to a constant arterial pressure during these phases. Careful examination of the arterial pulse during Valsalva's maneuver allows recognition of the changes in heart rate observed in normal individuals and their absence in heart failure. A more rigorous evaluation of all the hemodynamic effects of Valsalva's maneuver requires insertion of an indwelling needle or catheter connected to a blood pressure transducer and a recorder for examination of the tracing. Changes in intra-arterial pressure during Valsalva's maneuver in normal individuals can be summarized as follows: increase, decrease, further decrease, and recovery, for phases 1, 2, 3, and 4, respectively. Since the increased (phase 1) and decreased (phase 3) blood pressures that accompany initiation and termination of respiratory effort are also present in patients with heart failure, while blood pressure changes of phases 2 and 4 are absent, the tracing in cardiac failure resembles a "square wave." That is, blood pressure increases with initiation of the maneuver and remains elevated as long as the expiratory effort is sustained, and decreases with discontinuation of forced expiration in patients with heart failure.

214 How can exercise testing determine that dyspnea is of cardiac origin but not of respiratory origin?

❑ The response to exercise in patients with cardiac dyspnea is as follows: Exercise capacity is limited with decreased maximal $\dot{V}O_2$ and increased heart rate relative to work rate. In addition, oxygen uptake at all levels of exercise is increased, oxygen uptake per heart beat is decreased, but ventilatory response is normal.

215 How might the causes of dyspnea be conveniently classified from a clinical point of view?

❑ Dyspnea is a cardinal manifestation of respiratory and cardiac diseases. From a clinical standpoint, dyspnea might result from

(1) an increase in respiratory drive or effort necessary to overcome an imposed load, for example, obstructive or restrictive lung disease or pleural disease; (2) an increase in the proportion of respiratory muscle force required for breathing, for example, neuromuscular weakness or hyperinflation; and (3) an increase in ventilatory requirements, for example, oxygen deprivation of tissues, increased metabolic rate, anemia, hypoxemia, or pulmonary vascular disease.

216 Why is it important to differentiate pulmonary from cardiac dyspnea?

❑ Because treatment of each of these mechanisms of dyspnea is accomplished by the use of different diet regimens (ie, low-salt diet for cardiac dyspnea but not pulmonary dyspnea) and drugs (ie, bronchodilators for pulmonary dyspnea secondary to obstructed airways, digitalis and afterload-reducing agents for cardiac dyspnea), it is important to establish the pathogenesis of dyspnea in a given patient. Furthermore, patients with combined pulmonary and cardiac dyspnea for whom only one of the two components of dyspnea is recognized might remain short of breath despite successful treatment of the recognized cause of dyspnea. Failure to completely relieve the symptoms of such a patient frequently leads to the identification and treatment of the disease responsible for the previously unrecognized cause of dyspnea (pulmonary or cardiac).

217 Is the evaluation of circulation time (eg, arm to tongue) useful in the differentiation of pulmonary dyspnea from cardiac dyspnea? Is circulation time a sensitive parameter for the diagnosis of heart failure?

❑ Measurement of circulation time is not a sensitive test but remains as a useful tool (unfortunately, it is rarely done in some institutions) for the diagnosis of heart failure. This simple test helps to differentiate high-output from low-output heart failure, and pulmonary from cardiac dyspnea. The prolonged circulation time observed in patients with low-output cardiac failure is due to reduced velocity of blood flow and to dilution of the test substance (3 to 5 mL of 20% dehydrocholic acid [Decholin]) by the increased blood volume within the congested venous systems in the systemic and pulmonary circulations.

218 Describe how a bedside evaluation of circulation time helps to differentiate pulmonary from cardiac dyspnea. Explain this test in detail.

❑ Normal values of arm-to-tongue circulation time (9 to 16 seconds) are observed in patients with pulmonary dyspnea. In contrast, cardiac dyspnea caused by low-output heart failure is characterized by a prolonged circulation time (>16 seconds). The test is performed by rapidly injecting 3 to 5 mL of dehydrocholic acid in a vein of the antecubital fossa and measuring the time between the start of the injection and the appearance of a bitter taste sensed by the patient. This time-honored test, less commonly used nowadays, is of special value when the etiology of dyspnea is difficult to determine. It is also of value in assessing the relative contribution of pulmonary and cardiac dyspnea in patients with both diseases. Circulation time is normal or even reduced in patients with high-output heart failure. Consequently, this test fails to differentiate pulmonary dyspnea from the cardiac dyspnea of patients with high output heart failure.

219 How might the use of diuretics help to establish whether dyspnea is caused by pulmonary disease or heart failure?

❑ Improvement of dyspnea after a diuretic-induced weight loss that exceeds 2 kg (about 4 lb) supports that fluid overload due to heart failure has been responsible for the respiratory symptoms. Conversely, the lack of effects of a diuretic regimen on dyspnea suggests another pathogenesis for this symptom, including pulmonary diseases. It should be recognized that amelioration of the shortness of breath after the administration of diuretics simply indicates that fluid overload due to any cause (eg, heart failure, renal failure) was responsible for the symptom but is not a specific response observed in heart failure.

Part II: Pathophysiology of Respiratory Failure

9. Main Types of Respiratory Failure

RESPIRATORY PUMP FAILURE AND HYPOXEMIC RESPIRATORY FAILURE: OVERVIEW

220 What is the role of arterial blood gas (ABG) determination in the diagnosis of respiratory failure?

❑ The diagnosis of respiratory failure cannot be made on the basis of only the patient's history or physical examination but requires ABG measurements. Levels of PaO_2 lower than 55 mm Hg and $PaCO_2$ higher than 50 mm Hg are used for the diagnosis of respiratory failure. However, these values do not represent absolute criteria, as an increase in $PaCO_2$ does not necessarily imply respiratory failure. Therefore, it is imperative to evaluate the arterial blood pH, because a secondary increase in $PaCO_2$ is the expected response to metabolic alkalosis in the absence of respiratory failure. In fact, $PaCO_2$ of 86 mm Hg has been documented in a patient with metabolic alkalosis who was free of any respiratory disease. In addition, it is important to evaluate the arterial blood pH and serum bicarbonate level ($[HCO_3^-]$) to help determine whether respiratory acidosis is acute or chronic. As a rule of thumb, the secondary response (commonly referred to, inappropriately, as *compensatory response*) to hypercapnia is accompanied by a change in arterial blood pH, which falls by 0.08 unit and 0.03 unit in acute and chronic hypercapnia, respectively, for an increase in $PaCO_2$ of 10 mm Hg. The term *compensatory response* to a primary acid-base disorder should be discarded in favor of the less approbatory term *secondary response* because it has been demonstrated that in several conditions such response is maladaptive (ie, worsens the primary acid-base disorder).

221 What are the main causes of hypoxemia?

❑ The main causes of hypoxemia are (1) decreased partial pressure of oxygen in the inspired gas (PiO_2), (2) alveolar hypoventilation,

(3) diffusion impairment at the alveolar-capillary level (see below), (4) ventilation-perfusion abnormalities ($\dot{V}/\dot{Q}$ defects), and (5) right-to-left blood shunting. The specific conditions and diseases that can induce hypoxemia through one or more of these mechanisms are examined in the answers to pertinent questions. It must be recognized that hypoxemia caused by a diffusion impairment at the alveolar-capillary level, although of great theoretical interest, does not play a role in the development of hypoxemia in any disease state.

222 What are the determinants of the association of hypercapnia and hypoxemia in respiratory failure?

❑ The simplified form of the alveolar gas equation dictates that at sea level, and when breathing room air,

$$P_{A}O_2 = 150 - 1.25\ PaCO_2$$

where $P_{A}O_2$ is alveolar oxygen tension in millimeters of mercury. Reasoning from this relationship, it becomes apparent that the major threat to life from carbon dioxide retention in patients breathing room air is the associated obligatory hypoxemia. In the absence of supplemental oxygen, patients in respiratory arrest develop critical hypoxemia within a few minutes, long before severe hypercapnia ensues. The constraints of the alveolar gas equation establish that patients breathing room air cannot reach $PaCO_2$ levels much higher than 80 mm Hg, because the degree of hypoxemia that would develop at higher values is incompatible with life. Therefore, extreme hypercapnia occurs only during oxygen therapy, and indeed severe carbon dioxide retention is often the result of uncontrolled oxygen administration.

223 Is the association of hypercapnia and hypoxemia a constant feature in all forms of respiratory failure? What is the relationship between the severity of the hypoxemia and the level of $PaCO_2$ in patients with respiratory failure?

❑ No. The relationship between the severity of the hypoxemia and the level of $PaCO_2$ differs in the two major clinical forms of respiratory insufficiency. When respiratory acidosis results from "respiratory pump failure," a pattern of "pure alveolar hypoventilation" develops, in which the alveolar-arterial gradient for oxygen (P_A-aO_2) remains normal and the increment in $PaCO_2$ is accompanied by an equivalent decrement in PaO_2. This type of respiratory pump failure results from disorders without parenchymal lung disease, in which the alveolar gas exchange is normal. In contrast with respiratory pump failure, abnormalities in the lung parenchyma produce the so-called hypoxemic respiratory failure. In the latter condition, the reduction in PaO_2 is substantially greater than the simultaneous increment in $PaCO_2$, and the P_A-aO_2 widens. In fact, if sufficient ventilatory reserve is still present, lung disease frequently results in substantial hypoxemia in the company of normal or even low values of $PaCO_2$.

224 What are the major types of respiratory failure?

❑ The major types of respiratory failure are ventilatory pump failure, inefficient gas exchange (ie, hypoxemic respiratory failure), or a combination of these processes. Ventilatory pump failure may be secondary to reduced respiratory center drive, mechanical defects of the chest wall, and respiratory muscle fatigue. In turn, hypoxemic respiratory failure can be caused by abnormalities in functional residual capacity (FRC), ventilation-perfusion mismatch, and intrapulmonary shunt. Bedside calculation of the P_A-aO_2 gradient is useful for differentiating the two major types of respiratory failure because it will be normal with pure alveolar hypoventilation (ie, ventilatory pump failure) and increased with diseases associated with inefficient gas exchange (ie, $\dot{V}_A/\dot{Q}$ mismatch).

225 Outline the main features and causes of ventilatory pump failure.

❑ Ventilatory pump failure results in alveolar hypoventilation that is caused by decreased minute ventilation ($\dot{V}_E$). A reduction in alveolar ventilation ($\dot{V}_A$) secondary to decreased $\dot{V}_E$ will cause an increase in $PaCO_2$, provided that carbon dioxide production remains unchanged, as follows:

$$PCO_2 \approx \frac{\text{Carbon dioxide production}}{\dot{V}_A}$$

Overall $\dot{V}_E$ consists of two components: ventilation distributed to the gas-exchange units of the lungs ($\dot{V}_A$) and ventilation wasted in dead space ($\dot{V}_D$). Thus, $\dot{V}_A$ may decrease because of either a reduction in $\dot{V}_E$ (hypoventilation) or an increase in $\dot{V}_D$ secondary to ventilation-perfusion ($\dot{V}_A/\dot{Q}$) inequality. The main causes of ventilatory pump failure are reduced respiratory center drive, mechanical defects of the chest wall, and respiratory muscle dysfunction.

226 What specific conditions are associated with hypoxemia caused by alveolar hypoventilation?

❑ The specific conditions that might cause alveolar hypoventilation and thereby hypoxemia as well as carbon dioxide retention are conveniently classified as acute and chronic forms of hypercapnic respiratory failure. In addition, these acute and chronic conditions may be further divided into those associated with normal airways and lungs and those with abnormal airways and lungs. This classification is identical to that described for the causes of carbon dioxide retention (ie, acute and chronic respiratory acidosis). These causes are briefly reviewed in the answers to the following questions.

227 Compare the principal pathophysiologic abnormality of the two forms of respiratory failure (ie, hypoxemic and hypercapnic).

❑ Respiratory failure is characterized by the presence of hypoxemia, hypercapnia, or both abnormalities. Hypoxemic respiratory failure may result from hypoventilation, but is more commonly caused by ventilation: perfusion inequality or intrapulmonary shunting. On the other hand, hypercapnic respiratory failure results primarily from alveolar hypoventilation, although $\dot{V}A/\dot{Q}$ inequality can play a contributing role.

228 Why do patients with "hypoxemic respiratory failure," as opposed to those with "respiratory pump failure," commonly have arterial hypocapnia?

❑ As previously indicated, the nearly linear shape of the dissociation curve of carbon dioxide over the physiologic range allows for greater than normal carbon dioxide excretion (due to hypoxemia-induced enhanced ventilation) from areas of the lungs with relatively preserved gas exchange, thereby offsetting the effects of simultaneous carbon dioxide retention occurring in areas of the lung that are consolidated or underventilated. Conversely, the shape of the oxyhemoglobin dissociation curve accounts for the fact that hyperventilation of lung areas in which hemoglobin is already maximally saturated with oxygen will not offset the right-to-left shunting of hypoxic blood perfusing capillaries in underventilated areas. As a consequence, arterial hypoxemia in association with hypocapnia is commonly observed with "hypoxemic respiratory failure," but eucapnia and even hypercapnia can also develop.

RESPIRATORY PUMP FAILURE: PRIMARY HYPERCAPNIA (RESPIRATORY ACIDOSIS)

229 Define respiratory acidosis and explain its relationship with respiratory failure.

❑ Respiratory acidosis is the acid-base disturbance initiated with an increase in PCO_2 of body fluids. The terms *respiratory acidosis* and *primary hypercapnia* are synonymous. The secondary response involves an increased plasma bicarbonate concentration ($[HCO_3^-]_p$). During acute hypercapnia, a small increment in

$[HCO_3^-]_p$ that results from titration of the body's non-HCO_3^- buffers is observed. When hypercapnia is sustained, renal adjustments yield a much larger secondary increment in $[HCO_3^-]_p$. Respiratory acidosis is most commonly caused by decreased alveolar ventilation and therefore, indicates the presence of respiratory failure.

230 What is the major threat to life from carbon dioxide retention in patients breathing room air?

❑ The simplified form of the alveolar gas equation dictates that, at sea levels and when breathing room air,

$$P_{AO_2} = 150 - 1.2\ PaCO_2$$

Reasoning from this relationship, it becomes apparent that the major threat to life from carbon dioxide retention in patients breathing room air is the associated obligatory hypoxemia. Furthermore, in the absence of supplemental oxygen, patients in respiratory arrest develop critical hypoxemia within a few minutes, long before severe hypercapnia ensues.

231 Explain further the concepts of primary hypercapnia and secondary hypercapnia.

❑ Primary hypercapnia, also known as *respiratory acidosis,* is that acid-base disturbance initiated by an elevation in carbon dioxide tension of body fluids. Conversely, the hypercapnia observed in metabolic alkalosis is a secondary hypercapnia that should be viewed as an integral part of this primary metabolic disorder. Secondary hypercapnia develops as a physiologic response to alkalemia of metabolic origin.

232 Does the diagnosis of respiratory acidosis always require demonstration of $PaCO_2$ levels higher than normal?

❑ No. Although primary hypercapnia is usually recognized by the presence of $PaCO_2$ levels at rest and at sea level higher than

45 mm Hg, lower levels might be observed in special circumstances. For example, in patients with metabolic acidosis, the presence of normal $PaCO_2$ levels is indicative of the concomitant presence of primary hypercapnia, for the expected secondary response to the metabolic disorder is the development of hypocapnia. Another example is the presence of arterial eucapnia or even hypocapnia in the company of severe venous hypercapnia in patients having an acute, profound decrease in cardiac output; in this instance, the decreased pulmonary perfusion in association with relatively preserved pulmonary ventilation lead to reduction in carbon dioxide excretion and, thus, net retention of carbon dioxide in body fluids.

233 Explain the development of respiratory acidosis that results from an impaired alveolar gas exchange.

❑ A reduction in the effective alveolar ventilation ($\dot{V}_A$) leads to respiratory acidosis in the presence of normal or even increased total minute ventilation ($\dot{V}_E$). The defect responsible for this condition is an increased dead space ventilation resulting from alveoli that remained ventilated but not perfused and from alveoli with excessive ventilation with respect to their perfusion; in both instances, there exists an increased $\dot{V}_A/\dot{Q}$ ratio. Advanced chronic obstructive pulmonary disease (COPD) is the most typical condition in which this pathophysiologic defect dominates the carbon dioxide retention observed. The maintenance of eucapnia in patients with less advanced disease results from an increased minute ventilation, which compensates for the inefficiency of the carbon dioxide excretion imposed by the $\dot{V}_A/\dot{Q}$ mismatch. Should airway resistance increase (because of bronchial spasm, edema of the bronchial wall, or retention of secretions), however, or if the minute ventilation required to maintain eucapnia is too high, the $PaCO_2$ will rise, possibly because of respiratory muscle fatigue; under these circumstances, total ventilation might still be normal, yet inadequate to excrete the carbon dioxide load in the presence of a severe $\dot{V}_A/\dot{Q}$ mismatch.

234 Elaborate on the changes in blood pH and $[HCO_3^-]_p$ observed in respiratory acidosis.

❑ Hypercapnia acidifies body fluids and elicits an immediate small increment in $[HCO_3^-]_p$ because of titration of the body's nonbicarbonate buffers to the acid direction. Sustained hypercapnia produces a much larger secondary increment in $[HCO_3^-]_p$ that is accounted for by the renal acidification responses to carbon dioxide retention. The increased $[HCO_3^-]_p$ level resulting from primary hypercapnia diminishes the severity of the acidemia but falls short of fully correcting the decreased pH.

235 Is the acidemia (decreased blood pH) of respiratory acidosis accompanied by changes in intracellular and cerebrospinal pH?

❑ Yes. Hypercapnia acidifies body fluids and the decreased pH is evident in both intracellular and extracellular fluids. The intracellular pH during acute hypercapnia decreases in skeletal muscle and kidney by a magnitude similar to that in the extracellular compartment; yet, in other tissues including cardiac muscle, cerebral cortex, and liver, smaller changes in intracellular pH have been reported. Differences in physicochemical buffering, transmembrane ionic fluxes of hydrogen ions, and production of endogenous acids account for the different responses of intracellular pH in the various tissues. Changes in the electrolyte composition of the cerebrospinal fluid (CSF) take place in respiratory acidosis. A prompt increase in CSF hydrogen ion concentration is observed with increases in $PaCO_2$, because of diffusion of carbon dioxide across the blood-brain barrier. A progressive increase in CSF bicarbonate concentration occurs when hypercapnia persists, and the steady-state pH decrements in the blood and CSF compartments are virtually identical.

236 How is the diagnosis of ventilatory failure established?

❑ Information obtained from the clinical history, physical examination, and ancillary laboratory data, including ABGs, is required to properly establish the presence of respiratory acidosis and its pathogenesis. Accurate laboratory data are a prerequisite for making the diagnosis of ventilatory failure and whenever this disorder is suspected, ABGs should be measured. Yet, the demonstration of hypercapnia by ABG analysis is in itself insufficient to establish the presence of primary hypercapnia. ABG data should be evaluated in the context of the patient's history. Part or all of the rise in PCO_2 might reflect an adaptive response to metabolic alkalosis rather than being simply respiratory acidosis. If the patient's acid-base profile reveals hypercapnia in association with acidemia, at least an element of respiratory acidosis must be present. A normal or even an alkaline blood pH might accompany the carbon dioxide retention, however, if additional acid-base disorders are simultaneously present.

237 What are the mechanisms responsible for primary hypercapnia or respiratory acidosis?

❑ A positive carbon dioxide balance develops whenever carbon dioxide excretion is insufficient to match carbon dioxide production ($\dot{V}CO_2$). Thus, decreased carbon dioxide elimination, increased $\dot{V}CO_2$, or both, might generate primary hypercapnia or respiratory acidosis. It should be recognized that increased $\dot{V}CO_2$ does not induce hypercapnia unless the mechanics of breathing, the V_D/V_T ratio, or the control of ventilation is abnormal. In most clinical settings, the development of hypercapnia is multifactorial, and recognition of each one of the underlying mechanisms of carbon dioxide retention permits efficient patient management. Five factors may participate in the pathogenesis of respiratory acidosis: abnormalities in the gas-exchange function of the lung parenchyma (eg, altered V_D/V_T and $\dot{V}/\dot{Q}$), disturbances in the mechanics of breathing, abnormalities in respiratory muscles, alterations in the control of pulmonary ventilation, and increased $\dot{V}CO_2$.

238 What elements of the respiratory system must be defective to produce carbon dioxide retention?

❑ Defects within any element of the respiratory system including the central and peripheral nervous systems, the respiratory muscles, the thoracic cage, the pleural space, the airways, and the lung parenchyma can lead to carbon dioxide retention. Thus, primary hypercapnia can develop in patients with normal as well as abnormal airways and lungs. Not infrequently, more than one cause contributes to the development of primary hypercapnia in a given patient.

239 Describe the causes of increased carbon dioxide production that might result in respiratory acidosis.

❑ Excessive $\dot{V}CO_2$ is seldom, if ever, the sole cause of carbon dioxide retention because enhanced $\dot{V}CO_2$ stimulates ventilation, thus increasing carbon dioxide excretion. Yet, patients with marked reduction in pulmonary reserve and those receiving constant mechanical ventilation might develop respiratory acidosis as a result of increased $\dot{V}CO_2$. Relevant clinical conditions characterized by an increased $\dot{V}CO_2$ include physical activity, increased work by the respiratory muscles, seizures, shivering, fever, a large carbohydrate load, and hyperthyroidism. The effect of hyperthermia might be very substantial considering that $\dot{V}CO_2$ increases by 13% for each increase in body temperature of 1°C above the normal value. The administration of large carbohydrate loads, orally or parenterally, represents a potentially significant cause of enhanced $\dot{V}CO_2$ in patients with hypercapnic respiratory failure or when such patients are being weaned from ventilatory support. Under these circumstances, the use of a larger proportion of fat in the diet might properly supplement the caloric intake without imposing the carbon dioxide burden that results from the intake of carbohydrates. Additional causes of carbon dioxide loading include the infusion of bicarbonate-containing solutions, hemodialysis with sorbent regenerative cartridge systems, and insufflation of the peritoneum with carbon dioxide during endoscopic procedures.

240 Give a practical classification of causes of respiratory pump failure leading to respiratory acidosis.

❑ The causes of respiratory pump failure leading to respiratory acidosis might be classified in two broad categories, namely, acute and chronic respiratory acidosis. It is practical to classify them further into causes with normal airways and lungs and those with abnormal airways and lungs.

---

241 What are the causes of acute respiratory pump failure (ie, acute hypercapnic respiratory failure) in patients with normal airways and lungs?

❑ The causes of acute respiratory pump failure included in this category are (1) *central nervous system (CNS) depression* due to general anesthesia, sedative overdosage, head trauma, cerebrovascular accident, central sleep apnea, cerebral edema, brain tumor, or encephalitis; (2) *neuromuscular impairment* resulting from high spinal cord injury, Guillain-Barré syndrome, status epilepticus, botulism, tetanus, crisis in myasthenia gravis, hypokalemic myopathy, familial periodic paralysis or drugs or toxic agents (ie, curare, succinylcholine, aminoglycosides, and organophosphorus); (3) *ventilatory restriction* caused by rib fractures with flail chest, pneumothorax, hemothorax, or impaired diaphragmatic function (ie, peritoneal dialysis, ascites); and (4) *iatrogenic events* including misplacement or displacement of the airway cannula during anesthesia or mechanical ventilation, bronchoscopy-associated hypoventilation or respiratory arrest, and increased carbon dioxide production with constant mechanical ventilation (ie, due to high-carbohydrate diet or sorbent-regenerative hemodialysis).

---

242 What are the causes of acute respiratory pump failure (ie, acute hypercapnic respiratory failure) in patients with abnormal airways and lungs?

❑ Abnormalities in the airways and lungs that might cause acute respiratory pump failure include (1) *upper-airway obstruction* due to coma-induced hypopharyngeal obstruction, aspiration of a foreign body or vomitus, laryngospasm, angioedema, obstructive sleep apnea, or laryngeal obstruction after intubation; (2) *lower-airway obstruction* caused by generalized bronchospasm, severe episode of asthma, or bronchiolitis in infants and adults; (3) *alveolar filling defects* as a result of severe bilateral pneumonia or bronchopneumonia, acute respiratory distress syndrome (ARDS), or severe pulmonary edema; and (4) *pulmonary perfusion defects* including cardiac arrest, severe circulatory failure, massive pulmonary thromboembolism, and fat or air pulmonary embolism.

---

243 What are the causes of chronic respiratory pump failure (ie, chronic hypercapnic respiratory failure) in patients with normal airways and lungs?

❑ The causes of chronic respiratory pump failure included in this category are (1) *CNS depression* caused by sedative overdosage, methadone/heroin addiction, central alveolar hypoventilation syndrome, brain tumor, or bulbar poliomyelitis; (2) *neuromuscular impairment* caused by poliomyelitis, multiple sclerosis, muscular dystrophy, amyotrophic lateral sclerosis, diaphragmatic paralysis, myxedema, or myopathic disease (eg, polymyositis); and (3) *abnormal chest wall mechanics* due to kyphoscoliosis, ankylosing spondylitis, obesity, fibrothorax, or hydrothorax.

---

244 What are the causes of chronic respiratory pump failure (ie, chronic hypercapnic respiratory failure) in patients with abnormal airways and lungs?

❑ Abnormalities in the airways and lungs that might result in chronic respiratory pump failure include (1) *upper-airway obstruction* including tonsillar and peritonsillar hypertrophy, paralysis of the vocal cords, tumor of the cords or of the larynx, stenosis of airways after prolonged intubation, thymoma, and aortic aneurysm; (2) *lower-airway obstruction* due to chronic bronchitis, bronchiolitis, bronchiectasis, or emphysema; and (3) *disorders involving the pulmonary alveoli* caused by severe chronic pneumonitis, diffuse infiltrative disease (eg, alveolar proteinosis), or interstitial fibrosis.

245 What elements allow the differential diagnosis of acute hypercapnia from its chronic form?

❑ Differentiation between acute and chronic hypercapnia can be a difficult task. A major element that helps to make this distinction is the clinical history. Neither the level of hypercapnia nor the magnitude of the associated hypoxemia are particularly helpful. The acid-base parameters themselves can be of assistance if the presence of complicating acid-base disorders can be excluded. Acute hypercapnia is associated with a lower $[HCO_3^-]_p$ and blood pH than is chronic hypercapnia of the same magnitude. Yet, for a number of reasons, the levels of $[HCO_3^-]_p$ and blood pH are of limited help for the differentiation of acute and chronic hypercapnia. Such reasons include individual variability in the secondary response to hypercapnia, differences in the degree of expression of the adaptive responses due to disparities in the time elapsed from the onset of hypercapnia, and the possible coexistence of additional acid-base disorders. Once more, the most important information might be obtained from the patient's history.

246 What are the manifestations of carbon dioxide retention in acute respiratory failure? Describe the most commonly observed neurologic and cardiovascular signs and symptoms of hypercapnia.

❑ The major manifestations of hypercapnia are those that affect the CNS and to a lesser degree, the cardiovascular system. Acute hypercapnia can cause anxiety, dyspnea, confusion, transient psychosis, and coma. However, coma is uncommon in patients breathing room air, as the level of $PaCO_2$ necessary to cause coma is usually associated with a PaO_2 that is incompatible with life. Motor disturbances, including tremors, myoclonic jerks, asterixis, and seizures, frequently occur. Intracranial pressure can rise from the vasodilating action of carbon dioxide and can cause headache or papilledema. In addition, focal signs mimicking a cerebrovascular accident or tumor can occur. The cardiovascular features of hypercapnia are largely caused by the vasodilator and sympathetic stimulant effects of carbon dioxide. These effects include warm flushed skin, diaphoresis, and a bounding pulse; blood pressure may be normal or low. It must be pointed out that these clinical features are neither sensitive to nor specific for the development of hypercapnia. The pathophysiologic basis for these features, although not fully understood, is probably multifactorial in origin and depends on the rapidity and magnitude of the increase in $PaCO_2$ and on the severity of accompanying acidosis and hypoxemia.

RESPONSE TO PRIMARY HYPERCAPNIA

247 What is the secondary physiologic response to primary carbon dioxide retention (primary hypercapnia or respiratory acidosis)?

❑ Hypercapnia decreases the pH of body fluids due to accumulation of carbonic acid. A secondary adaptive increase in $[HCO_3^-]_p$ that originates from titration of body nonbicarbonate buffers is observed immediately and ameliorates the acidemia. During sustained hypercapnia, a much larger secondary increment in $[HCO_3^-]_p$ develops because of renal adaptive mechanisms.

248 Elaborate on the mechanisms of the secondary response to acute hypercapnia. Describe the expected change in the metabolic component of acid-base status during acute carbon dioxide retention.

❑ During acute hypercapnia, approximately one-third of the total buffering response can be ascribed to red blood cell and extracellular fluid buffering, the remaining two-thirds being attributed to tissue buffering. The kidney does not make a measurable contribution to the acute increment in $[HCO_3^-]_p$ elicited by acute hypercapnia; yet, changes in the bicarbonate reabsorption rate and in the urine composition are detectable within minutes after induction of hypercapnia. $[HCO_3^-]_p$ increases by approximately 0.1 mEq/L for each 1 mm Hg acute increment in $PaCO_2$, and this adjustment in bicarbonate levels due to buffering is completed within 5 to 10 minutes. Thus, the overall increment in $[HCO_3^-]_p$ is quite small, amounting to only 3 to 4 mEq/L even when $PaCO_2$ is increased to 80 or 90 mm Hg. The modest increase in $[HCO_3^-]_p$ observed during acute carbon dioxide equilibration in vivo contrasts sharply with the large increase obtained during in vitro carbon dioxide equilibration of whole blood over the same range of carbon dioxide tensions (see answer to pertinent question).

249 What accounts for the substantially larger increase in $[HCO_3^-]_p$ observed during in vitro carbon dioxide equilibration of whole blood in comparison with the results obtained during acute carbon dioxide equilibration in vivo (ie, intact subject developing acute respiratory acidosis)?

❑ As explained elsewhere in this book, an increase in PCO_2 in a blood sample in vitro as well as in an intact individual initiates the following reaction: Hydration of carbon dioxide generates carbonic acid (H_2CO_3), which subsequently dissociates, producing H^+ and a HCO_3^-. The H^+ is, to some extent, bound by the nonbicarbonate buffers; thus, the reaction is further sustained, resulting in an increment in $[HCO_3^-]_p$ as follows:

$$CO_2 + H_2O \Leftrightarrow H_2CO_3 \Leftrightarrow HCO_3^- + H^+$$

$$HCO_3^- + H^+ + Buf^- + X^+$$

$$\Leftrightarrow Buf\,H^+ + HCO_3^- + X^+ \text{ (mostly } Na^+)$$

This reaction is best known as the *interaction reaction* of body buffers and is responsible for the rise in $[HCO_3^-]_p$ during acute hypercapnia. Under in vitro conditions the newly formed bicarbonate fully remains in the compartment where it was generated; because blood is rich in the nonbicarbonate buffer hemoglobin, in vitro equilibration of blood with carbon dioxide produces a large increase in $[HCO_3^-]_p$. Under in vivo conditions the effects are quite different; acute hypercapnia acting on the intravascular and cellular compartments, rich in nonbicarbonate buffers, results in the production of significant quantities of new bicarbonate, increasing the concentration of bicarbonate in these compartments. Carbon dioxide, a rapidly diffusible gas, increases its tension to a similar degree in the interstitial fluid, which, as opposed to the intravascular and intracellular fluids, is practically devoid of nonbicarbonate buffers. Because there is no generation of bicarbonate in the interstitial compartment, the concentration of this ion initially remains unchanged. The new concentration gradient for bicarbonate among the body fluid compartments leads to the migration of bicarbonate from the intravascular, and possibly from the intracellular, to the interstitial compartment. Thus, the smaller rise in $[HCO_3^-]_p$ during acute hypercapnia under in vivo as compared to in vitro conditions (as well as the base deficit observed in vivo) is the result of the loss of bicarbonate from the blood to the interstitial fluid.

250 Does moderate hypoxemia and other conditions alter the adaptation to chronic hypercapnia? Do these factors modify the recovery from chronic hypercapnia?

❑ The adaptation to acute and chronic hypercapnia is not altered appreciably by the coexistence of moderate hypoxemia. In contrast to the lack of effect of chloride deprivation in the adaptive response to persistent hypercapnia, the return of body bicarbonate stores to normal during recovery from this disorder is hampered by chloride unavailability. Under these circumstances, $[HCO_3^-]_p$ remains elevated following restoration of a normal $PaCO_2$, because the chloride losses that developed during the adaptive process cannot be replenished. As a result, a state of "posthypercapnic metabolic alkalosis" develops.

251 Describe the expected secondary responses (ie, metabolic responses) to acute and chronic hypercapnia.

❑ In the case of primary respiratory acid-base disorders, the secondary response elicited is a change in $[HCO_3^-]_p$ in the same direction as the change in the PCO_2 level. Thus, respiratory acidosis induces secondary hyperbicarbonatemia, and respiratory alkalosis induces secondary hypobicarbonatemia. On average, $[HCO_3^-]_p$ increases by 0.1 mEq for each 1 mm Hg acute increment in PCO_2. As a result, $[H^+]_p$ increases 0.75 nEq/L for each 1 mm Hg rise in PCO_2. This adaptation is completed within 5 to 10 minutes of the rise in $PaCO_2$, but the response to chronic hypercapnia requires 3 to 5 days for its completion. On average, $[HCO_3^-]_p$ increases 0.3 mEq/L for each 1 mm Hg chronic increment in PCO_2; as a result $[H^+]_p$ rises 0.3 nEq/L for each 1 mm Hg rise in PCO_2.

---

252 Describe the expected secondary responses (ie, respiratory responses) or mean ''whole-body'' response equations for simple metabolic acid-base disturbances.

❑ In the case of primary metabolic acid-base disorders, the secondary response involves a change in the PCO_2 level in the same direction as the change in $[HCO_3^-]_p$. Thus, metabolic acidosis induces secondary hypocapnia and metabolic alkalosis induces secondary hypercapnia. The $\Delta PCO_2/\Delta[HCO_3^-]_p$ is approximately 1.2 mm Hg/mEq/L of $\Delta[HCO_3^-]_p$ in metabolic acidosis, and 0.7 mm Hg/mEq/L of $\Delta[HCO_3^-]$ in metabolic alkalosis. The maximum level of adaptation results in a PCO_2 as low as 10 mm Hg in metabolic acidosis and as high as 55 mm Hg or more (eg, a $PaCO_2$ of 86 mm Hg has been reported, although this level should be considered most unusual) in metabolic alkalosis.

---

253 Elaborate on the relationship between chloride intake and the adaptation to chronic hypercapnia as well as recovery from it.

❑ During adaptation to hypercapnia, the increment in $[HCO_3^-]_p$ is associated with increased chloruresis and a negative chloride balance. The level of dietary electrolyte intake has no significant relevance with respect to the adaptation to chronic hypercapnia. The recovery from chronic hypercapnia, however, is greatly influenced by dietary chloride intake. Animals and humans recovering from chronic hypercapnia promptly eliminate the secondary metabolic response in the presence of adequate chloride intake. The adequate chloride intake replaces the depressed chloride stores and allows the kidney to excrete bicarbonate. If the patient recovering from hypercapnia is not given adequate chloride intake, posthypercapnic metabolic alkalosis will develop and carbon dioxide retention due to the metabolic disturbance is added to the basic pulmonary abnormality.

10. Obstructive Airway Diseases

CHRONIC OBSTRUCTIVE PULMONARY DISEASE

254 What is COPD? How common is this condition and what are the most significant risk factors?

❑ *COPD* refers to a condition characterized by persistent airway obstruction or airflow limitation caused by emphysema, chronic bronchitis, or some combination of these disorders. There are at least 15 million patients with COPD in the United States. Incidence, prevalence, and mortality rates for COPD increase with age and are higher in males than in females and among the white than the nonwhite population. The single greatest risk factor for the development of COPD is cigarette smoking. Alpha-1-protease inhibitor (API) deficiency is another risk factor for COPD, especially emphysema, and this deficiency accounts for approximately 1% of patients with COPD in the United States. Occupations where atmospheres are polluted with dust or chemical fumes (eg, coal miners, grain handlers, copper smelter workers, workers exposed to granite dust, cotton, and other pollutants, fire fighters) can aggravate COPD and increase mortality arising from this disease.

255 What is pulmonary emphysema? How is the diagnosis established?

❑ *Emphysema* is the condition characterized by an abnormal enlargement of the airway distal to the terminal bronchioles associated with destruction of alveolar walls and septa. Although this definition is strictly anatomic, the clinical diagnosis of emphysema is made on the basis of indirect information that supports the presence of this disease without direct tissue examination. The clinical diagnosis of emphysema is based on information derived from the patient's history (eg, cigarette smoking, shortness of breath, absence of bronchial hypersecretion), physical and radiologic examination (ie, decreased vascular markings, presence of bullae), and pulmonary function tests (ie, obstructive ventilatory defect, decreased pulmonary diffusing capacity).

256 What are the causes of emphysema?

❑ Emphysema is most often caused by cigarette smoking and the resulting lung destruction is generally attributed, at least in part, to the effects of neutrophil elastase on lung matrix proteins. A less common cause of this disease, accounting for about 1% of patients with emphysema, is alpha-1-antitrypsin deficiency, which represents an autosomal codominant disorder. The risk of emphysema in patients with alpha-1-antitrypsin deficiency increases as serum levels of alpha-1-antitrypsin fall below a protective threshold of 80 mg/dL (normal, 150 to 350 mg/dL).

257 How does cigarette smoking produce lung injury leading to the development of COPD?

❑ Pathogenetic mechanisms of COPD including cigarette smoking involve protease-antiprotease imbalances in the lung parenchyma. Cigarette smoke directly blocks the inhibitory capacity of API and promotes accumulation of neutrophils in the alveolar structure. The blood-derived neutrophils release elastases that are capable of destroying the elastin fibers of the lung. Cigarette smoking is also associated with goblet cell metaplasia and bronchiolitis, which contribute to obstruction of the small airways.

258 How is the diagnosis of emphysema caused by alpha-1-antitrypsin deficiency established?

❑ Pulmonary and extrapulmonary manifestations of alpha-1-antitrypsin deficiency should be investigated in the patient and his or her family. The pulmonary manifestations include a family history of emphysema, especially an early-onset presentation (before age 50) of the disease, as well as hyperlucency in the lower lung areas detected by chest radiologic examination (which differs from the upper lung zone hyperlucency more commonly detected with smoking-related centriacinar emphysema). Extrapulmonary manifestations include personal and family history of panniculitis, neonatal jaundice, chronic hepatitis, cryptogenic cirrhosis, or hepatoma. The diagnosis is established by measuring the serum level of alpha-1-antitrypsin in association with phenotyping by isoelectric focusing when the level is below 120 mg/dL (16.5 μmol/L).

259 What are the structural and functional defects in emphysema? How is this disease defined?

❑ The structural defect in pulmonary emphysema consists of the loss of the alveolar walls, causing permanent airspace enlargement beyond the terminal bronchiole accompanied by destructive changes of the alveolar walls. The functional defect includes airflow limitation, increased pulmonary compliance, and a decreased diffusing capacity for carbon monoxide (DLCO); the latter defect reflects the loss of alveolar-capillary units. Airflow limitation is caused by reduced tethering and radial traction on the airways resulting in dynamic airway collapse, and gas trapping. Partial reversibility of airflow obstruction by inhaled bronchodilators is observed in up to two-thirds of patients with emphysema. The structural defect in emphysema explained above defines this disease.

260 What is chronic bronchitis? How is the diagnosis established?

❑ Chronic bronchitis is a condition characterized by persistent cough accompanied with hypersecretion of the lower airways. These symptoms must be present most days for 3 consecutive months or longer for at least 2 consecutive years, to satisfy the minimum requirements for reaching the diagnosis of chronic bronchitis. Thus, the patient's clinical history is the only element for the diagnosis of chronic bronchitis.

261 What are the structural and functional defects in chronic bronchitis? How is this disease defined?

❑ The structural defects in chronic bronchitis consist of narrowing of small airways, enlargement of mucus-secreting glands in bronchial walls, accumulation of mucus as well as bacterial colonization of the airways (eg, *Streptococcus pneumoniae, Haemophilus influenzae, Moraxella catarrhalis*), mucosal inflammation of the large central airways, cartilage atrophy, and smooth-muscle hyperplasia. The functional defect in this disease consists of expiratory airway obstruction. The definition of chronic bronchitis refers to the clinical picture and this disease is present in patients having persistent cough and sputum production on most days for 3 months of at least 2 consecutive years.

262 What is the most important functional defect in patients with COPD?

❑ The most important functional defect with respect to the mechanics of breathing in patients with COPD stems from airflow limitation and dynamic airway collapse, rather than increased airway resistance. In the past it was considered that increased airway resistance was the dominant defect in COPD, but this concept is now considered incorrect.

263 Briefly review the pathophysiology of respiratory failure in COPD. Might hypercapnia represent an adaptive response?

❑ COPD is associated with characteristic abnormalities in pulmonary mechanics, respiratory muscle function, pulmonary gas exchange, and respiratory control of ventilation. The abnormalities in pulmonary mechanics are caused, at least in part, by stimulation of airway sensory receptors by inhaled irritants or the release of inflammatory mediators producing increased airway resistance. A reduction in elastic recoil pressure, as in emphysema, decreases driving expiratory pressure and maximum flows.

Decreased lung elasticity also causes airflow limitation, as elastic recoil pressure normally exerts radial traction on the airways. Abnormalities in respiratory muscle function develop with lung hyperinflation, as the muscles operate at an unfavorable position on their length-tension curve, and elastic recoil of the chest wall is directed inward, thereby causing an extra elastic load; and breathing takes place at the upper, less compliant portion of the lung pressure-volume curve. Abnormalities in pulmonary gas exchange are primarily the result of hypoventilation and ventilation-perfusion mismatch. Although patients with COPD and hypercapnia display a decrease in the ventilatory response when rebreathing carbon dioxide, most of these patients have an elevated resting respiratory drive. However, the increased drive is insufficient to achieve a minute ventilation that normalizes $PaCO_2$. Other factors that may contribute to hypercapnia in patients with COPD include an inherited reduction in drive, influence of associated hypoxemia, increased work of breathing, ventilation-perfusion mismatch, and respiratory muscle dysfunction. Abnormalities in respiratory control leading to hypoventilation and carbon dioxide retention might reflect the wisdom of the ventilatory controlling mechanism. Hypoventilation and the consequent decrease in the work of breathing might reflect an adaptive response that takes priority over lowering the $PaCO_2$. The resulting increase in P_ACO_2 allows the body to get rid of more carbon dioxide for a given level of ventilation.

---

264 What are the ventilatory and energy demands of patients with COPD? Compare their values with those observed in healthy subjects.

❑ Under resting conditions, patients with COPD have a slightly increased minute ventilation, approximately 9 L/min, compared with healthy subjects, 6 L/min. The work and energy cost of breathing, however, are elevated markedly with COPD because of the increased airway resistance and hyperinflation (respiratory system compliance being decreased at high lung volumes). The oxygen cost of breathing increases from about 2.5 in healthy subjects to 30 mL/min in patients with COPD (that is, about 1% to 2% and 15% of the total body oxygen consumption, respectively). In addition, ventilatory reserve is markedly diminished in these patients, such that resting ventilation constitutes about 40% of maximum ventilatory capacity compared with about 5% in healthy subjects. Although expiratory airflow is severely limited, the increased work of breathing is performed primarily by the inspiratory muscles. As a result, the accessory muscles of respiration usually are recruited to aid with the task.

265 Compare the ventilatory response to hypoxia and hypercapnia in patients with COPD with that of normal subjects. Is the respiratory drive decreased in COPD?

❑ Patients with COPD have a reduced ventilatory response to hypoxia and hypercapnia that is caused by abnormalities in pulmonary mechanics (not by decreased respiratory center output, as considered in the past). Although respiratory drive is increased in hypercapnic patients, it is insufficient to achieve a normal $PaCO_2$. Factors that may contribute to the development of hypercapnia in patients with COPD include increased work of breathing, ventilation-perfusion mismatch, influence of associated hypoxemia, the metabolic milieu, and respiratory muscle dysfunction.

266 What factors contribute to decrease the respiratory muscle strength and endurance of patients with COPD? What is the role of nutrition, electrolytes, drugs, abnormal blood gases, and lung hyperinflation on the function of respiratory muscles?

❑ Factors that contribute to debilitate the respiratory and nonrespiratory muscles of patients with COPD include the presence of hypoxemia, hypercapnia, malnutrition, steroid-induced myopathy, abnormalities in body content and serum levels of electrolytes (potassium, calcium, magnesium, phosphate), and decreased oxygen delivery to the muscles. In addition, lung hyperinflation has multiple detrimental effects on respiratory muscle function that are caused by shortened muscle fibers, decreased diaphragmatic curvature and decreased zone of apposition, medial orientation of diaphragmatic fibers, horizontal ribs, and thoracic-cage elastic recoil directed inward, and possibly impaired blood supply.

267 What conditions other than COPD might lead to carbon dioxide retention in the presence of normal or even increased total minute ventilation ($\dot{V}_E$)?

❑ The expanded V_D observed in patients with advanced pulmonary disease of different causes, pulmonary thromboembolism, and shock results in ratios of $\dot{V}_D/\dot{V}_E$ and V_D/V_T (dead space–to–tidal volume) that might be twice the normal value of 0.3; such ratios are frequently associated with carbon dioxide retention. But just like increased carbon dioxide production, increased V_D/V_T is not a primary cause of hypercapnia.

268 Describe common causes of acute respiratory failure in patients with COPD. What factors other than a respiratory tract infection can precipitate this syndrome?

❑ In patients with advanced COPD, acute respiratory failure commonly occurs as the final event in a progressively downhill clinical course. However, life-threatening acute respiratory failure can also occur in less severe stages of COPD when an inciting event, such as viral or bacterial pneumonia, exacerbates the patient's underlying obstructive disease and overwhelms the respiratory system. The most common cause of acute respiratory failure in patients with COPD is respiratory tract infection, which is usually caused by a virus, *H. influenzae,* or *S. pneumoniae*. However, administration of sedatives or narcotic analgesics, the development of a pneumothorax, rib fracture secondary to trauma or excessive coughing, pulmonary embolism, congestive heart failure, and surgery can also precipitate episodes of acute respiratory failure.

269 What are the clinical manifestations of acute respiratory failure complicating COPD?

❑ The clinical manifestations of acute respiratory failure complicating COPD are conveniently classified in three categories: (1) features of the precipitating illness, (2) manifestations caused by worsening COPD (eg, increased bronchial secretions, dyspnea), and (3) signs and symptoms of carbon dioxide retention (eg, somnolence, flapping tremor). Additional information is provided in the answers to other related questions.

270 A 56-year-old man consults because of persistent cough with sputum production, shortness of breath walking a short distance, and leg swelling. These symptoms had been present for a minimum of 18 months. Past history is significant for heavy cigarette smoking for at least 30 years. Physical examination reveals scattered expiratory wheezes, normal findings on cardiac evaluation, and pitting edema in both feet. Chest x-ray films appear normal. Spirometry reveals severe airflow obstruction without response to inhaled bronchodilators.

What is the most likely diagnosis? What should be the initial management of this patient?

❑ The long history of cigarette smoking, dyspnea, cough with sputum production, and airway obstruction (ie, clinical and pulmonary function testing data) indicate the presence of COPD with a major component of chronic bronchitis. Pertinent recommendations in the initial management include measurement of ABGs (to establish baseline values and assess the need for oxygen supplementation), counseling on smoking cessation, and prescribing an inhaled anticholinergic agent (eg, ipratropium bromide, drug with effective bronchodilator properties). Oral administration of corticosteroids is not indicated until other therapy has been tried and failed in a patient who appears to be in a relatively chronic situation (ie, as opposed to an acute COPD exacerbation in which early therapy with systemic corticosteroids can be useful). Although this patient has peripheral edema, a likely manifestation of cor pulmonale, diuretics may not be necessary initially because fluid retention may favorably respond to the treatment of the underlying disease (ie, COPD). Persistence or worsening of fluid retention despite adequate therapy for COPD should prompt the clinician to prescribe diuretic therapy.

---

271 A 65-year-old man with COPD and chronic hypercapnia receives supplemental oxygen therapy at home and bronchodilators for more than 6 months. He had remained stable up to 5 days ago when he developed progressive dyspnea. The patient requests immediate transfer by ambulance to the hospital because of his very poor medical condition. The rescue team found him with intense dyspnea and cyanosis, gave him supplemental oxygen at 6 L/min, and transferred the patient to the medical center. On arrival to the hospital the patient exhibits severe confusion, asterixis, intense bilateral wheezing, and diaphoresis. Initial treatment consists of inhalation of a beta-adrenergic agonist and parenteral administration of corticosteroids, in addition to administration of supplemental oxygen by nasal cannula at 6 L/min. Blood gas analysis 30 minutes later reveals a PO_2 of 148 mm Hg, $PaCO_2$ of 96 mm Hg, pH 7.03, and $[HCO_3^-]$ of 25 mEq/L.

Why does this patient have severe confusion, asterixis, and intense carbon dioxide retention (hypercapnia)?

❑ Uncontrolled oxygen administration (ie, 6 L/min resulting in PaO_2 of 148 mm Hg) to a patient with COPD and chronic mild hypercapnia (eg, $PaCO_2$ of 50 mm Hg) commonly leads to severe carbon dioxide retention and hypercapnic encephalopathy (ie, anxiety, transient psychosis, confusion, asterixis, tremors, seizures, coma, papilledema). Oxygen therapy should be provided to patients with COPD and respiratory failure in a controlled manner, adjusting carefully the FiO_2 and monitoring the clinical response. The increase in PCO_2 is slight (about 1 to 5 mm Hg for a 10 mm Hg increase in PO_2) in most patients as long as PaO_2 is corrected to approximately 60 mm Hg. The baseline $PaCO_2$, pH, or bicarbonate levels are not predisposing factors of acute carbon dioxide retention with oxygen therapy. Conversely, a low baseline PaO_2 and a large increase in PaO_2 with oxygen therapy correlate with the development of major hypercapnia during oxygen supplementation.

EFFECTS OF HYPERINFLATION

272 What is the effect of airway obstruction on the function of the diaphragm? What is Hoover's sign?

❑ Hyperinflation of the lungs in the course of airway obstruction, whether acute or chronic, impairs the effectiveness of the respiratory muscles and may contribute to respiratory muscle fatigue. This primarily results from hyperinflation, which causes shortening of the respiratory muscles, which in turn decreases the pressure generated for a given level of neural stimulation. In addition, flattening of the diaphragm requires the generation of greater tension within the muscle to achieve a similar tidal volume. In states of severe pulmonary overinflation, contraction of the diaphragm causes inward movement of the lower part of the rib cage during inspiration, which is known as *Hoover's sign.*

273 What is the level of alveolar pressure at the end of expiration? Does airway obstruction have any effect on this parameter?

❑ Alveolar pressure is normally zero at the end of expiration, but a positive value is commonly observed in patients with obstructive lung disease (COPD), especially if they have tachypnea. This positive pressure is termed *auto-PEEP* or *intrinsic PEEP* (positive end-expiratory pressure).

274 Explain how abnormalities in the geometry of the chest and respiratory muscles can lead to ventilatory failure caused by respiratory muscle dysfunction.

❑ Several factors can alter the geometric arrangement of the respiratory muscles, resulting in ineffective force generation. Tachypnea is common in patients with severe pulmonary disease, and the resulting shortening in expiratory time reduces lung emptying, leading to dynamic hyperinflation. Adverse effects of hyperinflation include the following: The respiratory muscles operate at an unfavorable position on their length-tension relationship; flattening of the diaphragm increases the radius of curvature, and according to Laplace's law, tension within the muscle is less effectively translated into transdiaphragmatic pressure; the "bucket-handle" movement of the lower rib cage is reduced as a result of a decrease in the zone of apposition and by the switch from an axial to a medial orientation of diaphragmatic muscle fibers; and the inwardly directed elastic recoil of the chest wall poses an additional elastic load. Abnormalities in respiratory muscle geometry can also occur as a result of asynchronous and paradoxical motion of the rib cage and abdomen. In a study employing quantitative assessment of asynchrony and paradox, patients who failed a weaning trial displayed significantly greater asynchrony and paradox of the rib cage and abdomen than did patients who were successfully weaned from the ventilator. Such a manner of breathing is extremely inefficient and poses a marked increase in the energy costs for a given level of ventilation.

275 Explain the concept of dynamic (pulmonary and thoracic) hyperinflation. What factors promote the development of dynamic hyperinflation?

❑ Normally, the lung volume at end-expiration approximates the relaxation volume of the respiratory system (ie, the lung volume determined by the static balance between the opposing elastic recoil of the lung and chest wall). However, in patients with airflow limitation, the end-expiratory volume may no longer be determined by an equilibrium between static forces. Instead, end-expiratory lung volume may exceed predicted FRC, because the rate of lung emptying is slowed and expiration is interrupted by the next inspiratory effort before the patient has exhaled to the static relaxation volume. This is termed *dynamic hyperinflation,* and the factors that determine its development include increased tidal volume, prolonged time constant (resistance times compliance) for emptying the respiratory system, and a shortened expiratory time (ie, increased respiratory rate).

276 What are the adverse effects of dynamic hyperinflation?

❑ Dynamic hyperinflation has several adverse effects that include (1) operation of the respiratory muscles at an unfavorable position on their length-tension curve; (2) elastic recoil of the chest wall directed inward, thereby causing an extra elastic load; and (3) breathing at the upper, less compliant portion of the pressure-volume curve of the lung. These factors cause a decrease in the efficiency of force generation by the respiratory muscles, an increase in the work of breathing, and development or intensification of dyspnea.

277 Why do patients with lung hyperinflation and severe respiratory compromise have an increased work of breathing during assisted ventilatory support?

❑ Patients with COPD and severe respiratory compromise commonly experience an augmented ventilatory workload as a result of dynamic hyperinflation and auto-PEEP. To initiate airflow during assisted ventilatory support, alveolar pressure needs to be decreased below ambient pressure. Normally, this is accomplished by only a small decrease in pleural pressure. However, in the presence of hyperinflation (eg, COPD), a much greater decrease in pleural pressure is required to decrease alveolar pressure below ambient pressure, resulting in a proportional increase in the work of inspiration.

278 What are the consequences of the increased lung volume (hyperinflation) in COPD on inspiratory muscle function?

❑ For the diaphragm to function as an effective inspiratory pump, it must be curved, with its convexity directed upward. Contraction of the diaphragmatic muscle fibers generates a tangential tension (Tdi) within the muscle, which in turn is translated into a pressure difference between the abdominal and pleural surfaces of the diaphragm (transdiaphragmatic pressure, Pdi). The importance of diaphragmatic curvature is best understood in terms of Laplace's law: Pdi = 2 Tdi/Rdi, where Rdi represents the radius of curvature of the diaphragm. Tension developed in a tightly curved diaphragm (low Rdi), therefore, is converted more effectively into transdiaphragmatic pressure than is the tension developed in a flattened diaphragm. In fact, a completely flattened diaphragm, with an infinite radius of curvature, is incapable of generating any useful inspiratory pressure. Indeed, in this case, diaphragmatic contraction draws inward the lower part of the rib cage, so it functions as an expiratory muscle, and its action is clinically detected as Hoover's sign.

279 What is the role of the abdominal muscles during inspiration and expiration of patients with COPD? How effective are the expiratory muscles in augmenting expiratory flow in COPD?

❑ When healthy subjects face a large ventilatory challenge, they commonly recruit the abdominal muscles during expiration. This facilitates the action of the inspiratory muscles through a number of mechanisms. Abdominal muscle contraction during expiration causes lung volume to decrease below the passively determined end-expiratory volume, pushing the diaphragm cephalad toward the rib cage, stretching its fibers and allowing them to function over a more favorable portion of the length-tension curve. Abdominal muscle contraction also makes the diaphragm more curved and the resulting decrease in the radius of curvature improves its mechanical efficiency on the basis of Laplace's law. In addition, elastic energy is stored in the abdominal muscles during expiration, which can be used to assist with the subsequent inspiratory effort. Unfortunately, these beneficial effects do not occur in patients with COPD, because the development of airway collapse prevents any reduction in end-expiratory volume. Forced expiration is effort dependent only in its early portion, and once airway collapse has occurred, further expiratory effort only produces more airway collapse, with no improvement in expiratory airflow but with an increase in the energy cost of breathing.

---

280 What are the causes of the increased work of breathing in patients with asthma?

❑ Airway obstruction and hyperinflation are the main determinants of the increased work of breathing in patients with asthma. Airway resistance is increased two to three times the normal value in asthmatic patients during a remission, and it is increased 5 to 15 times the normal level during an acute attack. The capacity of the inspiratory muscles to deal with this load is impaired by the concomitant hyperinflation. The FRC in normal subjects is approximately 50% of predicted total lung capacity (TLC), but the FRC rises in asthma to 70% of predicted TLC during remission and to 100% during an acute attack. This degree of hyperinflation is sufficient to cause marked decreases in maximum inspiratory airway pressure (Pimax), because the muscles are operating at an unfavorable position of the length-tension curve. The hyperinflation of asthma not only is caused by gas trapping behind obstructed airways, but also is determined by contraction of the inspiratory muscles in the postinspiratory period. The increased energy cost of breathing, combined with impaired function of the respiratory muscles, places them at risk of respiratory muscle fatigue. The respiratory muscles eventually will fatigue if they are required to generate 60% of Pimax with each breath, and breathing at 75% of TLC rather than at normal FRC (ie, 50% of TLC) markedly increases this likelihood. Thus, the combination of airway obstruction and hyperinflation during an acute attack lead the patient to exceed the critical pressure, with each breath fostering the development of fatigue.

11. Muscle Dysfunction

RESPIRATORY MUSCLE DYSFUNCTION AND CHEST WALL DISORDERS

281 How does a shallow and rapid breathing pattern predispose to carbon dioxide retention?

❑ A mechanism leading to an increased $\dot{V}_D$ is a decreased tidal volume accompanied by increased respiratory rate, a combination that occurs whenever rapid shallow breathing develops. The total minute ventilation in this condition might be normal or increased, but alveolar ventilation is curtailed.

282 What are the effects of decreased lung compliance and increased airway resistance on the work of breathing?

❑ To move gas to and from the alveoli, work must be performed by the respiratory muscles. In engineering terms, work is calculated as force times distance, which in the respiratory system is equivalent to pressure times volume. Disease processes associated with stiffer lungs such as pulmonary infiltration or edema increase the force that opposes lung expansion, leading to a decrease in lung compliance; consequently, a higher inflating pressure is required for a given change in lung volume. Similarly, increases in airway resistance caused by bronchospasm, kinking of an endotracheal tube, or increased resistance of a ventilator circuit necessitate an increase in the inflating pressure to achieve a given tidal volume. Unlike the pressure increase required to overcome decreased compliance, the pressure increase necessary to secure a given tidal volume with airway narrowing is considerably higher at elevated flow rates. The increase in inflating pressure associated with both airway narrowing and decreased compliance leads to an increase in the work of breathing. In addition, alveolar diseases aggravate the patient's condition by interfering with gas exchange.

283 Elaborate on abnormalities in the mechanics of breathing as causes of respiratory acidosis.

❑ Inadequate ventilation leading to carbon dioxide retention might occur whenever the respiratory bellows fail to adequately propel air through the respiratory conduits, in spite of a normal respiratory drive, and in the absence of lung disease. Primary disorders of the respiratory muscles and of the motoneurons responsible for pulmonary ventilation are classic examples of this pathophysiologic mechanism. There is, however, an even larger and heterogeneous group of patients in whom fatigue of the respiratory muscles might play a critical role in the development of respiratory acidosis. Such respiratory muscle fatigue might be observed in states of poor nutrition, certain electrolyte disorders, an obligatory high level of ventilation, decreased compliance of the respiratory system, increased resistance to airflow, and alterations in the thoracic configuration (eg, COPD, kyphoscoliosis).

284 What are the major abnormalities of the breathing pattern with respect to rib cage–abdominal motion?

❑ During normal breathing, both the rib cage and the abdomen expand on inspiration and decrease toward the resting position during expiration. Since the size of excursion with normal breathing is virtually identical for the two compartments, an X-Y plot of rib cage–abdominal motion shows the formation of a closed loop. Three major patterns of abnormal rib cage–abdominal motion are recognized: (1) asynchrony, in which the size of excursion of the rib cage motion differs from the abdominal motion, causing a widened loop of the X-Y plot; (2) paradox, in which the two compartments move in opposite directions, resulting in a negative slope on the X-Y plot; and (3) increase in the breath-to-breath variation of the relative contribution of the rib cage and abdominal motion to tidal volume, caused by recruitment and derecruitment of different respiratory muscles.

285 What abnormalities in pulmonary function are observed in patients with neuromuscular disease? How is the respiratory dysfunction first detected in these patients?

❑ Patients with respiratory muscle weakness due to neuromuscular disease typically present with a "restrictive" pattern on pulmonary function testing: markedly decreased vital capacity (VC) (40% to 70% of predicted), reduced TLC and FRC, and relatively normal residual volume (RV) and FEV_1/VC ratio. Many patients show a greater than expected loss in vital capacity because of an associated decrease in the compliance of both the lungs and the chest wall. The cause of the decrease in pulmonary compliance is unknown, but probably is related to the presence of diffuse microatelectasis. Diffusing capacity (when factored to lung volume) and gas exchange are relatively normal, unlike in patients with a restrictive pattern caused by infiltrative lung disease. Respiratory muscle weakness in patients with neuromuscular disease frequently goes undetected until the precipitation of ventilatory failure by aspiration pneumonia or the development of cor pulmonale. Ventilatory failure arises because impaired skeletal muscle function prevents patients from exceeding their limited ventilatory capacity and because respiratory muscle weakness often is greater than the level of general muscle weakness.

286 Describe the breathing pattern and ABG abnormalities in neuromuscular disease. When might hypercapnia develop?

❑ The breathing pattern in patients with respiratory muscle weakness is characterized by rapid shallow breaths and infrequent sighs. The tachypnea may be caused by afferent signals arising in the weakened respiratory muscles, intrapulmonary receptors stimulated by microatelectasis, or decreased respiratory compliance. Expiratory muscle weakness causes a decrease in the effectiveness of cough because of impairment in cough-induced dynamic compression, leading to a reduction in the velocity of airflow. Pulmonary gas exchange usually is well maintained with a relatively normal $P_{A\text{-}a}O_2$. $PaCO_2$ may be reduced early in the disease, but an elevated $PaCO_2$ becomes likely when respiratory muscle strength falls to 30% or less of the predicted normal value.

---

287 Compare the ventilatory impairment of patients with severe cervical cord lesions (ie, motor paralysis of limbs) involving the high (C1–C2), middle (C3–C5), and low (C6–C8 and T1–T6) areas. Do all spinal cord lesions impair cough and clearance of bronchial secretions?

❑ *High cervical* cord lesions (C1–C2) cause paralysis of the diaphragm, intercostal, scalene, and abdominal muscles. Patients develop hypertrophy of their sternomastoid and trapezius muscles, which are spared because they are innervated by the eleventh cranial nerve. In addition, phasic inspiratory electromyographic activity may be observed in the muscles of the neck and the floor of the mouth (eg, platysma, mylohyoid, and sternohyoid muscles) in such patients, who can be conditioned to breathe for hours using only these muscles or by employing the technique of glossopharyngeal breathing (ie, frog breathing). Ventilation can also be sustained by a diaphragmatic pacemaker because the phrenic nerve motoneuron pool (C3–C5) is spared. Lesions of the *middle cervical* cord (C3–C5) destroy the phrenic motoneurons, causing diaphragmatic paralysis that is unresponsive to phrenic pacing. The prognosis is better in patients with more caudal lesions: 40% of patients with a C3 lesion remain dependent on a ventilator compared with 14% and 11% of patients with C4 and C5 lesions, respectively. Injuries of the *lower cervical* (C6–C8) and upper thoracic (T1 and T6) regions of the cord denervate the intercostal and abdominal muscles, but leave the diaphragm and neck muscles intact. Ventilatory endurance is not a problem and few patients require prolonged mechanical ventilation because the diaphragm is functional. Respiratory muscle strength is impaired, the extent depending on the level of the lesion. All muscles of expiration are paralyzed in patients with spinal cord lesions (high, middle, and low) with the result that cough is defective and clearance of bronchial secretions impaired.

288 Is there any involvement of the respiratory muscles in patients who develop hemiplegia (caused by a stroke or cerebrovascular accident)?

❑ Yes. Hemiplegia is generally associated with a striking reduction in electromyographic activity of the diaphragm and parasternal intercostal muscles on the paralyzed side. The reduction in diaphragmatic activity is less than that of the intercostal muscles. Such involvement may contribute to the development of ineffective cough and bronchopulmonary infections in these patients.

289 What are the most important motor end-plate neuromuscular disorders leading to respiratory failure? Does myasthenia gravis commonly lead to respiratory failure?

❑ Respiratory muscle involvement is rare early in the course of myasthenia gravis (1% to 4%) but eventually becomes significant in 50% to 60% of patients. Ventilatory failure may be precipitated by surgery or inappropriate use of cholinergic medications in patients with myasthenia gravis. Ventilatory failure also develops in patients with the Lambert-Eaton myasthenic syndrome, a neurologic condition that alters the neuromuscular junction and occurs in association with either malignancies (eg, small-cell carcinoma of the lung) or autoimmune diseases. In addition to these disease states, a number of pharmacologic agents (eg, curare-related drugs, aminoglycosides) are known to interfere with neuromuscular transmission and are particularly likely to impair the respiratory muscles in patients recovering from anesthesia and those with preexisting myasthenia.

290 What ventilatory defect can develop in patients with ankylosing spondylitis? How common is the presence of respiratory failure in this thoracic cage disorder?

❑ Patients with ankylosing spondylitis display a marked reduction in chest wall compliance, associated with decreased rib cage movement and a greater than normal excursion of the diaphragm during breathing. In contrast to other causes of thoracic deformity, FRC is elevated in more than half of these patients. The elevated FRC is thought to occur because the stiffer rib cage displaces the equilibrium position of the respiratory system (FRC) toward the resting position of the rib cage, which has a volume about 1 L larger than normal FRC. Patients with ankylosing spondylitis rarely if ever develop ventilatory failure, unless there is superimposed pulmonary disease.

291 What are the consequences of the diaphragmatic dysfunction observed in some patients following upper abdominal surgery?

❑ Patients undergoing upper abdominal surgery frequently develop a marked reduction in lung volumes associated with bilateral diaphragmatic elevation and lower-lobe atelectasis. Diaphragmatic dysfunction has long been invoked as a possible mechanism. A series of studies performed in patients undergoing upper abdominal surgery (usually cholecystectomy) demonstrated diaphragmatic dysfunction as reflected by decreases in inspiratory pressure swings, the ratio of changes in gastric to esophageal pressures, and the ratio of abdominal to rib cage excursion. This diaphragmatic dysfunction may partially reverse within 24 hours or may persist for a week. It is not caused by general anesthesia as it is not observed after lower abdominal surgery. It is not caused by pain because it is not modified by the use of opiate epidural analgesia. It is currently considered that the diaphragmatic dysfunction is caused by a reflex mediated by stimulation of visceral or somatic afferent pathways during surgery that causes inhibition of phrenic nerve output. Indeed, mechanical stimulation of the gallbladder in dogs causes inhibition of diaphragmatic contraction.

292 Explain further the possible development of respiratory muscle dysfunction in conditions other than primary neurologic or muscular diseases.

❑ Malnutrition, electrolyte disorders, diseases of the chest wall, and chronic airway obstruction can lead to respiratory failure, possibly as a result of respiratory muscle dysfunction. Hypercapnia due to failure of the respiratory muscles occurs when the ventilatory demand consumes a large fraction of the respiratory reserve (maximal level of voluntary ventilation). Structural and functional changes in the respiratory muscles, as well as depletion of their energy stores, are observed with malnutrition. Potassium and phosphate depletion are the most common electrolyte abnormalities that are known to decrease contractility of the respiratory muscles. Diseases of the chest wall, the pleura, and other disorders that decrease compliance of the respiratory system (eg, kyphoscoliosis, obesity) are also major causes of diaphragmatic dysfunction. When the airway pressure levels required to maintain eucapnia consistently exceed 50% to 70% of the maximal level that the respiratory muscles can generate, they become fatigued and hypercapnia develops. Dysfunction of the respiratory muscles can also occur because of carbon dioxide retention itself, decreased oxygen saturation, anemia, and low cardiac output. Thus, attempts at correcting as many of these disorders as possible should improve the function of the respiratory muscles.

---

293 Enumerate metabolic, endocrine, and drug-induced disorders that predispose patients to develop respiratory muscle pump failure.

❑ Metabolic abnormalities such as hypophosphatemia, hypokalemia, hypocalcemia, and hypomagnesemia can adversely affect respiratory muscle function. Endocrine disturbances such as hypothyroidism, hyperthyroidism, and adrenal hyperfunction can impair respiratory muscle function, as can corticosteroid therapy. Drug-induced disorders (eg, aminoglycosides), especially in patients who recently received neuromuscular blockade, can result in prolonged respiratory muscle weakness after the agent has been discontinued.

---

294 What physiologic mechanisms might lead to respiratory muscle fatigue?

❑ The major physiologic mechanisms leading to respiratory muscle fatigue include inhibition of neural drive, impaired transmission across the neuromuscular junction (as in myasthenia gravis), excessive force and duration of contraction, insufficient muscular blood supply, and impaired excitation-contraction coupling (as in hypokalemic periodic paralysis). Depletion of muscle energy stores and failure of the contractile machinery (resulting from destructive changes that develop in muscle dystrophies or disuse atrophy) can also contribute to fatigue.

295 What is the role of respiratory muscle dysfunction in the development of hypercapnic respiratory failure? Explain the concept of hypercapnia caused by either increased respiratory load or decreased neuromuscular capacity.

❑ Hypercapnic respiratory failure results from the development of alveolar hypoventilation, which in turn is largely caused by impaired respiratory neuromuscular function. The balance between neuromuscular capacity of the respiratory muscles and the load being imposed on them is the critical determinant of the development of respiratory muscle dysfunction. Since repetitive contraction of the respiratory muscles is essential to maintain an adequate level of ventilation, the strength and endurance qualities of these muscles are of particular importance in guarding against the development of acute hypercapnia. Respiratory muscle dysfunction results when the neuromuscular capacity of the respiratory muscles is insufficient to meet the demands being placed on them. A variety of disease states can produce respiratory muscle dysfunction, and from a clinical perspective, it is useful to consider these conditions in terms of those that result from decreased neuromuscular capacity (eg, Guillain-Barré syndrome) and those caused by increased respiratory load (eg, status asthmaticus).

RESPIRATORY PUMP FAILURE: CLINICAL CASES

296 A 60-year-old man with a smoking history of 100 packs/yr and chronic bronchitis during the last 15 years had been previously known to have severe COPD. He had been followed in the outpatient pulmonary clinic and was known to have chronic hypercapnia. His steady-state PCO_2 had been approximately 60 mm Hg and he had been stable until 1 week prior to admission. At that time he developed a flulike syndrome, an increase in shortness of breath and sputum production (yellow-green in color at presentation), and subjective fever. The patient was brought to the hospital by ambulance; he was in an altered mental state and had confusion alternating with episodes of profound sleepiness. On physical examination, the patient had myoclonic jerks, flapping tremor of both hands, and extensor plantar responses. Eye ground examination revealed papilledema. Cardiovascular examination revealed that he was diaphoretic and had a blood pressure of 170/95 mm Hg, warm skin, and bounding pulse. There was moderately severe central and peripheral cyanosis. He had distant heart sounds, best heard in the tricuspid area, where a third sound (S_3) was also heard. He also had jugular venous distention, hepatomegaly, and 2+ pitting edema. Laboratory data included a hematocrit of 58%, blood urea nitrogen (BUN) level of 32 mg/dL, and creatinine concentration of 1.4 mg/dL. ABG values and serum electrolyte levels on arrival were:

pH	7.22
PCO_2	80 mm Hg
PO_2	75 mm Hg
$[Na^+]$	141 mEq/L
$[K^+]$	4.3 mEq/L
$[Cl^-]$	98 mEq/L
$[HCO_3^-]$	32 mEq/L
Anion gap	11 mEq/L

What would the acid-base diagnosis be?

❑ This patient's history indicates severe COPD due to chronic bronchitis that is responsible for his earlier diagnosis of chronic hypercapnia. The history and physical examination are consistent with aggravation of his ventilatory status as well as symptoms of respiratory failure (hypercapnia, hypoxemia). The laboratory data indicate substantial acidemia and hypercapnia, a moderate increment in [HCO_3^-]; the remaining electrolyte levels are normal. This pattern is compatible with acute respiratory acidosis superimposed on chronic respiratory acidosis.

297 What are the mechanisms involved in the development of hypercapnia in this patient?

❑ This patient's main problem was an abnormality in the lungs that led to a reduction in effective alveolar ventilation, even in the presence of either normal or increased minute ventilation. Disturbances in the mechanics of breathing are also important in this patient's carbon dioxide retention. The obligatory high level of minute ventilation, the increased resistance to airflow, and the alteration in the thoracic configuration might have resulted in respiratory muscle fatigue (although strongly suspected, there is no conclusive evidence that muscle fatigue occurs in these patients). Hyperinflation of the lungs results in flattening of the diaphragm so that a higher pressure gradient (between alveoli and mouth) may be needed to achieve a given change in pulmonary volume and airflow. Alterations in the control of pulmonary ventilation may also have been impaired in this patient, as respiratory drive might have been diminished by correction of the hypoxemia. Finally, the increased work of the respiratory muscles may have resulted in increased carbon dioxide production. In addition, he had myoclonic jerks as well as fever. A patient's carbon dioxide production increases by 13% for every 1°C increase in body temperature above the normal value.

298 What is the evidence that this patient's hypoxemia had been partially corrected?

❑ Examination of the simplified form of the alveolar gas equation provides the answer. This equation establishes that, at sea level and when breathing room air,

$$P_AO_2 = 150 - 1.25\ PaCO_2$$

where P_AO_2 is the alveolar oxygen tension in millimeters of mercury. By examining this relationship it becomes apparent that the major threat to life from carbon dioxide retention, in patients breathing room air, is the associated obligatory hypoxemia. If this patient had been breathing room air, his expected P_AO_2 would have been

$$\begin{aligned} P_AO_2 &= 150 - (1.25 \times 80) \\ &= 150 - 100 \\ &= 50 \text{ mm Hg} \end{aligned}$$

Assuming a minimum P_A-aO_2 gradient of 10 mm Hg, his maximum possible PaO_2 should have been 40 mm Hg instead of 75 mm Hg. If the P_A-aO_2 gradient was 30 mm Hg—thc average value in patients with an acute exacerbation of COPD—his PaO_2 would have been 20 mm Hg, a value incompatible with life. Thus, the patient must have been receiving oxygen supplementation when the arterial blood was drawn for analysis.

299 Comment on this patient's CNS signs and symptoms in the presence of respiratory acidosis.

❑ Several clinical manifestations in this patient arose from disturbed function of the CNS; they are collectively known as *hypercapnic encephalopathy.* Their development is a function of the magnitude of the hypercapnia, the rapidity with which it develops, the severity of the acidemia, and the degree of accompanying hypoxemia. This symptom complex may progress to carbon dioxide narcosis and coma; thus, consideration must be given to airway intubation and mechanical ventilation before these more advanced stages of carbon dioxide encephalopathy are reached.

300 What are hypercapnic encephalopathy and carbon dioxide narcosis? Describe their signs and symptoms including the so-called pseudotumor cerebri.

❑ The term *hypercapnic encephalopathy* includes all clinical manifestations arising from the effects of respiratory acidosis on the CNS. Factors that play a role in the pathophysiology of this entity are the magnitude of the hypercapnia, the rapidity with which it develops, the severity of the acidemia, and the degree of attendant hypoxemia. Important manifestations include irritability, inability to concentrate, mental cloudiness, apathy, confusion, incoherence, combativeness, headache, and anorexia. A transient psychosis can occur, as well as hallucinations and delirium. A progressive narcosis and coma might develop in patients receiving oxygen therapy, especially those with an acute exacerbation of chronic respiratory insufficiency in whom $PaCO_2$ levels up to 100 mm Hg or even higher might develop. Drowsiness that results from the so-called carbon dioxide narcosis is frequently seen with even lower $PaCO_2$ levels. Motor disturbances, including myoclonic jerks, flapping tremor identical to that observed in liver failure, and seizures, are not uncommon manifestations. Depressed reflexes are usually observed with severe hypercapnia, but deep tendon reflexes can be increased in mild to moderate respiratory acidosis. The plantar response can be extensor. The pupils are usually constricted and equal. Frank papilledema and other manifestations of increased intracranial pressure that are collectively named *pseudotumor cerebri* are occasionally observed in patients with either acute or chronic hypercapnia.

301 Elaborate on the mechanisms responsible for carbon dioxide narcosis.

❑ When healthy persons breathe carbon dioxide, most lose consciousness when the $PaCO_2$ rises above 100 mm Hg. Patients usually maintain mental clarity if the $PaCO_2$ is less than 80 mm Hg and the pH is higher than 7.30. Mental disturbances are almost invariably present if the $PaCO_2$ exceeds 120 mm Hg and the pH is lower than 7.10. However, patients receiving long-term oxygen therapy may function satisfactorily with a $PaCO_2$ of more than 110 mm Hg. This finding suggests that the acidosis and hypoxemia are probably the major factors that account for the clinical manifestations of carbon dioxide narcosis rather than $PaCO_2$ per se.

302 Comment on this patient's cardiovascular signs and symptoms in relationship with his respiratory acidosis.

❑ The hemodynamic consequences of respiratory acidosis include (1) direct depression of myocardial contractility, (2) systemic and cerebral vasodilation by a direct action on vascular smooth muscle, (3) vasoconstriction in the pulmonary and renal circulations (the latter might be caused by increased sympathetic activity), and (4) sympathetic stimulation resulting in elevated plasma catecholamine levels; however, acidemia blunts the receptor responsiveness to catecholamines. The composite hemodynamic effect observed in mild to moderate hypercapnia consists of an increased cardiac output, normal or increased blood pressure, bounding pulse, warm and flushed skin, and diaphoresis. These cardiovascular manifestations might be substantially modified if considerable hypoxemia is present or hypercapnia is severe; decreases in both cardiac output and blood pressure might be observed under such circumstances. The hemodynamic response to respiratory acidosis might be further modified by the presence of severe hypoxemia, congestive heart failure, as well as concomitant therapy with vasoactive medications. Cardiac arrhythmias, particularly those of supraventricular origin with ventricular rates between 120 and 160 beats/min, are frequently seen in these patients. They are usually not associated with major hemodynamic compromise and respond poorly to antiarrhythmic medications, including digitalis. The disturbed heart rhythm is not primarily due to the elevated PCO_2 but rather to the associated hypoxemia, sympathetic discharge, concomitant medications (bronchodilators), electrolyte abnormalities, and underlying cardiac disease. Rapid and complete correction of hypercapnia is known to trigger cardiac arrhythmias as well as generalized convulsions.

---

303 A 65-year-old man with a history of cigarette smoking of 60 pack years, 10 years of chronic bronchitis, and severe COPD documented with pulmonary function tests was admitted to the hospital because of an altered mental status and increasing cyanosis. During the physical examination the patient was obtunded and had papilledema and asterixis. The room-air blood gas values and other laboratory data, on admission, were as follows:

pH	7.29
PCO_2	82 mm Hg
$[HCO_3^-]_p$	39 mEq/L
PO_2	39 mm Hg
Hematocrit	62%

How should this patient's acid-base abnormality be characterized?

❑ The acid-base data are internally consistent, as, in accordance with the Henderson equation, the estimated $[H^+]$ is approximately equal to that expected for this pH. Since $[H^+] = 24 \times PCO_2/[HCO_3^-]$, for this patient estimated $[H^+] = 24 \times 82/39 = 51$, and $[H^+]$ of 51 nEq/L represents pH 7.29. The history, the physical examination, and the ABG values are all indicative of respiratory acidosis. In addition, the historical data are consistent with a chronic acid-base disturbance. The relationship between hypercapnia and hyperbicarbonatemia differs in acute and chronic hypercapnia. If the patient's HCO_3^- level resulted from an acute change in PCO_2 from 40 to 82 mm Hg, the expected $[HCO_3^-]_p$ should be approximately 28 mEq/L (24 + 4 mEq/L for acute response). If the patient's $[HCO_3^-]_p$ resulted from a chronic elevation in PCO_2 of the same magnitude, then the expected $[HCO_3^-]_p$ should be approximately 37 mEq/L (24 + 13 mEq/L for a chronic response). These values were calculated considering that for every 10 mm Hg increase in PCO_2, $[HCO_3^-]_p$ increases by 1 mEq/L in acute hypercapnia and by 3 mEq/L in chronic hypercapnia.

---

304 The patient's airway was intubated and mechanical ventilation was performed. A new set of ABG measurements obtained 30 minutes later showed the following:

pH	7.48
PCO_2	50 mm Hg
$[HCO_3^-]_p$	36 mEq/L
PO_2	160 mm Hg (FiO_2 = 0.40)

Is the new acid-base disorder a posthypercapnic alkalosis, also called *posthypercapnic metabolic alkalosis*?

❑ No. The patient has simply an elevated $[HCO_3^-]_p$ due to respiratory acidosis, which is now vanishing. Because a period of days is required to build a secondary response to chronic hypercapnia, it will take a day or more to obliterate it. This special combination of high $[HCO_3^-]_p$ with a simultaneous decreased PCO_2 produces alkalemia. If the supply of electrolytes is adequate, the secondary metabolic response to hypercapnia will disappear within 2 to 3 days. Note that if these acid-base data were examined in the absence of the clinical history previously mentioned, one might be tempted to characterize this acid-base disturbance as primary metabolic alkalosis.

---

305 Three days later the patient was breathing spontaneously and the following room-air ABG values were obtained:

pH	7.42
PCO_2	55 mm Hg
$[HCO_3^-]_p$	35 mEq/L
PO_2	65 mm Hg

How should this patient's acid-base disorder be characterized?

❑ Since the patient has hypercapnia and a high-normal pH, he does not fit the diagnosis of primary hypercapnia. In addition, he does not fit the diagnosis of metabolic alkalosis as a simple (single) disturbance because of the clinical history and the excessive hypercapnia for the level of hyperbicarbonatemia. The expected PCO_2 as a respiratory response to metabolic alkalosis with a $[HCO_3^-]_p$ equal to 35 mEq/L is approximately 48 mm Hg, considering that PCO_2 increases 0.7 mm Hg for each milliequivalent per liter of increased $[HCO_3^-]$ (ie, $[HCO_3^-]$ is 11 mEq/L higher than normal value of 24 mEq/L, and multiplying 11×0.7 we obtain 7.7 or approximately 8 mm Hg of increased PCO_2). Thus, the patient has a mixed acid-base disorder that includes respiratory acidosis plus a posthypercapnic metabolic alkalosis. As 3 days have elapsed since the partial correction of the hypercapnia, the kidney should have already corrected the secondary response. The lack of correction of the hyperbicarbonatemia several days after the stimulus for bicarbonate retention has disappeared indicates the existence of an additional acid-base disorder: a posthypercapnic metabolic alkalosis.

306 Because the patient was capable and willing to eat, a generous dietary NaCl intake was given. Two days later, the following acid-base data were obtained:

pH	7.36
PCO_2	50 mm Hg
$[HCO_3^-]_p$	27 mEq/L

A review of the patient's old chart reveals that the above ABG values are comparable to his baseline values at discharge from the previous hospitalization.

Explain the determinants of the improved ABG values.

❑ The posthypercapnic metabolic alkalosis has been corrected by the administration of the chloride (Cl^-) salts. The disappearance of the metabolic alkalosis removes its inhibitory effect on alveolar ventilation and is reflected in the improvement of the hypercapnia. The values of the pH changed from the high-normal to the low-normal range.

---

307 Describe the role of chloride (Cl^-) intake in the recovery phase of respiratory acidosis.

❑ If the patient's chloride intake remains adequate, the secondary hyperbicarbonatemia due to the now vanished primary hypercapnia will disappear in 1 to 3 days; the acid-base condition present during this period, although commonly referred to as *posthypercapnic metabolic alkalosis,* is not strictly a variety of metabolic alkalosis. On the other hand, lack of correction of the hyperbicarbonatemia, for a period in excess of 3 days or longer, allows a diagnosis of posthypercapnic alkalosis to be made since sufficient time has elapsed for correction of the secondary metabolic adjustment. Unavailability of chloride is the usual culprit responsible for the presence of metabolic alkalosis in patients with chronic hypercapnia. Failure to recognize and correct a superimposed metabolic alkalosis in patients with underlying pulmonary dysfunction can have important clinical consequences; relative or absolute alkalemia can depress alveolar ventilation in such patients. If plasma acid-base values are diagnostically inconclusive, a measurement of urine chloride concentration might help to exclude the presence of the most common forms of metabolic alkalosis. In the absence of recent diuretic administration, the finding of abundant urinary chloride indicates that chloride-sensitive alkalosis is not present.

12. Noncardiogenic and Cardiogenic Edema

HYPOXEMIC RESPIRATORY FAILURE: PULMONARY EDEMA

308 What factors protect the lung against edema?

❑ The lung possesses several mechanisms that prevent the development of edema: (1) an effective lymphatic system, (2) low hydraulic permeability of the pulmonary capillaries, (3) very low diffusivity of proteins across the capillary walls, and (4) very low electrolyte conductance of the epithelial barrier.

309 Explain the role of lung lymphatic vessels in the pathogenesis of pulmonary edema.

❑ The lymphatics play a critical role in removing fluid from the interstitial space (ISF). The rate of fluid accumulation in the lung can be theoretically estimated as the difference between the net fluid flow from the pulmonary capillaries (pc) to the interstitium [$\dot{Q}$ (pc → ISF)] and the lymphatic flow ($\dot{Q}$ lymph) from the pulmonary tissue to the systemic circulation as follows:

$$\text{Rate of fluid accumulation} = \dot{Q}\ (\text{pc} \rightarrow \text{ISF}) - \dot{Q}\ \text{lymph}$$

The pulmonary lymphatic flow in a normal man at rest is about 20 mL/hr and can increase up to 10-fold with stimulation (eg, pulmonary hypertension, lung inflammatory process). Consequently, the large lymphatic reserve plays a major role in protecting the lung from developing pulmonary edema. The lymphatic flow is facilitated by the additive effects of active contraction of lymphatic capillaries that have valves, which allow unidirectional fluid transport, and compression of lymphatic vessels secondary to respiratory movements and vascular pulsations. The pulmonary lymph drains into the thoracic duct, which empties into the systemic venous system. Consequently, increased systemic venous pressure secondary to right-sided heart failure opposes lymph drainage and facilitates the development of pulmonary edema.

310 Provide a classification of pulmonary edema according to its pathogenesis.

❑ Pulmonary edema might be caused by (1) an imbalance of Starling's forces (eg, increased pulmonary capillary pressure, as in heart failure, or decreased oncotic pressure, as in hepatic failure with hypoalbuminemia, or both); (2) increased alveolar-capillary membrane permeability as in ARDS; and (3) insufficiency of pulmonary lymphatic drainage as might be observed after lung transplantation, with lymphangitis carcinomatosis, or in fibrosing lymphangitis. Pulmonary edema caused by heart failure can occur with myocardial failure (eg, cardiomyopathy) or without it (eg, mitral stenosis). It should be recognized that pulmonary edema can be initiated or exacerbated in individuals with a mild or moderate increase in pulmonary capillary pressure (eg, heart failure) who concomitantly have decreased plasma oncotic pressure (hypoalbuminemia due to hepatic failure or nephrotic syndrome), ''leaky'' alveolar-capillary membranes, or pulmonary lymphatic insufficiency.

311 Can hypoalbuminemia in the absence of other cofactors cause pulmonary edema?

❑ No. Although hypoalbuminemia favors the exit of fluid from the vascular into the perivascular space of all body capillaries (pulmonary as well as systemic) due to decreased intravascular colloid osmotic pressure, it does not cause pulmonary edema in the absence of other cofactors. The increased rate of fluid loss from pulmonary capillaries augments the net amount of fluid collected by pulmonary lymphatics for return to the systemic circulation. Unless other factors intervene, significant pulmonary fluid accumulation does not occur. Factors that might have additive effects to hypoalbuminemia to cause pulmonary edema include increased pulmonary capillary hydrostatic pressure as well as conditions such as infections that cause ''leaky'' alveolar-capillary membranes.

312 Name conditions that can cause pulmonary edema due to increased permeability of the alveolar-capillary membrane. How are these conditions related to ARDS?

❑ Pulmonary edema due to increased permeability of the alveolar-capillary membrane (also called *noncardiogenic pulmonary edema*) can be caused by (1) infections (eg, bacterial, viral), (2) inhaled irritants (eg, aspiration of gastric contents, toxic substances contained in inspired air such as phosgene), (3) blood-borne endogenous or exogenous substances (eg, histamine, bacterial endotoxins, snake venoms), (4) exogenous physical factors (eg, trauma, radiation pneumonitis), (5) blood disorders (eg, disseminated intravascular coagulation), (6) hypersensitivity-immunologic reactions, and (7) circulatory catastrophes (eg, acute hemorrhagic pancreatitis). Despite the variety of underlying causes, the clinical and pathophysiologic sequence of events is remarkably similar among most patients, producing the condition known as *ARDS*.

313 Describe the three stages of fluid accumulation in the lung leading to pulmonary edema (cardiogenic and noncardiogenic types).

❑ Stage 1 of pulmonary edema is an exaggeration of the normal physiologic process of fluid leaving the pulmonary capillaries and entering the pulmonary interstitial space. This fluid subsequently returns to the vascular compartment by way of pulmonary lymphatics. The exaggerated fluid flow observed in stage 1 might be due to either an imbalance of Starling's forces favoring exit of fluid from capillaries (increased hydrostatic pressure or decreased oncotic pressure within pulmonary capillaries) or damage of alveolar-capillary membranes. The augmented fluid traffic of stage 1 prevents significant fluid accumulation in the interstitial space. In stage 2, the traffic of fluid and proteins exceeds the maximum rate of lymphatic drainage, causing expansion of the interstitial space. Because the negative pressure and compliance of the peribronchial and perivascular interstitial spaces are larger than those of the interstitial space surrounding alveoli, fluid accumulation (edema) within bronchi and small blood vessels precedes that developing around alveoli. This fluid accumulation causes compression of small airways and blood vessels in the lung. Stage 3 is the state of alveolar flooding that can occur (1) directly from the surrounding alveolar interstitial space and caused by high pressures that disrupt the alveolar membrane or (2) indirectly due to overflow of fluid from the peribronchiolar and perivascular space into alveoli with intact structure of their walls (ie, normal alveolar-capillary barrier). It must be recognized that the indirect mechanism is the most common seen in clinical practice (eg, pulmonary edema due to heart failure or fluid overload). When alveolar flooding occurs in the presence of intact alveolar membranes as with the indirect mechanism, reversal of pulmonary edema can be achieved more promptly and completely.

314 What lung zones are examined in the course of hemodynamic evaluations aimed at assessing pulmonary vascular resistance and pulmonary capillary wedge pressure?

❑ Zone 3 is considered to be the exclusive area for a meaningful measurement of pulmonary capillary wedge pressure and calculation of pulmonary vascular resistance. In zone 3, increases in pulmonary arterial pressure in the apex-to-base direction are offset by nearly identical increases in venous pressure so that gravity-dependent effects on the pulmonary circulation are minimized as compared to areas 1 and 2 of the lung.

315 What is vascular redistribution of pulmonary blood perfusion? How is this abnormality recognized?

❑ In normal humans in the upright position, blood perfusion is greater in the pulmonary bases than in the apical areas. Any deviation from this gravity-dependent pattern of pulmonary blood perfusion is known as *vascular redistribution.* Thus, an increase in apical perfusion in association with a reduction in the perfusion of the bases is present in vascular redistribution of pulmonary blood flow. This phenomenon occurs because of compression of capillaries at the lung bases due to pulmonary edema and to hypoxia-induced constriction of pulmonary arterioles in this area. Vascular redistribution is diagnosed by radiologic examination (ie, chest x-ray films) and is not an early sign of pulmonary edema because it occurs after the onset of alveolar edema, when auscultatory findings are already present.

316 Why does pulmonary edema first appear at the lung bases as opposed to the lung apices?

❑ The gravity-dependent distribution of pulmonary edema is due to the greater effects of gravity on blood flow of different lung zones in comparison with its effects on airway flow or pressures. The effective perfusion pressure in the pulmonary capillaries increases by about 1 cm H_2O/cm of vertical distance from apex to base, whereas pleural pressures increase by only about 0.25 cm H_2O/cm of vertical distance. However, alveolar pressure does not differ in the pulmonary base as compared to its apex. Consequently, gravity has no effect on alveolar pressure, a small effect on pleural pressure, and a large effect on capillary perfusion pressure. These differences explain why pulmonary edema is first evident at the lung bases (see also answers to other related questions for additional explanations of the concept). Thus, the higher hydrostatic pressure within the pulmonary capillaries at the basilar compared to the apical areas is the main reason for detection of alveolar rales first at the lung bases of patients with pulmonary edema.

317 What is the so-called high-altitude pulmonary edema?

❑ High-altitude pulmonary edema (ie, acute mountain sickness) is a syndrome that can develop shortly after rapid ascent to altitudes in excess of 2700 m. It occurs mostly in adolescents and young adults who engage in demanding physical activity before they become acclimatized to high altitude. Symptoms include cough, dyspnea, chest pain, and tachycardia and usually develop within a day of ascent. Physical examination reveals cyanosis, bilateral pulmonary rales, and patchy infiltrates scattered throughout both lung fields as seen on chest x-ray films. Administration of high oxygen concentration or returning the patient to a lower altitude reverses the syndrome within 1 or 2 days. Acetazolamide, a diuretic that inhibits carbonic anhydrase, is effective in ameliorating the symptoms of acute mountain sickness. Nitrates and nifedipine also have been used in the management of this condition. Preventive measures include avoidance of vigorous exercise for the first 2 to 3 days at high altitude and gradual ascent if possible. The pathogenesis of this syndrome is still unknown. Hemodynamic evaluation of patients with high-altitude pulmonary edema reveals pulmonary artery hypertension and near-normal pulmonary capillary wedge pressure.

318 What is neurogenic pulmonary edema? What patients might develop this condition?

❑ *Neurogenic pulmonary edema* refers to a form of lung edema that occurs in patients with major neurologic disorders such as head trauma or grand mal seizures in the absence of other common causes of pulmonary edema. The pathogenesis of this entity includes both an imbalance of Starling's forces in the pulmonary capillaries and increased permeability of these vessels. The intense and sustained sympathetic discharge observed in these neurologic disorders might be responsible for the pulmonary edema according to the following mechanisms: (1) constriction of arterioles and veins in the systemic circulation that produces hypertension with increased left ventricular afterload and shifts of blood from the systemic to the pulmonary circulation, thereby increasing hydrostatic pressure in the pulmonary capillaries and favoring exit of fluid from the vasculature due to abnormal Starling's forces; and (2) increased permeability of the capillaries due to direct effects or constriction of vessels including the veins in the pulmonary circulation. In experimental models of this disorder, the pulmonary edema that follows severe injury of the CNS can be completely prevented by sympathectomy. Thus, it appears that neurogenic pulmonary edema is caused by a combination of a neurally mediated increase in the hydrostatic pressure and the permeability of pulmonary capillaries.

319 Describe the acute pulmonary edema secondary to overdose of narcotics (ie, opium derivatives and related compounds).

❑ Overdose of heroin, morphine, methadone, and dextropropoxyphene can cause pulmonary edema by mechanisms incompletely understood. Increased permeability of pulmonary capillaries due to narcotic-induced release of histamine has been proposed as the pulmonary capillary pressure is normal and the edema fluid is rich in protein.

320 What is the pathogenesis of pulmonary edema observed following general anesthesia?

❑ A large positive fluid balance (fluid administration significantly exceeds urine output and other fluid losses) in the course of general anesthesia, especially in patients with heart disease, might precipitate pulmonary edema. Reduction of pulmonary lymphatic drainage due to general anesthesia might explain the development of pulmonary edema when fluid overload and left ventricular dysfunction are absent.

321 What is the pathogenesis of pulmonary edema seen after cardioversion?

❑ Several mechanisms have been implicated in the pathogenesis of pulmonary edema seen after cardioversion. Possible determinants include ineffective left atrial function immediately following cardioversion (ie, patients with atrial fibrillation), left ventricular dysfunction, and activation of neural pathways in a manner comparable to that occurring in neurogenic pulmonary edema.

---

322 Explain the mechanisms responsible for pulmonary edema observed with the use of cardiopulmonary bypass.

❑ Possible pathogenetic mechanisms for this type of pulmonary edema include anaphylactic reactions to the infusion of fresh-frozen plasma and loss of alveolar surfactant due to prolonged lung collapse during the procedure.

---

323 What are the mechanisms responsible for the acute pulmonary edema observed with eclampsia?

❑ The massive sympathetic discharge and hypervolemia observed with eclampsia are implicated in the acute systemic hypertension, which leads to left ventricular failure and secondary pulmonary edema. Hypoalbuminemia due to renal losses also contributes to fluid accumulation in the lungs and elsewhere. In addition, disseminated intravascular coagulation might play a pathogenetic role in the pulmonary edema of eclampsia.

---

324 Compare the pathogenesis of acute pulmonary edema due to pulmonary embolism with large thrombi (massive) to that observed with multiple small emboli (microemboli). Provide clinical examples of these forms of pulmonary embolism.

❑ Acute pulmonary edema in patients with massive pulmonary embolism is due to backward failure of the left ventricle secondary to encroachment of its cavity by the interventricular septum (displaced because of distention of the right ventricle) as well as due to myocardial depression resulting from associated profound hypoxemia. Examples of this form of pulmonary embolism include those secondary to displacement of thrombi originating in the lower extremities, pelvic veins, renal veins, and right atrium. A different pathogenesis has been proposed for the pulmonary edema secondary to microemboli. In this case, intravascular coagulation generates thrombin that causes platelet aggregation, complement activation, and degradation of fibrinogen and fibrin, which eventually leads to pulmonary edema secondary to increased permeability of the alveolar-capillary membrane. An example of microemboli-induced pulmonary edema is that present in patients with endocarditis involving the right side of the heart (eg, tricuspid endocarditis).

325 Explain how pulmonary embolism can lead to respiratory acidosis.

❑ Patients with acute pulmonary embolism who previously had a limited ventilatory reserve (due to lung disease, abnormalities in the mechanics of breathing, or alterations in the control of ventilation), or those receiving constant mechanical ventilation, can develop carbon dioxide retention due to the acute increase in $\dot{V}_A/\dot{Q}$ ratio that results from obstruction in the pulmonary circulation. A mechanism that tends to preserve the normalcy of the $\dot{V}_A/\dot{Q}$ ratio in pulmonary embolism is constriction of the airways due to the low $PaCO_2$ in areas of the lung that are not perfused; this change reduces the obligatory increase in dead space ventilation ($\dot{V}_D$) that accompanies this circulatory catastrophe.

13. Primary Hypocapnia

RESPIRATORY ALKALOSIS

326 Define respiratory alkalosis and explain its relationship with respiratory failure.

❑ *Respiratory alkalosis* is the acid-base disturbance initiated with a decrease in carbon dioxide tension of body fluids. The term *primary hypocapnia* is synonymous with respiratory alkalosis. It should be recognized that these two terms imply the presence of the expected secondary metabolic response. The secondary hypocapnia that develops in metabolic acidosis is an integral part of this metabolic disorder and should not be confused with respiratory alkalosis. Respiratory alkalosis may be secondary to hypoxemia and therefore, represents the most commonly observed acid-base disorder that accompanies so-called hypoxemic respiratory failure (eg, ARDS).

327 How common and life-threatening is respiratory alkalosis?

❑ Primary hypocapnia is probably the most frequent acid-base disturbance encountered. In critically ill patients breathing spontaneously, its presence might be a grave prognostic sign, especially if $PaCO_2$ levels are below 20 to 25 mm Hg. Furthermore, respiratory alkalosis is the most common acid-base abnormality in patients hospitalized in intensive care units, occurring either as the simple disorder or as a component of mixed disturbances. In sharp contrast with respiratory acidosis, which always reflects a serious condition, some causes of respiratory alkalosis are benign. As blood pH levels do not exceed 7.55 in most patients with primary hypocapnia, severe manifestations of decreased systemic acidity are usually absent. Severe alkalemia, however, might be produced, especially with the use of the ventilator set at inappropriate parameters, with some psychiatric conditions, and with lesions involving the CNS.

328 Elaborate on the changes in blood pH and $[HCO_3^-]_p$ observed in respiratory alkalosis (also known as *primary hypocapnia*).

❑ Primary hypocapnia alkalinizes all body fluids and elicits a prompt and modest reduction in $[HCO_3^-]_p$ that originates mainly from titration of the body's nonbicarbonate buffers. A much larger secondary decrement in $[HCO_3^-]_p$ is observed in chronic hypocapnia and results from the adaptive acidification response of the kidney. The decreased $[HCO_3^-]_p$ that results from the metabolic adjustment to hypocapnia diminishes the magnitude of the pH rise, yet alkalemia is characteristically found in uncomplicated acute and chronic hypocapnia.

329 Is the alkalemia (increased blood pH) of respiratory alkalosis accompanied by changes in intracellular and cerebrospinal pH?

❑ Yes. The acute decrement in $PaCO_2$ has been shown to decrease not only the extracellular acidity but also the intracellular acidity. The change in the intracellular pH in acute hypocapnia, however, appears to be significantly smaller than that in the extracellular fluid. There are no data available for chronic hypocapnia. Because the acidity of the CSF (at equilibrium with the brain interstitial fluid) plays a critical role in the regulation of respiration, the changes in pH in this fluid have been the subject of intensive investigation. CSF bicarbonate and hydrogen ion concentrations fall during acute hypocapnia in parallel with arterial blood values. The reduction in cerebral blood flow associated with acute hypocapnia might explain a relatively high PCO_2 in the CSF (yet lower than the level found in eucapnia), which results in a widening of the CSF-arterial PCO_2 difference. A reduction in both CSF bicarbonate and hydrogen ion concentrations of similar magnitude to those of arterial blood has been also reported in chronic hypocapnia.

330 What are the effects of hypocapnia on cerebral blood flow and on intracranial pressure? What are the medical applications of those effects?

❑ Acute hypocapnia decreases cerebral blood flow and produces decreased acidity in all body fluids, hypocalcemia, hypokalemia, and a pH-induced shift of the oxyhemoglobin dissociation curve; all these alterations have been implicated as determinants of the clinical manifestations of this acid-base disorder. The acute hypocapnia-induced reduction in cerebral blood flow might reach values lower than 50% of normal, resulting in an increased lactate output by the brain due to cerebral hypoxia. A reduction in intracranial pressure, which is generally not harmful, and electroencephalographic changes consisting of generalized slowing and high-voltage waves are also present in acute respiratory alkalosis. The effects of acute hypocapnia on the cerebral circulation have been used in the treatment of brain edema resulting from neurosurgical procedures, head trauma, meningitis, or encephalitis. Unfortunately, the hypocapnia-induced reduction in intracranial pressure is short-lasting, and blood flow returns to normal in sustained hypocapnia.

331 What are the effects of hyperventilation, leading to primary hypocapnia, on the cardiovascular system? Compare the hemodynamic and biochemical effects of active and passive hyperventilation.

❑ The cardiovascular manifestations of respiratory alkalosis might be also very prominent. A major reduction in cardiac output accompanied by arteriolar vasoconstriction, tissue hypoperfusion, and a large increment in plasma lactate concentration is frequently attributed to severe acute hypocapnia. This syndrome is typically observed in surgical patients under general anesthesia or those having depression of the CNS and receiving mechanical ventilation; in all likelihood, it reflects the effects of passive hyperventilation. Normal volunteers with active hyperventilation do not develop the prominent cardiovascular manifestations observed in patients receiving passive hyperventilation. Patients with ischemic heart disease might develop occasional cardiac arrhythmias, ischemic electrocardiographic changes, and even angina pectoris during acute hypocapnia. Yet, normal volunteers do not exhibit clinical manifestations of coronary insufficiency or cardiac arrhythmias. None of the previously described hemodynamic effects seem to be present in uncomplicated chronic hypocapnia.

332 What are the mechanisms responsible for primary hypocapnia or respiratory alkalosis?

❑ Hypocapnia might result from increased alveolar ventilation, decreased carbon dioxide production, or a combination of these mechanisms. A negative carbon dioxide balance with the expected hypocapnia might also result from the extrapulmonary elimination of carbon dioxide by a dialysis device or extracorporeal circulation (eg, heart-lung machine). In the majority of patients, however, primary hypocapnia reflects pulmonary hyperventilation due to increased ventilatory drive.

333 What are the physiologic mechanisms leading to primary hypocapnia caused by hyperventilation?

❑ Primary hypocapnia might result from an increased alveolar ventilation secondary to signals arising from the lungs, the peripheral chemoreceptors (carotid and aortic), the brain stem chemoreceptors, or influences originating in other centers of the brain. The normal response to carbon dioxide of the brain stem chemoreceptors can be augmented by systemic diseases (eg, sepsis and liver disease), pharmacologic agents, anxiety, volition, and other influences. Hypoxemia is also a major stimulus to pulmonary ventilation, but PaO_2 values lower than 60 mm Hg are required to consistently elicit this effect. In mechanically ventilated patients a reduction in physical activity (eg, sedation, skeletal muscle paralysis) or in the basal metabolic rate (eg, hypothermia) might result in respiratory alkalosis because the $\dot{V}_E$ effected by the ventilator is excessive for the patient's metabolic needs (ie, decreased $\dot{V}CO_2$). In states of severe circulatory failure, arterial hypocapnia might coexist with venous and, therefore, tissue hypercapnia; in such circumstances, there has been enrichment of the body's carbon dioxide stores, and respiratory acidosis rather than respiratory alkalosis is present (''pseudorespiratory alkalosis'').

334 How is the diagnosis of respiratory alkalosis established?

❑ Evaluation of the patient's clinical history, physical examination, and ancillary laboratory data is required to establish the diagnosis of respiratory alkalosis. Careful observation can detect abnormal breathing patterns in some patients, yet marked hypocapnia can be present without a clinically evident increase in respiratory effort. Therefore, ABG values should be obtained to diagnose primary hypocapnia because the physical examination is unreliable in detecting the presence of this acid-base disorder. Caution should be exercised in the interpretation of altered blood gas values, as the electrolyte pattern of hyperchloremic hypobicarbonatemia is present in chronic respiratory alkalosis and in normal anion gap metabolic acidosis. Examination of plasma potassium concentration ($[K^+]_p$) might help to differentiate these two disorders; whereas a normal potassium concentration is observed with chronic respiratory alkalosis, hypokalemia or hyperkalemia often accompanies the various types of hyperchloremic metabolic acidosis. If alkalemia is present in a patient with hypocapnia, an element of respiratory alkalosis must be present. Primary hypocapnia, however, might be associated with normal or increased plasma acidity as a result of the concomitant presence of another acid-base disturbance. A high-normal blood pH is commonly observed in patients with mild chronic respiratory alkalosis. Since hypocapnia might reflect an adaptive response to metabolic acidosis, it is imperative to establish that the decreased $PaCO_2$, or part of it, is the initial acid-base derangement. Determination of the cause of respiratory alkalosis is as important as making the diagnosis of this disorder.

335 Enumerate the major causes of pulmonary hyperventilation.

❑ Pulmonary hyperventilation might result from signals arising from the lung, the peripheral chemoreceptors (carotid and aortic), the brain stem chemoreceptors, or influences originating in other centers of the brain. The response to carbon dioxide of the brain stem chemoreceptors can be augmented by systemic diseases (eg, sepsis, liver diseases), pharmacologic agents, anxiety, volition, and other influences. Hypoxemia is a major stimulus to pulmonary ventilation but PaO_2 values less than 60 mm Hg are required to consistently elicit this effect.

336 Outline a useful classification of the causes of respiratory alkalosis.

❑ The various causes of respiratory alkalosis can be arranged in five major categories: (1) hypoxemia or tissue hypoxia, (2) stimulation of chest wall and intrapulmonary receptors, (3) CNS stimulation, (4) drugs or hormones, and (5) miscellaneous.

337 What conditions can lead to the primary hypocapnia mediated by activation of arterial chemoreceptors?

❑ Stimulation of ventilation through activation of arterial chemoreceptors is observed with a decreased inspired PO_2, bronchopulmonary diseases with $\dot{V}A/\dot{Q}$ mismatching, cyanotic heart diseases, and decrements in oxygen-delivering capacity of hemoglobin. In all these conditions, tissue hypoxia occurs in spite of the presence of adequate blood perfusion. Tissue hypoperfusion also stimulates alveolar ventilation as a result of oxygen deprivation; yet, it might produce "pseudorespiratory alkalosis" characterized by a distinct pattern of blood gases, in which arterial hypocapnia and alkalemia are associated with venous (and tissue) hypercapnia and acidemia (see details in answers to pertinent questions).

338 What specific conditions are associated with hypoxemia caused by decreased PO_2 in inspired air?

❑ Common conditions responsible for this category of hypoxemia, also known as *hypoxic hypoxemia,* include exposure to high altitude (eg, skiing trip to the mountain, visitors and permanent residents of those areas), flying in a nonpressurized or inadequately pressurized airplane, confinement within a small and airtight closed space, and subjects trapped in a burning building.

339 Describe the specific causes of respiratory alkalosis that result from hypoxemia or tissue hypoxia.

❑ Stimulation of ventilation through activation of arterial chemoreceptors is observed with a decreased inspired PO_2, bronchopulmonary diseases with $\dot{V}_A/\dot{Q}$ mismatching, cyanotic heart diseases, and decrements in oxygen-delivering capacity of hemoglobin. In all these conditions, tissue hypoxia occurs despite the presence of adequate blood perfusion to peripheral tissues. Tissue hypoperfusion also stimulates alveolar ventilation due to oxygen deprivation, yet it might produce pseudorespiratory alkalosis characterized by a distinct pattern of blood gases, in which arterial hypocapnia and alkalemia are associated with venous (and tissue) hypercapnia and acidemia.

340 Name the conditions and diseases that can cause respiratory alkalosis as a result of hypoxemia or tissue hypoxia.

❑ The conditions and diseases leading to primary hypocapnia due to hypoxemia or tissue hypoxia include decreased inspired PO_2; high altitude; ARDS; bacterial or viral pneumonia (and many other pulmonary diseases); aspiration of food, foreign body, or vomitus; angioedema; laryngospasm; drowning; cyanotic heart disease; severe anemia; left-shift deviation of hemoglobin-oxygen curve; hypotension; severe circulatory failure; and pulmonary edema.

341 Name the conditions and diseases that can cause respiratory alkalosis as a result of stimulation of the CNS.

❑ The conditions and diseases that can cause respiratory alkalosis as a result of stimulation of the CNS include voluntary hyperventilation, pain, anxiety, psychoneurosis, psychosis, fever, subarachnoid hemorrhage, cerebrovascular accident, meningoencephalitis, brain tumor, and head trauma.

342 Describe the specific causes of respiratory alkalosis that result from stimulation of the CNS.

❑ CNS-mediated respiratory alkalosis can result from a variety of causes. The anxiety hyperventilation syndrome is a benign, commonly observed form. By contrast, several neurologic diseases due to vascular, infectious, traumatic, or neoplastic processes can produce more serious forms of primary hypocapnia by enhancing stimulatory inputs to pulmonary ventilation, or by interrupting normal inhibitory pathways. Central hyperventilation is a distinct respiratory pattern accompanying neurologic injury in the midbrain and upper pontine area that is characterized by an increase in both the respiratory rate and the depth of breathing. Because these neurologic lesions are usually lethal, the presence of central hyperventilation is of grave prognostic significance. Other ventilatory patterns observed with some diseases of the brain are equally serious, including lesions at a low pontine level and in the medulla, which produce apneustic and irregular breathing, respectively. A distinct ventilatory pattern, known as *Cheyne-Stokes respiration,* is included within this category of causes of respiratory alkalosis.

343 Describe the specific causes of respiratory alkalosis that result from stimulation of receptors located in the chest wall and lung parenchyma.

❑ The diseases leading to primary hypocapnia as a result of stimulation of chest receptors include pneumonia, asthma, pneumothorax, hemothorax, flail chest, acute respiratory distress syndrome, heart failure, noncardiogenic pulmonary edema, pulmonary embolism, and pulmonary fibrosis.

344 What are the mechanisms and the receptors responsible for the development of hyperventilation and respiratory alkalosis in patients with pulmonary diseases?

❑ Mechanisms leading to respiratory alkalosis in patients with pulmonary diseases include, in addition to any hypoxic drive, the local stimulation of receptors by irritants (nociceptive receptors), pulmonary expansion or collapse (stretch receptors), and pulmonary capillary congestion (juxtacapillary or J-receptors).

345 List the drugs and hormones that might cause hyperventilation and primary hypocapnia (respiratory alkalosis).

❑ Causes of primary hypocapnia due to drugs and hormones include nikethamide, ethamivan, doxapram, progesterone, medroxyprogesterone, xanthines, salicylates, catecholamines, angiotensin II, vasopressor agents, dinitrophenol, and nicotine.

346 Describe the specific causes of respiratory alkalosis that result from the effect of drugs or hormones (eg, "respiratory stimulants" for possible use in patients with respiratory depression).

❑ Respiratory alkalosis is commonly observed as an adverse effect of medication. Aspirin and other salicylates in doses exceeding a few grams per day might produce significant hyperventilation by direct action on CNS chemoreceptors. In patients with salicylate intoxication, metabolic acidosis due to an accumulation of organic acids can complicate the primary hypocapnia. Several other substances are known to stimulate pulmonary ventilation in normal subjects. Some of these respiratory stimulants have been used to increase pulmonary ventilation in the treatment of carbon dioxide retention (ie, nikethamide, ethamivan, doxapram, and progesterone), but they have not influenced patient outcome; these agents are no longer commonly used. The action of nikethamide is complex and includes direct stimulation of the respiratory center, increase in the center's sensitivity to carbon dioxide, and activation of peripheral chemoreceptors. Several other agents including dinitrophenol, nicotine, xanthines, and catecholamines also stimulate pulmonary ventilation.

347 Describe other specific causes of respiratory alkalosis commonly observed in clinical practice that might be included in the miscellaneous category.

❑ Other causes of hyperventilation leading to primary hypocapnia that are commonly referred to as a miscellaneous group are pregnancy, gram-positive septicemia, gram-negative septicemia, hepatic failure, mechanical hyperventilation, heat exposure, and recovery from metabolic acidosis. Hepatic failure is a common and important cause of primary hypocapnia. The severity of hypocapnia correlates with the blood level of ammonia (NH_3) and has prognostic significance. Systemic infections arising from gram-positive and gram-negative bacteria are also major causes of respiratory alkalosis. Direct stimulation of central chemoreceptors by bacterial toxins from gram-negative organisms explains, at least in part, the hyperventilation observed in some patients with sepsis. Thus, unexplained respiratory alkalosis in a hospitalized patient calls for evaluation for the presence of sepsis, especially that resulting from gram-negative organisms.

348 Name possible causes of decreased carbon dioxide production that can lead to respiratory alkalosis.

❑ A reduction in physical activity (eg, sedation, skeletal muscle paralysis) or in the basal metabolic rate (eg, hypothermia) can result in respiratory alkalosis due to decreased carbon dioxide production in the presence of constant carbon dioxide excretion effected by mechanical ventilation. Because patients breathing spontaneously adjust their pulmonary ventilation to match carbon dioxide production, a reduction in the latter does not cause respiratory alkalosis.

349 Describe the adaptation to acute hypocapnia.

❑ A reduction in PCO_2 results in a prompt fall in hydrogen ion concentration ($[H^+]$) because of a decrease in the carbonic acid concentration of the body fluids. Adaptation to acute hypocapnia is characterized by an immediate decrement in $[HCO_3^-]$ that results from nonrenal mechanisms and is accounted for principally by alkaline titration of the nonbicarbonate body buffers. This adaptation is completed within 5 to 10 minutes after the onset of hypocapnia, and assuming no further changes in $PaCO_2$, no additional, detectable changes in acid-base equilibrium occur for a period of several hours. $[HCO_3^-]$ falls, on average, by approximately 0.2 mEq/L for each 1 mm Hg acute decrement in $PaCO_2$. Consequently, $[H^+]$ decreases by approximately 0.75 nEq/L for each 1 mm Hg reduction in $PaCO_2$. Acute adaptation to a $PaCO_2$ of 20 mm Hg in a subject who initially had a normal acid-base composition ($PaCO_2$ of 40 mm Hg, $[HCO_3^-]$ of 24 mEq/L, and $[H^+]$ of 40 nEq/L or pH 7.40) will result on average in a $[HCO_3^-]$ of 20 mEq/L and $[H^+]$ of 24 nEq/L or pH 7.62.

350 Describe the adaptation to chronic hypocapnia.

❑ In comparison with acute hypocapnia, a larger decrement in $[HCO_3^-]$ occurs in chronic hypocapnia, which reflects the renal adaptation to the acid-base disorder. This renal adaptation involves suppression of the mechanisms of urine acidification in both proximal and distal tubules. The body bicarbonate stores are reduced by a transient decrease in net acid excretion that occurs in the first few days of hypocapnic exposure; the persistent suppression of bicarbonate reabsorption maintains the hypobicarbonatemia of chronic hypocapnia. Completion of the adaptation requires 2 to 3 days. [HCO_3^-] decreases, on average, by about 0.4 mEq/L for each 1 mm Hg chronic decrement in $PaCO_2$ and, as a consequence, plasma [H^+] decreases by approximately 0.4 nEq/L for each 1 mm Hg reduction in $PaCO_2$. Chronic adaptation to a $PaCO_2$ of 20 mm Hg results on average in a [HCO_3^-] of 15 mEq/L and [H^+] of 32 nEq/L (pH 7.49).

CLINICAL CASES OF PRIMARY HYPOCAPNIA

351 A 32-year-old woman presents with acute respiratory distress after a near-drowning accident. Analysis of ABGs while breathing 100% oxygen by face mask reveals PaO_2 of 36 mm Hg, $PaCO_2$ of 26 mm Hg, and pH 7.32. Hemoglobin (Hb) is 8 gm/dL. These data led the physician to initiate mechanical ventilation and insert a pulmonary artery catheter for monitoring of tissue oxygenation and hemodynamic parameters. The following data were obtained:

SaO_2 (arterial oxygen saturation)	81%
PaO_2	46 mm Hg
$S\bar{v}O_2$ (mixed venous oxygen saturation)	59%
$\dot{Q}t$ (cardiac output)	5.2 L/min
Pulmonary artery wedge pressure	20 mm Hg

Estimate the transport of oxygen to the tissues based on the above information from this patient with hypoxemic respiratory failure.

❑ The transport of oxygen to the tissues is estimated as the product of arterial oxygen content (CaO_2) and cardiac output. Arterial oxygen content is calculated as follows:

$$
\begin{aligned}
CaO_2 &= (Hb \times 1.34 \times SaO_2/100) + (0.0031 \times PaO_2) \\
&= (8 \times 1.34 \times 81/100) + (0.0031 \times 46) \\
&= 8.68 + 0.14 \\
&= 8.8 \text{ mL}/100 \text{ mL} \\
&= 88 \text{ mL/L}
\end{aligned}
$$

Consequently, 88 mL/L × 5.2 L/min = 458 mL/min, the latter value being the estimated amount of oxygen transported to the tissues. The previous calculations demonstrate that dissolved oxygen accounts for a very small fraction of the total amount of oxygen transported in the blood. In fact, the major determinants of systemic oxygen transport are cardiac output, hemoglobin concentration, and arterial oxygen saturation. A blood transfusion generally produces a greater improvement in tissue oxygenation of patients with anemia than do supplemental oxygen or inotropic or vasoactive drugs. Mixed venous oxygen saturation is not used for the calculation of systemic oxygen delivery (transport).

---

352 A 63-year-old woman had multiple episodes of urinary tract infection during the previous 20 years and required hospitalization for this problem on three occasions. The week prior to her visit to the emergency room, she had a fever as high as 39.9°C, shaking chills, and generalized malaise. She remained with intermittent high fever and was brought by her family to the emergency room; at that time she was severely weak and obtunded and was immediately admitted to the hospital. Positive findings on physical examination included fever (40.3°C), a borderline low blood pressure of 92/56 mm Hg, and a heart rate of 120 beats/min; signs of peripheral circulatory failure were absent. Laboratory evaluation revealed a white blood cell count of 14,000/μL with 87% polymorphonuclear leukocytes and 8% band forms. Examination of a fresh urine sediment revealed many white blood cells in clumps as well as white blood cell casts; many gram-negative rods were seen. Arterial blood acid-base data and serum electrolytes were as follows:

pH	7.55
PCO_2	19 mm Hg
$[HCO_3^-]_p$	16 mEq/L
PO_2	105 mm Hg
$[Na^+]$	140 mEq/L
$[K^+]$	3.8 mEq/L
$[Cl^-]$	110 mEq/L
Anion gap	14 mEq/L

Describe this patient's acid-base disorder.

❑ The acid-base data are internally consistent. The patient's history demonstrates the presence of a febrile syndrome that most likely results from a urinary tract infection and possible urosepsis. The most commonly observed acid-base disorder in this condition is primary hypocapnia (respiratory alkalosis). Hypoxemia is not responsible for the respiratory alkalosis because the PO_2 is not significantly depressed. The composition of arterial blood reveals significant alkalemia and hypocapnia, findings consistent with the presumptive diagnosis of respiratory alkalosis. The reduction in $[HCO_3^-]_p$ might be explained mainly by a secondary metabolic response to respiratory alkalosis (the observed PCO_2 is 21 mm Hg below normal, and this value multiplied by 0.4 mEq/L/mm Hg of decreased PCO_2 [ie, the expected metabolic response to sustained hypocapnia] predicts a decrease in $[HCO_3^-]_p$ of 8.4 mEq/L below normal). Since the measured $[HCO_3^-]_p$ is 16 mEq/L and the expected decrease in $[HCO_3^-]_p$ is 8 mEq/L, the addition of these two figures allows reconstruction of a normal $[HCO_3^-]_p$ prior to her illness. The plasma anion gap is 14 mEq/L; this borderline high-normal value might be explained by a small rise in plasma lactate, as well as other organic acids in response to alkalemia.

353 What other laboratory data might be relevant to establish the cause of primary hypocapnia in this 63-year-old woman?

❑ The results of blood cultures obtained at the time of admission disclosed gram-negative rods in all bottles. Bacteremia due to gram-negative organisms is an important and well-established cause of respiratory alkalosis.

354 What are the mechanisms responsible for the development of primary hypocapnia or respiratory alkalosis, including the hypoxemia-induced type?

❑ Hypocapnia might result from increased alveolar ventilation, decreased carbon dioxide production, or a combination of these mechanisms. The hypoxemia-induced respiratory alkalosis is secondary to increased alveolar ventilation. A negative carbon dioxide balance with the expected hypocapnia might also result from the extrapulmonary elimination of carbon dioxide by a dialysis device or extracorporeal circulation (eg, heart-lung machine) or from mechanical ventilation with inappropriate settings. In the great majority of patients, however, primary hypocapnia reflects pulmonary hyperventilation due to increased ventilatory drive.

14. Miscellaneous Topics

ELECTROLYTES IN PRIMARY HYPERCAPNIA AND HYPOCAPNIA

355 What are the expected changes in plasma electrolyte composition in acute and chronic hypercapnia?

❑ Whereas $[Cl^-]_p$ is not substantially changed in acute hypercapnia, hypochloremia is consistently found with chronic hypercapnia and reflects the loss of urinary chloride during the adaptive process, and the shift of chloride into red cells. The $[Na^+]_p$ rises 1 to 3 mEq/L in acute and chronic hypercapnia. Plasma lactate, pyruvate, and total unmeasured anions decrease with acute hypercapnia but are not significantly altered with chronic hypercapnia. A very mild increase in $[K^+]_p$ of only 0.1 mEq/L for each 0.1-unit fall in pH, due to a shift of this ion out of cells, occurs during acute hypercapnia; appreciable changes in $[K^+]_p$ are not observed in chronic hypercapnia. Similar to the change in K^+ levels, a rise in $[HCO_3^-]_p$ is characteristic of acute hypercapnia but is not observed in chronic hypercapnia. Consistent changes in $[Ca^{++}]_p$ and $[Mg^{++}]_p$ have not been noted during respiratory acidosis.

356 Describe the alterations in plasma electrolyte composition in acute and chronic hypocapnia.

❑ Significant and characteristic changes in the plasma electrolyte composition are observed with acute and chronic respiratory alkalosis. A prompt, but small decrement in $[HCO_3^-]_p$ develops in acute hypocapnia, as noted already. In addition, small rises in $[Cl^-]_p$, lactate, and other unmeasured anions balance the decrement in $[HCO_3^-]_p$ that occurs in acute respiratory alkalosis. Plasma lactate increases very modestly in acute hypocapnia, by only 0.5 to 1.5 mEq/L. Changes in other electrolytes include decreases in $[Na^+]_p$ (1 to 3 mEq/L), in $[K^+]_p$ (0.2 mEq/L for each 0.1-unit rise in pH), and in phosphorus. A larger decrement in

$[HCO_3^-]_p$ is observed in chronic hypocapnia in association with changes in other electrolytes. A rise in $[Cl^-]_p$ accounts for about two-thirds of the fall in $[HCO_3^-]_p$, the remainder being offset by an increase in plasma unmeasured anions. Appreciable changes in $[Na^+]_p$, $[K^+]_p$, lactate, or phosphorus do not occur in chronic hypocapnia.

357 Explain the effects of changes in the acidity (eg, respiratory acidosis and alkalosis) of body fluids on $[K^+]_p$. Describe a major determinant of potassium release from cells during respiratory acidosis and other acidemic states.

❑ Acidemia is generally associated with potassium release from intracellular fluid, increasing $[K^+]_p$. Conversely, alkalemia generally shifts potassium into cells, thereby decreasing $[K^+]_p$. Intracellular proteins interact with potassium by electrostatic binding and the approximately 55 mEq/L of anionic proteins within skeletal muscle cells are balanced by K^+. The ion-binding sites of proteins have preference for H^+ over other ions; however, other ions can compete only if their concentration is considerably higher than that of H^+. This requisite is amply satisfied in the cytosolic fluid by potassium because its concentration is six orders of magnitude higher than that of H^+ ($[K^+]_i = 10^{-1}$ M; $[H^+]_i = 10^{-7}$ M). Nevertheless, when cell pH decreases ($[H^+]_i$ increases) hydrogen ions (H^+) displace potassium from the proteins that are known to have substantial buffer value. The diminished binding of potassium by intracellular proteins in acidosis will alter the electrochemical gradient for this ion favoring the cellular exit of K^+.

358 Describe the expected change in serum $[K^+]$ in acute respiratory acidosis and alkalosis, and compare with the response to metabolic acid-base disturbances.

❑ Acute acidemia is usually associated with a rise in serum $[K^+]$ while acute alkalemia has the opposite effect. The quantitative relationship between the altered acidity and extracellular $[K^+]$ is properly expressed as the $\Delta[K^+]_p/\Delta pH$. The corresponding values for each acid-base disturbance are as follows: (1) respiratory acidosis, −1 mEq/L/pH unit; (2) respiratory alkalosis, −2 mEq/L/pH unit; (3) metabolic acidosis, −7 mEq/L/pH unit; and (4) metabolic alkalosis, −4 mEq/L/pH unit. It is evident that the changes in serum $[K^+]$ in acute respiratory acid-base disorders are very modest as compared to those of metabolic disorders.

359 How persistent and severe is hyperkalemia resulting from redistribution (eg, stress of patients with asthma or COPD, beta-adrenergic agonists) of body potassium stores?

❑ Hyperkalemia resulting from potassium redistribution is usually short-lasting, and if this process occurs in the presence of normal renal potassium excretion, its severity is from mild to moderate. However, hyperkalemia due to redistribution might occasionally be severe and even lethal.

360 Explain what significance changes in the intracellular concentration of bicarbonate ($[HCO_3^-]_i$) have in the release of potassium from cells during respiratory acidosis.

❑ In respiratory acidosis $[HCO_3^-]_i$ increases, contrasting with its decrease in metabolic acidosis. In addition, potassium is released from intracellular proteins due to the buffering of hydrogen ions (H^+) in respiratory acidosis; the displaced potassium can be electrostatically balanced by the anionic equivalency resulting from the simultaneous generation of $[HCO_3^-]$. Consequently, in respiratory acidosis there is not a substantial release of cellular potassium that is known to occur in metabolic acidosis due to the differential response in $[HCO_3^-]$ (in metabolic acidosis $[HCO_3^-]_i$ decreases, while in respiratory acidosis, $[HCO_3^-]_i$ increases).

361 What is the effect of respiratory alkalosis on the K^+-binding capacity of proteins and bicarbonate within intracellular fluid?

❑ In a comparable manner to metabolic alkalosis, the diminished $[H^+]_i$ observed in respiratory alkalosis induces proteins to release H^+, increasing their anionic equivalency. Hence, intracellular potassium binds to protein sites previously occupied by hydrogen ions. The simultaneous presence of a diminished $[HCO_3^-]_i$ will decrease the K^+-binding capacity of this anion. Consequently, the change in potassium bound by cytosolic bicarbonate in respiratory alkalosis occurs in association with an opposite change in the K^+-binding properties of the intracellular proteins. The net effect is a milder hypokalemic response to respiratory alkalosis compared to the one elicited by metabolic alkalosis.

362 Compare the immediate and sustained response of renal potassium (K^+) excretion in respiratory acidosis and alkalosis.

❑ The immediate response of renal potassium excretion in acidosis (respiratory and metabolic) is a decreased kaliuresis, while in alkalosis (respiratory and metabolic), there is an increased kaliuresis. This response is short-lasting. The sustained response in acidosis, respiratory and metabolic, is a greater than normal potassium excretion, leading to a K^+ deficit that is mild in respiratory acidosis and moderate in metabolic acidosis. In respiratory alkalosis, potassium excretion promptly returns to normal so that a significant K^+ deficit does not develop in this condition. In contrast with respiratory alkalosis, a larger K^+ deficit develops in metabolic alkalosis, due to a sizable kaliuresis. The increased potassium excretion observed in chronic respiratory acidosis is elicited by an increased delivery of sodium to the distal nephron, which enhances kaliuresis, overriding the expected renal potassium retention due to acidosis.

RESPIRATORY AND MIXED DISTURBANCES. PSEUDORESPIRATORY ALKALOSIS

363 Name the simple acid-base disorders.

❑ The simple acid-base disorders are respiratory acidosis, respiratory alkalosis, metabolic acidosis, and metabolic alkalosis.

364 Categorize the various acid-base disturbances. Explain the concepts of a single and a mixed acid-base disorder.

❑ The various acid-base disorders are properly categorized as simple and mixed disorders. A simple acid-base disorder is characterized by a primary or initiating abnormality in either the respiratory component (PCO_2 levels) or the metabolic component (plasma $[HCO_3^-]$) accompanied by a secondary change in the other component. Thus, the primary abnormality coupled with the secondary physiologic response constitute the simple disorder. The term *mixed acid-base disorders* denotes the simultaneous presence of two or more acid-base disturbances. Such association might comprise two or more simple (cardinal) acid-base disorders, two or more entities of a single simple disorder that have different pathogenesis or time course, or a combination of the previous two forms. The secondary or adaptive response to a simple acid-base disorder cannot be taken as one of the components of a mixed disorder.

365 Define the terms *acidemia* and *acidosis,* as well as *alkalemia* and *alkalosis,* and contrast the meaning of each pair of terms.

❑ *Acidemia* indicates a decreased pH level (or increased $[H^+]$) in the blood. *Acidosis* is a pathophysiologic process characterized by either a primary acid gain or a primary alkali loss. Acidosis is usually associated with acidemia; however, a normal blood pH or even alkalemia might accompany this process (ie, mixed disturbance). *Alkalemia* indicates an increased pH level (or decreased $[H^+]$) in the blood. *Alkalosis* is a pathophysiologic process characterized by either a primary acid loss or a primary alkali gain. Alkalosis is usually associated with alkalemia; however, a normal pH or even acidemia might accompany this process (ie, mixed disturbance).

366 Provide an example of the correct terminology to describe an acid-base disorder with an abnormal PCO_2 that represents a secondary response.

❑ Considering the following acid-base data from a patient with cholera—pH 7.15, ($[H^+]$ of 71 nmol/L), PCO_2 of 18 mm Hg, and $[HCO_3^-]_p$ of 6 mEq/L—the correct terminology to describe it would be "metabolic acidosis." An alternative terminology might be "metabolic acidosis with the expected respiratory response." Incorrect terminology would be "metabolic acidosis with respiratory alkalosis" as well as "metabolic acidosis with secondary respiratory alkalosis," because the respiratory response (ie, secondary hypocapnia) to metabolic acidosis should not be identified with the name of a primary disorder (ie, respiratory alkalosis).

367 What are the respiratory acid-base disorders? Are these abnormalities in acid-base status commonly present in isolation from other disturbances of body acidity?

❑ Respiratory acid-base disorders are those abnormalities in acid-base equilibrium initiated by a change in carbon dioxide tension of body fluids. Very frequently, however, acid-base disturbances of metabolic nature are superimposed on either respiratory acidosis or alkalosis; effective patient care requires the proper recognition and management of these mixed acid-base disorders.

368 What is pseudorespiratory alkalosis?

❑ *Pseudorespiratory alkalosis* is characterized by a distinct pattern of blood gases, in which arterial hypocapnia and alkalemia are associated with venous (and tissue) hypercapnia and acidemia. Consequently, sole examination of ABGs leads to the mistaken diagnosis of respiratory alkalosis or primary hypocapnia in a patient who has elevated body carbon dioxide stores (thereby respiratory acidosis is the correct diagnosis). This acid-base pattern is observed in many patients with severe circulatory failure.

369 How does pseudorespiratory alkalosis develop?

❑ Concerning the pathogenesis of this disorder, an isolated severe reduction in cardiac output in the presence of constant production of carbon dioxide will result in a diminished excretion of carbon dioxide as well as a proportional widening of the arteriovenous difference in PCO_2 simply because of the longer transit time. Under these conditions, a greater than normal addition of carbon dioxide per unit of blood traversing the systemic capillaries will tend to generate venous hypercapnia. At the same time, increased removal of carbon dioxide per unit of blood traversing the pulmonary circulation results from the enlarged $\dot{V}/\dot{Q}$ ratio and creates relative arterial hypocapnia.

370 What measures must be taken to rule out pseudorespiratory alkalosis?

❑ To rule out pseudorespiratory alkalosis in a patient with circulatory failure and arterial hypocapnia, blood gas monitoring must include central venous blood sampling. In addition, measurement of end-tidal PCO_2 ($P_{ET}CO_2$) helps to assess whether arterial hypocapnia is a component of pseudorespiratory alkalosis, as follows: A significant decrement in $P_{ET}CO_2$ is observed in pseudorespiratory alkalosis because in this condition there is a reduction in pulmonary carbon dioxide excretion.

371 What are the most clinically relevant acid-base disturbances that might be associated with acute and chronic respiratory acidosis?

❑ The metabolic acidosis associated with respiratory acidosis, as well as the mixed disturbance that includes metabolic alkalosis with respiratory acidosis, are among the most clinically relevant mixed acid-base disturbances. In addition, chronic hypercapnia is commonly complicated with acute respiratory acidosis (acute hypercapnia).

372 Describe the characteristics of the mixed disturbance involving respiratory acidosis and metabolic acidosis.

❑ The combination of respiratory acidosis and metabolic acidosis is commonly observed in patients with cardiorespiratory arrest, COPD complicated by circulatory failure or sepsis, severe pulmonary edema, combined renal and respiratory failure, or diarrhea or renal tubular acidosis complicated by paralysis of respiratory muscles, and in patients poisoned with various toxic agents and drugs. The additive effects on plasma acidity of primary hypercapnia on the one hand and the bicarbonate deficit on the other might produce profound acidemia that requires prompt therapy. Whenever possible, the treatment should focus on both the respiratory and the metabolic components; mechanical ventilation and alkali therapy should be used, if necessary, for the management of these patients.

373 How important is the association of metabolic acidosis and respiratory alkalosis as a mixed acid-base disorder?

❑ Primary hypocapnia is frequently associated with other acid-base disturbances. Respiratory alkalosis in association with metabolic acidosis is one of the most important and is relatively common in critically ill patients. Patients with septicemia, particularly due to gram-negative organisms, might experience respiratory alkalosis plus metabolic acidosis, the latter being secondary to lactic acidosis or renal failure. Combined hepatic and renal failure represents another important clinical setting, in which this mixed acid-base disturbance might be observed. Patients with salicylate intoxication, as previously mentioned, commonly develop metabolic acidosis and respiratory alkalosis, reflecting the effects of salicylates on both cellular metabolism (uncoupling of oxidative phosphorylation) and ventilation (stimulation of central chemoreceptors). Patients undergoing hemodialysis, using an acetate bath with highly efficient systems, can develop primary hypocapnia due to rapid loss of carbon dioxide into the dialysate as well as metabolic acidosis. The dialysis-induced metabolic acidosis is secondary to the rapid removal of bicarbonate by the dialyzer, which might occur faster than the rate at which the body's alkali stores can be replenished by the metabolic conversion of circulating acetate.

---

374 What are the major causes of lactic acidosis? Describe the specific causes of lactic acidosis that result from tissue hypoxia.

❑ The most prominent causes of lactic acidosis are tissue hypoxia, metabolic disorders, drugs and toxins, and hereditary defects. Tissue hypoxia leading to lactic acidosis might result from (1) increased oxygen demand due to sepsis, seizures, and vigorous exercise; (2) diminished tissue perfusion due to low cardiac output or severe circulatory failure; and (3) diminished transport of oxygen in arterial blood due to extreme anemia, profound hypoxemia, or occupation of hemoglobin by carbon monoxide or other toxins.

---

375 Explain the changes in blood lactate levels in severe hypoxemia (eg, hypoxic lactic acidosis).

❑ As tissue oxygenation becomes inadequate, anaerobic metabolism begins and the cell produces lactate. However, interpretation of blood lactate levels is difficult. While an increase in blood lactate can occur with tissue hypoxia, it can be also seen with decreased liver metabolism of lactate, with alkalemia-induced increases in glycolysis, with vigorous muscular contraction (eg, seizures or rigors), or during fluid resuscitation of previously hypoperfused tissue (''washout'' phenomenon). In addition to the nonspecificity of a raised lactate level, it is an insensitive guide to tissue hypoxia. Indeed, it has been suggested that the blood lactate level is rarely significantly increased in states of hypoxemia unless there is a concomitant decrease in hepatic blood flow or severe impairment in liver function.

376 Describe the characteristics of the mixed disturbance involving respiratory acidosis and metabolic alkalosis.

❑ A deviation of plasma pH toward alkalinity, as opposed to the expected acidemia, is commonly observed in patients with respiratory acidosis because of several complicating events. Gastritis, peptic ulcer disease, and gastrointestinal bleeding occur very frequently in patients with COPD due to the intake of xanthines and corticosteroids, and possibly due to the underlying disease; thus, metabolic alkalosis resulting from absorbable antacid administration or vomiting is most prevalent. The renal effects of the chronic administration of corticosteroids might also result in potassium depletion and metabolic alkalosis. If cor pulmonale is present, the physician frequently prescribes diuretics to control fluid retention, and these agents might produce metabolic alkalosis through several mechanisms. Since potassium depletion is also common in patients with chronic respiratory acidosis (due to low potassium intake, treatment with corticosteroids, and diuretics), this electrolyte imbalance is also a significant contributor to metabolic alkalosis. Rapid correction of the carbon dioxide retention via mechanical ventilation or other means in patients with longstanding hypercapnia and secondary hyperbicarbonatemia might result in transient alkalemia. In the absence of a clinical history, simple observation of the blood gases might lead to an erroneous diagnosis of primary metabolic alkalosis.

377 The alkalemia that can occur immediately with reduction of PCO_2 in a patient with chronic hypercapnia has been previously discussed. We also discussed posthypercapnic metabolic alkalosis. Are there any other major causes of metabolic alkalosis in patients with chronic respiratory acidosis?

❑ Yes, there are at least three major reasons (analyzed in more detail elsewhere in this book) for the frequent development of metabolic alkalosis in these patients. First, administration of corticosteroids for the management of reactive-airway disease may cause metabolic alkalosis. Second, antacid administration and vomiting are most prevalent in these patients. Third, the development of fluid retention prompts the physician to prescribe diuretics.

378 How important is the association of metabolic alkalosis and respiratory alkalosis as a mixed acid-base disorder?

❑ The other major mixed acid-base disorder involving respiratory alkalosis results from the concomitant presence of metabolic alkalosis. The association of two primary alkalemic disorders might induce an extreme elevation of blood pH values. The increased excitability of both the CNS and the myocardium, in extreme alkalemia, is responsible for the grave prognosis of this condition. Patients with hepatic insufficiency commonly develop metabolic alkalosis due to vomiting and diuretics (among other causes), which can be superimposed on the chronic respiratory alkalosis characteristic of liver disease. Patients with other causes of primary hypocapnia, such as pregnancy, heart failure, and pulmonary diseases, can manifest this mixed acid-base disorder, if metabolic alkalosis develops. Effective correction of respiratory alkalosis in patients receiving mechanical ventilation can be achieved by changing the ventilator settings or mode.

379 Elaborate on the characteristics of the mixed disturbance in which chronic hypercapnia is complicated by acute hypercapnia.

❑ This clinical picture is commonly observed in patients with severe COPD who develop intercurrent pulmonary infections or cardiac failure, and those who have been medicated with sedatives or excessive oxygen administration, or both. These patients might have been fully adapted to a certain level of $PaCO_2$, only to experience a further rise in $PaCO_2$ due to deterioration of their effective alveolar ventilation. The blood acid-base composition in these patients will be intermediate between that typically observed in acute and that in chronic respiratory acidosis. It should be noted that an acid-base pattern identical to that present in patients with chronic hypercapnia complicated by acute hypercapnia might be observed in (1) patients with a stable degree of hypercapnia in whom a full secondary metabolic response has not yet occurred, (2) patients with chronic hypercapnia and a superimposed metabolic acidosis of mild to moderate severity, and (3) patients with metabolic alkalosis associated with acute respiratory acidosis. The therapy of chronic respiratory acidosis complicated by an acute increase in $PaCO_2$ is discussed in a subsequent question.

Part III: Clinical Picture of Respiratory Failure

15. Acute Lung Injury

ACUTE RESPIRATORY DISTRESS SYNDROME

380 What is the acute respiratory distress syndrome (ARDS)?

❑ ARDS is a life-threatening condition characterized by hypoxemic respiratory failure caused by acute lung injury (ALI), in which noncardiogenic pulmonary edema and diffuse lung infiltrates are typically present. Since ARDS is not limited to adults, the ''A'' of ARDS should not be taken as indicative of ''adult'' but signifies ''acute.'' This syndrome may develop in response to multiple conditions that are examined in the answers to pertinent questions.

381 Does the term *acute lung injury* represent the same condition as ARDS?

❑ No. The clinical spectrum of acute pulmonary diseases that alter oxygenation by mechanisms other than hydrostatic edema is very broad and includes ALI and ARDS. The latter term (ie, ARDS) is reserved for the most severe form of this spectrum of conditions. The current criteria for both ALI and ARDS according to a joint committee of European and North American experts (1994) include an acute pulmonary disease with bilateral infiltrates seen on a frontal chest radiograph, absence of clinical evidence of elevated left atrial pressure or pulmonary artery pressure equal to or less than 18 mm Hg (when measured), and a significant oxygenation defect (more severe in ARDS than in ALI). The ratio of arterial oxygen tension to fractional inspired oxygen (PaO_2/FiO_2) is equal or less than 300 in ALI but equal or less than 200 in ARDS, regardless of the positive end-expiratory pressure (PEEP). It becomes apparent on examination of the diagnostic criteria that all patients with ARDS have ALI, but the reverse is not true—not all patients with ALI have ARDS.

382 What is ALI? What are its causes?

❑ ALI recently was defined by a committee of European and North American experts (1994) as a syndrome of inflammation and increased permeability associated with clinical, radiologic, and physiologic abnormalities that cannot be explained by, but may coexist with, left atrial or pulmonary capillary hypertension. Conditions commonly associated with ALI (as well as ARDS) include sepsis syndrome, aspiration, primary pneumonia, and multiple trauma. ALI and ARDS are less commonly associated with cardiopulmonary bypass, multiple transfusions, fat embolism, and pancreatitis.

383 What conditions can lead to ALI and ARDS caused by direct lung injury?

❑ Direct lung injuries that can cause ALI and ARDS include (1) aspiration, (2) diffuse pulmonary infection (eg, bacterial, viral, *Pneumocystis*), (3) near-drowning, (4) toxic inhalation, and (5) lung contusion.

384 What conditions can lead to ALI and ARDS as a result of indirect injury?

❑ Indirect lung injuries that can lead to ALI and ARDS include (1) sepsis syndrome, (2) severe nonthoracic trauma, (3) multiple transfusions (ie, hypertransfusion) for emergency resuscitation, and (4) cardiopulmonary bypass (infrequently).

385 Name all the major conditions (ie, causative factors) that can lead to ARDS.

❑ Conditions that can lead to ARDS include (1) diffuse pulmonary infections (eg, viral, bacterial, fungal, *Pneumocystis*), (2) systemic reaction to extrapulmonary processes (eg, gram-negative septicemia, fat embolism, severe pancreatitis, amniotic fluid embolism), (3) nonthoracic trauma with hypotension, (4) exposure to drugs (eg, heroin, methadone, morphine, dextropropoxyphene, nitrofurantoin) and irritant or toxic inhalants (eg, high concentrations of oxygen, chlorine gas, NO_2, smoke, ozone), (5) aspiration (eg, water as with a near-drowning accident, gastric contents with Mendelson's syndrome), (6) immunologic disorders (eg, systemic lupus erythematosus, Goodpasture's syndrome), and (7) postcardiopulmonary bypass (also known as *postperfusion lung* or *pump lung syndrome*). More details with respect to the causes of ARDS are provided in the answers to pertinent questions.

386 Elaborate on the causes of ARDS according to the route of lung injury.

❑ The causes of ARDS have been conveniently classified according to the route of lung injury, as follows: (1) airway source (ie, aspiration of gastric contents, near-drowning, diffuse infectious pneumonia, smoke inhalation injury, irritant gas inhalation, oxygen toxicity), (2) vascular route (ie, sepsis, trauma, multiple transfusions, drug overdose, head injury, fat embolism, pancreatitis, shock, toxic shock syndrome, surface burns, drug idiosyncratic reaction, thrombotic thrombocytopenic purpura, leukemia, venous air embolism, amniotic fluid embolism, paraquat intoxication, cardiopulmonary bypass), and (3) direct or physical injury (ie, lung contusion, radiation, hanging).

387 What causes of ARDS are responsible for most of the episodes observed in clinical practice?

❑ More than 85% of episodes of ARDS are caused by one of the following eight conditions: aspiration, near-drowning, sepsis, trauma, multiple blood transfusions, drug overdose, head injury, and lung contusion. The average incidence of ARDS in patients with one of the aforementioned risk factors is 25% and doubles in patients with more than one risk factor (the highest risk is associated with sepsis and multiple transfusions for emergency resuscitation).

388 What are the early clinical and laboratory abnormalities of patients with ARDS?

❑ An increase in respiratory rate or dyspnea or both represent the early clinical manifestations of ARDS. Laboratory abnormalities observed in these patients include hypoxemia, increased alveolar-arterial difference for oxygen, and hypocapnia. Physical examination reveals either normal findings or few fine inspiratory rales. In addition, chest x-ray films either appear normal or demonstrate few small and scattered interstitial infiltrates.

389 What are the clinical and laboratory derangements of advanced ARDS?

❑ Clinical findings in severe ARDS include tachypnea, dyspnea, and obvious cyanosis (evident on examination of the tongue and extremities, known as *central* and *peripheral cyanosis,* respectively). Chest examination may reveal prominent bilateral crackles and tubular breath sounds (uncommon finding). Radiographic evaluation discloses interstitial and alveolar infiltrates that are diffuse and bilateral. There is minimal correction of hypoxemia after increasing the inspired PO_2. The lack of response to higher inspired oxygen is caused by the presence of right-to-left blood shunting through collapsed or filled alveoli in the late stage of ARDS. Application of mechanical ventilation with PEEP increases lung volume, which in turn can open collapsed alveoli (recruitment), decreasing shunting and ameliorating hypoxemia.

390 What are the main criteria to establish the diagnosis of the ARDS?

❑ Patients with ARDS have a severe form of diffuse lung injury associated with increased capillary permeability. Commonly used major criteria to establish the diagnosis of ARDS include the simultaneous presence of all of the following abnormalities: (1) severe hypoxemia (ie, ratio of PaO_2 over P_AO_2 <0.2), (2) normal pulmonary capillary wedge pressure (PCWP) (ie, <15 mm Hg) (see more information about the role of PCWP in the diagnosis of ARDS in the answers to other questions), (3) bilateral lung infiltrates documented on chest x-ray film, (4) appropriate risk factors for the development of ARDS, (5) exclusion of other pulmonary diseases (eg, chronic interstitial fibrosis), and (6) reduced total static thoracic compliance (ie, <50 mL/cm H_2O). The previously mentioned information is not always available for patients with a suspected diagnosis of ARDS. Consequently, the criteria presented above should be considered only as a useful guideline for the diagnosis of ARDS. In addition, there are quantitative criteria for the diagnosis of ARDS that consist of a scoring system described in the answer to another question.

---

391 What are the components and individual values of the lung injury score (described by Murray and coworkers) for the diagnosis and follow-up of patients with ARDS?

❑ The components and individual values of the lung injury score of ARDS are as follows: (1) chest radiograph (ie, absence of alveolar consolidation scores 0, and alveolar consolidation present in 1, 2, 3, and 4 quadrants score 1, 2, 3, and 4 points, respectively); (2) hypoxemia (ie, PaO_2/FiO_2 >300, from 225 to 299, from 175 to 224, from 100 to 174, and <100 score 0, 1, 2, 3, and 4 points, respectively); (3) PEEP when ventilated (ie, >5 cm H_2O, from 6 to 8 cm H_2O, from 9 to 11 cm H_2O, from 12 to 14 cm H_2O, and >15 cm H_2O score 0, 1, 2, 3, and 4 points, respectively); and (4) compliance of respiratory system, if available (ie, >80 mL/cm H_2O, from 60 to 79 mL/cm H_2O, from 40 to 59 mL/cm H_2O, from 20 to 39 mL/cm H_2O, and <19 mL/cm H_2O score 0, 1, 2, 3, and 4 points, respectively). The final value for the lung injury score is obtained by dividing the total score by the number of components that were used in the computation. The interpretation of the final value is as follows: (1) absence of lung injury corresponds to score 0; (2) mild to moderate lung injury, when the score is from 0.1 to 2.5; and (3) severe lung injury indicative of the presence of ARDS, when the score is higher than 2.5.

---

392 What is the rationale for the use of PaO_2/FiO_2 in the assessment of hypoxemia with the lung injury score? Why were scores not assigned for PEEP values up to 5 cm H_2O?

❑ The rationale for the use of PaO_2/FiO_2 in the assessment of hypoxemia with the lung injury score system stems from the routine availability of the information to calculate this parameter in patients with ARDS and from the fact that this ratio provides an adequate assessment of gas exchange comparable to PaO_2/P_AO_2, but PaO_2/FiO_2 is more simple to calculate than the other ratio. With respect to PEEP, a score is not assigned for PEEP values up to 5 cm H_2O because these levels are commonly used when ventilating patients with normal lungs (eg, drug overdosage, following major surgery), but in ARDS patients higher PEEP levels are usually applied.

---

393 What are the main determinants of the arterial hypoxemia and abnormal hemodynamic status of patients with ARDS? Does mechanical ventilation play a role in the abnormal hemodynamic status?

❑ Critically ill patients with ARDS develop significant arterial hypoxemia because of the presence of a right-to-left shunt (main defect), increased lung fluid, and a reduction in mixed venous oxygen level. An abnormal hemodynamic status is commonly observed in ARDS due to the increased intrathoracic pressure caused by mechanical ventilation and cardiac dysfunction (associated with either expanded or contracted intravascular volume). Arterial hypoxemia and abnormal hemodynamic status are simultaneously present in many patients and their management requires substantial dedication and expertise of the health care team.

394 Is pulmonary artery catheterization required for the diagnosis of ARDS?

❑ No. Although the diagnosis of ARDS requires the exclusion of heart failure as the cause of pulmonary edema, this task can be accomplished with noninvasive techniques (eg, two-dimensional echocardiography). Consequently, pulmonary artery catheterization is not required for the diagnosis of ARDS.

395 Explain the potential pitfalls for the use of pulmonary artery catheterization in the diagnosis of ARDS.

❑ Although pulmonary artery catheterization can help differentiate increased-permeability pulmonary edema from the cardiogenic type, this procedure has several limitations in the diagnosis of ARDS. Patients with cardiogenic pulmonary edema caused by a transient episode of myocardial ischemia may have a normal pulmonary wedge pressure at the time of measurement. Conversely, patients with ALI or ARDS may have a high pulmonary wedge pressure caused by the intravenous infusion of a large volume of fluids. Furthermore, a given patient can have pulmonary edema caused by both high-pressure and increased permeability mechanisms. Other pitfalls with the use of pulmonary artery catheterization include technical problems, complications of the procedure, and selection of patients unusually ill because they require monitoring of pulmonary artery pressure.

396 What is the role of pulmonary artery wedge pressure measurements in the differential diagnosis of cardiogenic and noncardiogenic pulmonary edema? Elaborate on the importance of the measurement of protein concentration in bronchial secretions.

❑ Measurements of pulmonary artery wedge pressure by means of a Swan-Ganz catheter help to determine the pathogenesis of pulmonary edema. This evaluation is the most useful diagnostic aid to help resolve this common medical dilemma. Pulmonary edema might be due to an imbalance of Starling's forces (cardiogenic type) or to abnormal permeability of pulmonary capillaries (noncardiogenic type of pulmonary edema). A cardiogenic origin of pulmonary edema (imbalance of Starling's forces) is most likely if the pulmonary capillary wedge or pulmonary artery diastolic pressure exceeds 25 mm Hg (if previous pressure levels were normal) or 30 mm Hg (if previous pressure levels were abnormally high). The protein concentration in bronchial secretions also helps to establish the pathogenesis of pulmonary edema. Finding protein levels in these secretions that are close to those of plasma is consistent with increased capillary permeability (and therefore consistent with noncardiogenic pulmonary edema), whereas a low protein concentration in bronchial secretions is typically found in cardiogenic pulmonary edema. Although theoretically appealing, the overlap in the results of individual patients has limited the value of measuring protein levels in bronchial secretions and plasma, and this test is rarely performed in the practice of medicine. The two forms of pulmonary edema are not mutually exclusive because a given patient might have elements of both cardiogenic and noncardiogenic pulmonary edema contributing to the disease.

397 What conditions lead to ARDS that develops rapidly and can resolve quickly and completely without sequelae?

❑ Patients with heroin-induced pulmonary edema, air embolism, fat embolism, pulmonary contusion, or some infectious pneumonias can fully recover pulmonary function promptly (within a few days) after the development of ARDS. Conversely, patients with ARDS associated with sepsis are more likely to have a more protracted course of lung injury that can lead to connective-tissue deposition and lung remodeling.

398 How might the future development of ARDS be predicted in a given patient? How likely is the development of ARDS in patients having one or more risk factors for this condition?

❑ Identification of diseases that commonly lead to ARDS (such as aspiration of gastric contents, sepsis, and trauma) is the most practical method of predicting the development of this condition in a given patient. The average incidence of ARDS is 25% in patients with one risk factor and it doubles in those with two or more risk factors. Sepsis is the most common cause of ARDS and a major risk factor, as 40% of patients with sepsis develop this form of respiratory failure. Various blood-borne mediators and markers of ALI are elevated in patients with ARDS; these markers, however, are also elevated in patients with similar clinical risk factors in the absence of ARDS. Consequently, none of these markers has been shown to predict consistently the likelihood for the development of ARDS in an individual patient.

399 What are the mechanisms of lung injury in ALI and ARDS?

❑ ALI and ARDS can develop because of a direct insult on lung tissue or indirectly as a component of an acute systemic inflammatory response. Both the lung endothelium and the epithelium are injured in ALI and ARDS. The mechanisms of lung injury possibly differ according to the specific cause of ALI or ARDS, but the inflammatory response includes both cellular and humoral components.

400 What are the morphologic abnormalities of the lungs observed in ARDS? Describe the early and late pulmonary lesions.

❑ The lungs in ARDS have an increased weight largely caused by edema and airless regions demonstrating atelectasis, consolidation, and hemorrhage. The early lesions detected on light microscopy include fluid accumulation (edema); vascular congestion; atelectasis; hyaline membrane deposition; and cellular infiltration (red blood cells, polymorphonuclear leukocytes, platelets) of interstitial areas, interalveolar septa, and alveolar spaces. In addition, loss of alveolar *type I* pneumocytes and hyperplasia/dysplasia of granular pneumocytes (also known as *type II*) may be detected. In patients with prolonged disease that exceeds 10 days, interstitial fibrosis can develop in association with the abnormalities observed in the early stage.

401 What are the factors that predispose to aspiration pneumonia?

❑ Predisposing factors for aspiration pneumonia include (1) *neurologic disorders* (ie, decreased level of consciousness caused by general anesthesia, drug overdose, alcoholism, stroke, head injury, and seizures; pseudobulbar palsy; Parkinson's disease; multiple sclerosis; myasthenia gravis; local anesthesia to the pharynx); (2) *gastrointestinal disorders* (ie, esophageal disease including achalasia, stricture, tumor, diverticulum, and tracheoesophageal fistula; gastric disease characterized by protracted vomiting, delayed gastric emptying, gastric distention due to diabetes mellitus, and sphincter incompetency; bowel obstruction); and (3) *pulmonary disorders* (ie, impaired mechanical barriers including endotracheal tube, tracheotomy tube, nasogastric tube, and incompetent larynx; impaired mucociliary clearance; and cellular defense mechanisms).

402 Briefly explain the pathophysiology of aspiration pneumonia.

❑ It has been generally assumed that inhalation of gastric juice with a pH higher than 2.4 does not cause significant lung injury. It is now known that aspiration of all types of gastric juice, of whatever pH, with or without foodstuff, can cause significant hypoxemia. If the inoculum is of a relatively high pH and is free of foodstuff, the insult is rapidly surmounted, whereas vomitus with a low pH causes parenchymal damage with inflammation, edema, and hemorrhage; aspiration of foodstuff causes an obliterative bronchiolitis with subsequent granuloma formation. The volume of gastric aspirate is an important determinant of lung injury, and at least 2 to 4 mL/kg is required to produce significant injury in experimental animals. The physiologic response to aspiration is dramatic, with a precipitous fall in PaO_2 that is thought to be due to the rapid development of atelectasis secondary to acid denaturation of surfactant. Later, there is massive exudation of fluid into the lung (noncardiogenic pulmonary edema, ARDS). While aspiration of gastric contents is not associated with immediate infection, it increases susceptibility to subsequent bacterial pneumonia.

403 What are the main clinical features of aspiration pneumonia?

❑ In the immediate period after the episode of aspiration, patients may display fever, tachypnea, diffuse crackles, severe hypoxemia, and an asthma-like reaction. The latent interval from the time of aspiration until the onset of symptoms is generally less than 1 hour. The initial chest x-ray film appears abnormal in the majority of the patients, but in some patients the radiograph is clear. In contrast to the radiographic pattern of pneumonia associated with aspiration of oropharyngeal contents, aspiration of gastric contents is not associated with characteristic radiographic findings, and the type of radiographic picture does not correlate with mortality. Most patients show progressive clearing of infiltrates within 2 to 16 days, and progressive worsening on the chest x-ray film, especially after 3 days or a period of improvement, suggests the development of bacterial pneumonia or ARDS. The subsequent course takes one of three patterns: A minority (12%) show progressive worsening of the clinical and radiographic picture and generally die within 24 hours; the majority (63%) show rapid clinical and radiographic improvement; and the remainder (25%) display a rapid initial improvement followed by clinical deterioration, with new or progressive infiltrates and signs of infection suggestive of a superimposed nosocomial pneumonia. Bacterial pneumonia develops in 36% to 45% of patients who aspirate gastric contents. This occurs within 2 to 10 days (usually 3 to 5 days) of the acute episode. It is an ominous development as the mortality rate is threefold higher in patients with infection as compared with noninfected cohorts. Diagnosis of pneumonia in this setting is fraught with difficulties.

404 Explain the fat embolism syndrome.

❑ The fat embolism syndrome is usually attributed to the release of neutral fat from the bone marrow secondary to bone injury. It is characterized by the development of ARDS associated with thrombocytopenia, deteriorating mental status, and the appropriate clinical setting. It occurs in less than 2% of patients with isolated tibial or femoral fractures and 5% to 10% of patients with multiple long-bone or pelvic fractures; the mortality rate is about 4% and 20% in these two settings, respectively. During the first 12 hours, fat globules cause mechanical obstruction of the end-organ vasculature; this may result in rapidly deteriorating oxygenation. After a latent interval of 24 to 72 hours, lipase hydrolyzes the neutral fat into free fatty acids such as oleic acid, which cause intense local inflammation and tissue damage.

405 What neurologic and hematologic abnormalities commonly develop in the fat embolism syndrome?

❑ Confusion commonly develops in the first 24 to 48 hours. Additional neurologic findings depend on the magnitude and site of embolization. Retinal exudates and hemorrhages are found in 50% to 60% of patients. Petechiae develop in 50% to 60% of patients but usually do not appear before 24 hours. These are typically found in the axillae, conjunctivae, mucous membranes, anterior part of the chest, neck, and shoulders. Multiple hematologic abnormalities may occur and include thrombocytopenia, platelet aggregation, and activation of the intrinsic coagulation cascade and the fibrinolytic system.

406 How is the diagnosis of fat embolism syndrome determined?

❑ Diagnosis of the fat embolism syndrome is made by exclusion because there is no single laboratory test that confirms its presence. The demonstration of fat in the urine or sputum is neither sensitive nor specific for the syndrome. Likewise, neither the demonstration of fat globules in the blood nor serum lipase activity are clinically useful. Recent data suggest that bronchoalveolar lavage may be helpful in the diagnosis of this condition.

407 What is amniotic fluid embolism? What are its manifestations?

❑ Amniotic fluid embolism is a catastrophic obstetric complication that occurs most commonly during delivery. Although uncommon (about 1 in 80,000 deliveries), this condition has a mortality higher than 80% in some series. Patients typically present with sudden dyspnea, profound hypotension, pulmonary edema (apparent on chest x-ray films in 70% of patients), seizures (in 10% to 20% of patients), bleeding diathesis (in 10% to 15% of patients), or cardiopulmonary arrest. Approximately half of the patients die within 1 hour of the onset of symptoms. The mechanisms of pulmonary edema include both a cardiogenic and a noncardiogenic component. Following the initial disturbances, about 40% to 50% of patients develop hemorrhagic manifestations secondary to disseminated intravascular coagulation (DIC) or uterine bleeding caused by atony of this organ. The management of amniotic fluid embolism is aimed at supporting oxygenation and the circulation, and reversing the coagulation disorder.

408 What are the main features of smoke inhalation injury? What is the mortality rate of this condition?

❑ The primary cause of smoke inhalation injury is the release of toxic products of incomplete combustion rather than the heat of the fire. Clinical presentation depends on the predominant form of injury. While thermal injury results in immediate inflammation, the deleterious effects of chemical injury have a delayed onset, which makes early diagnosis difficult. However, inhalation injury should be suspected in patients with facial burns, singed nasal hairs, hoarseness, stridor, wheezing, carbonaceous sputum, or phonation difficulties. The major pulmonary complications include asphyxia (mainly due to carbon monoxide intoxication), airway damage (upper-airway and bronchial obstruction), and parenchymal damage (ARDS). Smoke inhalation alone has a low mortality (5% to 10%) because the patient either dies immediately or gets better. However, the combination of smoke inhalation with cutaneous burns is particularly ominous, and the mortality (approximately 40% to 80%) is disproportionately higher than that predicted for the extent of the cutaneous burn.

409 What clinical features of smoke inhalation are dependent on toxic effects of the patient's hemoglobin?

❑ Smoke inhalation is the leading cause of carbon monoxide intoxication. Features associated with carbon monoxide intoxication include headache, nausea, fatigue, behavioral change, ataxia, and hypoxic damage of the heart or brain. Cherry-red coloration of the lips is usually absent unless the carboxyhemoglobin (COHb) concentration is higher than 40%; cyanosis due to depressed respiration is more common. An intoxicated person displays a normal PaO_2 because the oxygen dissolved in plasma remains unchanged. High levels of carbon monoxide interfere with the oxygen-carrying capacity of hemoglobin, and oxygen saturation is decreased. However, the oxygen saturation included in a routine arterial blood gas (ABG) report is calculated from the PO_2 by using the standard oxyhemoglobin dissociation curve and correcting for the effects of PO_2, pH, and temperature and thus, may be normal. Consequently, it is imperative to directly measure oxygen saturation by using a cooximeter. Despite severe oxygen desaturation, minute ventilation is not increased in carbon monoxide intoxication because the carotid body responds to PaO_2 rather than oxygen content; minute ventilation may increase if tissue hypoxia is severe, causing lactic acidosis. Confirmation of carbon monoxide intoxication is made by measurement of blood COHb: less than 2% in healthy subjects, 5% to 10% in cigarette smokers, and 30% to 50% in fire injury victims. The clinical features of carbon monoxide intoxication are relatively well correlated with the COHb level. Nomograms can be used to "backestimate" the COHb level at the time of exposure from a postexposure measurement. Patients displaying initial neurologic recovery may have a relapse up to 21 days after exposure, and this is associated with a poor prognosis. Carbon monoxide intoxication is the most frequent immediate cause of death in fire victims (accounting for >80% of deaths); burns cause only 11% of the early (<6 hours) mortality.

410 What is the pathophysiology of drowning and near-drowning?

❑ The pathophysiology of drowning and near-drowning in both freshwater and salt water is similar. Survival depends on the pulmonary insult, the amount of hypoxemic brain damage, and the degree of acidosis. A drowning victim responds initially by closing the glottis, and 10% of drowned victims aspirate no fluid but die of asphyxia. The remainder aspirate fluid, develop pulmonary edema and intrapulmonary shunt, and may progress to profound hypoxemia accompanied by a clinical picture identical to ARDS. The quantity of aspirated fluid is rarely sufficient to produce significant change in blood volume. Occasionally, however, near-drowning in hypotonic freshwater can cause transient hypervolemia, whereas hypovolemia may follow hypertonic saltwater aspiration. Alterations in hematocrit or serum electrolytes are rarely life-threatening and not different with saltwater or freshwater near-drowning. Metabolic acidosis develops in 70% of victims. Renal function remains normal in most patients, but some develop hemoglobinuria, albuminuria, or acute tubular necrosis. The cardiovascular system displays remarkable stability, and alterations are primarily a consequence of hypoxemia or acidosis. The likelihood of neurologic impairment depends on the duration of immersion and possibly, the temperature of the water. Recovery has been reported after submersion in very cold water for up to 40 minutes. This may be partly due to the diving reflex, which is initiated by facial immersion in cold water (<20°C) and results in severe bradycardia, and also due to the shunting of blood to the heart and brain in an attempt to limit hypoxic damage. Additionally, hypothermia lowers oxygen requirements and prolongs the tolerance of the brain and heart to severe hypoxemia.

411 What elements obtained from the clinical history, physical examination, and laboratory evaluation (eg, protein level in bronchial secretions) facilitate the differential diagnosis of cardiogenic from noncardiogenic pulmonary edema?

❑ The clinical history generally provides important information with respect to a previous disease that predisposes to the development of cardiogenic (eg, ischemic heart disease, uncontrolled hypertension) or noncardiogenic (eg, trauma, sepsis) pulmonary edema. In addition, an acute cardiac event (eg, atrial fibrillation) might be detected in the cardiogenic type, but is absent in noncardiogenic edema. The physical examination in cardiogenic pulmonary edema might reveal poor blood perfusion of the extremities, cardiomegaly, S_3 gallop, jugular vein distention, and pulmonary wet crackles. None of the previously mentioned physical examination findings are present in patients with noncardiogenic pulmonary edema. Laboratory evaluations that help differentiate the two main forms of pulmonary edema include (1) blood gases (that reveal small and large venous shunting in cardiac and noncardiac edema, respectively); (2) protein level in the fluid derived from the airways (eg, ratio of protein concentration from edema fluid to that of serum is <0.5 in cardiogenic and >0.7 in noncardiogenic edema)—it must be recognized that evaluation of this ratio is only of theoretical interest and has no practical value because the necessary measurements are almost never done; (3) PCWP is higher than 18 mm Hg in the cardiac type and lower than 18 mm Hg in the noncardiac type of edema; (4) chest radiographs that show perihilar distribution in cardiogenic edema and peripheral distribution in noncardiogenic edema; and (5) electrocardiogram and cardiac enzymes that might be abnormal in the cardiac type but normal in the noncardiogenic form of edema.

412 How can cardiogenic and noncardiogenic pulmonary edema be differentiated?

❑ The clinical setting in which pulmonary edema occurs is an important clue in differentiating cardiogenic from noncardiogenic causes. Patients with pulmonary edema associated with a history of heart disease or current signs and symptoms of heart failure (particularly acute) should be strongly suspected of having cardiogenic pulmonary edema. On the other hand, patients with conditions that can cause noncardiogenic pulmonary edema (eg, septic shock, inhaled toxins) without a history or evidence of heart disease should be suspected of having noncardiogenic pulmonary edema. Manifestations of left-sided heart failure including exertional dyspnea, orthopnea, paroxysmal nocturnal dyspnea, exercise intolerance, and weakness support a diagnosis of cardiogenic pulmonary edema. Elevated left-sided heart diastolic pressures detected by invasive monitoring would be supportive of a cardiogenic etiology for the pulmonary edema, whereas normal or low filling pressures would support a noncardiogenic cause. Although a high oncotic pressure of bronchial secretions is evidence for a disrupted alveolar-capillary membrane and therefore supports a noncardiogenic cause for the pulmonary edema, this information is not available in clinical practice.

413 What is the so-called vascular redistribution that can be observed on examination of a standard chest x-ray film of patients with pulmonary edema?

❑ *Vascular redistribution* refers to an accentuation of the vascular structures in the upper regions of the lung fields on a standard posteroanterior chest x-ray film that might be observed in conditions of pulmonary vascular congestion. Recognition of this important radiologic sign of pulmonary venous congestion is important in the routine care of outpatients and inpatients.

---

414 Recapitulate the mechanisms responsible for the vascular redistribution of blood in the pulmonary circulation in states of pulmonary venous congestion.

❑ The increased blood flow of the upper regions of the lung in individuals having vascular redistribution is caused by the partial collapse of pulmonary blood vessels in the lower regions of the lung as a result of increased perivascular pressure due to fluid accumulation in the latter regions. Blood flow in the lower areas of the lung is higher than that in the upper regions during sitting or standing in normal individuals as well as those with pulmonary edema. During the sitting or standing position, the gravity-related increase in hydrostatic pressure within pulmonary capillaries in the lower compared to the upper lung regions is larger than the increase in pressure of the interstitial space surrounding these capillaries. The lower pressure in the interstitial space as compared to the vascular space at the lung bases (occurring in health and disease) is due to a greater effect of the negative (subatmospheric) alveolar pressure during inspiration on the interstitium as compared to the vessels. It should be apparent that the net forces favoring exit of fluid from the pulmonary capillaries are larger in the lower compared to upper lung regions, dictating that pulmonary edema will occur first in the lower lung regions. This perivascular edema increases perivascular pressure, causing collapse of blood vessels. In addition, alveolar flooding decreases oxygen tension, leading to pulmonary arteriolar vasoconstriction in the lung bases.

---

415 Explain the chest x-ray findings observed with each level of increased pulmonary capillary pressure.

❑ The appearance of the lung fields on x-ray films correlates with the levels of pulmonary capillary pressure. When capillary pressure is normal, the lung apices receive less perfusion than the bases. Equal perfusion of apical and basal areas occurs when pulmonary capillary pressure is elevated to 15 to 20 mm Hg (normal values <10 mm Hg). With capillary pressures of 20 to 25 mm Hg, pulmonary veins in the upper lobes are more prominent than those in the lower lobes. Fluid accumulation in the lungs as interstitial edema, Kerley's B lines, alveolar edema, and pleural effusion might be seen with capillary pressures that exceed 25 mm Hg. Consequently, serial evaluation of chest x-ray films in patients with heart failure allows monitoring of the severity and progression or regression of disease and results of therapy.

416 What abnormalities on the chest x-ray film indicate interstitial edema and alveolar edema?

❑ Interstitial edema is the accumulation of fluid in the tissue surrounding both the pulmonary capillaries and the alveoli. It might produce the following radiologic abnormalities: (1) increased linear markings in central areas of the lung fields, (2) ill-defined blotchy areas with increased density and irregular distribution ("pulmonary clouding"), and (3) haziness and loss of sharp outline of pulmonary arteries and veins. Alveolar pulmonary edema is the accumulation of fluid in the alveolar spaces. Thus, alveolar edema is a more advanced form of pulmonary fluid accumulation than is interstitial edema. The radiologic findings of alveolar pulmonary edema include the following:

1. The "butterfly" or "bat" shadow or appearance on the chest x-ray film wherein the heart and mediastinal structures make the body of the butterfly or bat, and the bilateral symmetric infiltration of lung fields caused by pulmonary edema makes the wings. The shadows are more prominent in the central portions of the lungs and fade toward the periphery; the apices, bases, and lateral margins of the lungs are relatively spared (uninvolved). The butterfly or bat shadow is usually indicative of severe pulmonary edema.
2. In less severe cases, a one-winged butterfly shadow (right

side is more common), ill-defined areas of increased density, or nodular/miliary infiltrates.

3. Rarely, only one lobe or the upper lung fields have shadows indicative of alveolar edema.

It must be recognized that interstitial pulmonary edema and alveolar pulmonary edema might be caused by noncardiac causes so that their presence is not a specific indicator of heart failure.

417 How might pleural effusions caused by fluid overload appear on a chest x-ray film? Explain Kerley's lines.

❑ The radiologic appearance of a pleural effusion caused by fluid overload might include the following:

1. Free pleural fluid collection that blunts the costophrenic angle and is easily recognized in the upright position. It is located bilaterally in two-thirds of patients but if unilateral is most commonly on the right side.
2. Subpleural collection in which fluid accumulates in the subpleural space, resembling either paralysis of one hemidiaphragm (elevation of one leaf) or a free pleural fluid accumulation with blunting of the costophrenic sulci. Comparison of chest x-ray films obtained with the patient in the upright and recumbent or Trendelenburg (head-down) position allows differentiation between subpleural collections (fluid remains immobile) and free pleural collections (fluid migrates in response to gravity since it is located in the main intrapleural space).
3. Interlobar fissure thickenings that are sharp linear densities located predominantly in the lower portions of the lungs. Within this category are Kerley's A lines that extend peripherally from the hilum in the upper and middle portions of the lungs while Kerley's B lines are peripheral markings (most commonly horizontal lines) that project to the pleural space or over the diaphragm or both.

4. Pseudotumor which consists of fluid collections located in the interlobar spaces that might simulate pneumonia, tumor, or infarction of the lung.

418 What are the clinical manifestations of acute cardiogenic pulmonary edema?

❑ Patients experiencing this syndrome have extreme breathlessness and anxiety, elevated respiratory rate, and noisy breathing with gurgling sounds during inspiration and expiration. Cough and expectoration of pink, frothy sputum are characteristically present. The intense air hunger prompts patients to sit upright or stand, and accounts for the dilated nostrils and inspiratory depression of supraclavicular fossa and intercostal spaces (reflecting large negative intrapleural pressures). Cyanosis is evident, sweating is profuse, and the skin is cold and ashen due to sympathetic activation yielding poor perfusion. Auscultation of the lungs reveals rhonchi, wheezes, and crepitant rales (fine and moist). The latter appear first at the lung bases and extend upward as pulmonary edema worsens. Cardiac auscultation might disclose a third heart sound (S_3) and accentuation of the pulmonic component of the second sound (S_2). The loud respiratory sounds make cardiac auscultation difficult.

419 What are the clinical manifestations of chronic pulmonary edema?

❑ The clinical manifestations of chronic pulmonary edema (eg, tight mitral stenosis, severe diastolic dysfunction of the left ventricle, long-term elevation of left atrial pressure due to multiple causes) are qualitatively similar to those found in acute pulmonary edema but their intensity is greatly diminished. Thus, the difference in symptomatology between acute and chronic pulmonary edema is quantitative but not qualitative. Recruitment of multiple compensatory mechanisms explains the ameliorated intensity of clinical manifestations of chronic pulmonary edema.

16. Obstructive Airway Diseases

ASTHMA

420 What are the obstructive lung diseases?

❑ Obstructive pulmonary diseases include a variety of conditions characterized by an obstructive pattern on pulmonary function testing. The most important of these diseases in children and adolescents are bronchiolitis, asthma, and cystic fibrosis. The most important obstructive pulmonary diseases in adults are asthma and related conditions (eg, allergic bronchopulmonary aspergillosis), emphysema, chronic bronchitis, bronchiolitis, and bronchiectasis. The term *chronic obstructive pulmonary disease* (COPD) refers to emphysema and chronic bronchitis.

421 Name common causes of an obstructive ventilatory defect. How is this defect recognized?

❑ Common causes of an obstructive ventilatory defect include asthma, bronchiolitis, emphysema, and upper-airway diseases. It appears likely that chronic bronchitis without emphysema is not sufficient in itself to increase airway resistance. Obstruction of the upper airway may be due to edema, foreign bodies, stenosis, or tumors. Pulmonary function tests allow clinicians to establish the presence of an obstructive ventilatory defect. Additional information obtained from the clinical history and other laboratory tests allows one to establish the specific cause of the obstructive ventilatory defect.

422 Is the differential diagnosis of asthma, chronic bronchitis, and emphysema easily determined?

❑ Clearly distinguishing asthma, chronic bronchitis, and emphysema can be difficult because these diseases can have common clinical features (eg, phlegm production and reversibility of airflow obstruction with bronchodilators) and because affected patients may have more than one process. Nevertheless, recurrent or chronic dyspnea, wheezing, and phlegm production should readily suggest the presence of obstructive lung disease, even though recognition of the specific underlying disease responsible for the obstructive pattern may not be possible.

423 Define *asthma* and *status asthmaticus.* Compare the pathogenesis of these conditions.

❑ *Asthma* is a common disease affecting 3% of the population that is characterized by transient rapid increases in airway resistance. *Status asthmaticus* or *acute severe asthma* is defined as an acute episode of asthma of severe nature that fails to respond to treatment. The pathogenesis of acute asthma includes bronchospasm, mucus plugging of the airways, and inflammation of the bronchial walls. It is not known whether the pathogenesis of fulminant fatal asthma differs from that of a routine acute asthmatic attack.

424 What is cardiac asthma? Does cardiac asthma resemble bronchial asthma?

❑ The remarkable similarity of many clinical manifestations observed in patients having severe bronchial asthma (ie, acute asthma attack) and those with acute pulmonary edema accounts for the term *cardiac asthma* applied to the latter condition. Both entities might produce extreme dyspnea that forces an upright posture, diffuse wheezes that interfere with cardiac auscultation, and pulsus paradoxus (reduction in the amplitude of arterial pulse or disappearance with deep inspiration).

425 What are the main features of asthma? How can spirometry help its diagnosis?

❑ The main features of asthma are airway inflammation, nonspecific airway hyperreactivity, and airflow obstruction that is reversible with inhaled bronchodilators. If baseline spirometry findings are normal or the diagnosis is uncertain, the demonstration of bronchoconstriction after exposure to nonspecific stimuli (eg, methacholine, histamine, exercise, or cold-air inhalation) can help establish the diagnosis of asthma.

426 What are the symptoms of asthma? What other conditions can resemble this disease?

❑ Asthma can manifest as cough, wheezing, dyspnea, or chest tightness, any of which can be paroxysmal and can occur especially at night. Several entities can cause episodic wheezing and therefore mimic asthma, such as upper-airway obstruction (including a syndrome of episodic vocal cord dysfunction), congestive heart failure (which may be associated with increased airway responsiveness and is known as *cardiac asthma*), and COPD.

427 What is mild, moderate, and severe asthma?

❑ The main features of mild asthma are the presence of intermittent and brief (<1 hour) episodes of wheezing, cough, or dyspnea during rest or after exercise and infrequent (less than twice a month) nocturnal cough or wheezing. Patients with mild asthma are asymptomatic between episodes. Moderate asthma, a more serious clinical form of the disease, is characterized by symptoms that alter the patient's activity or sleep, last several days, and occur more than one or two times a week. Patients with moderate asthma occasionally require emergency care. Severe asthma, a disabling and more serious form of the disease, is characterized by continuous symptoms that limit the patient's activity, frequent exacerbations with nocturnal symptoms, and more than occasional need of hospitalization to relieve the condition.

---

428 What are the main features of patients with status asthmaticus? Are fatal asthma attacks potentially preventable? Does measurement of expiratory flow rate help to evaluate the risk of sudden death? What is "night dipping"?

❑ The hallmark of an acute severe attack of asthma (ie, status asthmaticus) is increasing consumption of bronchodilators with diminishing benefit. Most fatal attacks occur on a background of days or weeks of deteriorating respiratory function; consequently, death in these patients is potentially preventable. The unexpected nature of the fatal attack does not necessarily indicate the sudden development of airway obstruction. Sudden death in these patients reflects inadequate perception of the severity of airway obstruction by the patient as well as failure of the physician to assess and treat the patient adequately, without recognizing the minimal respiratory reserve of the patient to cope with even a slight increase in airway obstruction. Potentially avoidable factors are present in up to 80% of patients who die of asthma. Marked diurnal variability in pulmonary function also appears to predict an increased risk of sudden death. Healthy subjects display a diurnal variability in peak expiratory flow rate (PEFR) of about 8%, asthmatic patients show more than 20% variability, while asthmatic patients at risk of death show more than 50% variability. The greatest falls in PEFR often are observed during the night ("night dipping"), and the incidence of fatal attacks appears to be increased at this time.

---

429 What are the main signs and symptoms of acute severe asthma? Compare the correlation of PaO_2 and $PaCO_2$ with respect to the severity of the attack.

❑ Patients with acute severe asthma typically present with dyspnea, wheezing, diaphoresis, and difficulty in speaking, walking, lying recumbent, or sleeping. Although the patient's perception of the severity of an attack is better than that of a physician, some patients are unable to sense even marked airway obstruction. Wheezing is a characteristic feature of asthma, but it is not a good guide to the severity of airway obstruction; indeed, a fulminant attack may be associated with an almost silent chest. Tachycardia, tachypnea, pulsus paradoxus, and use of the accessory muscles of respiration (especially the sternomastoids) are considered characteristic findings in a patient with an acute asthmatic attack. However, in a recent study of patients with severe asthma (FEV_1 <1.0 L), 36% had a pulse rate less than 100 beats/min, 17% had a respiratory rate equal to or less than 20 breaths/min, and 33% had no pulsus paradoxus. Clinical examination should not be completely discredited, and abnormalities are useful when present; however, failure to detect "classic signs" should not lead to underestimation of the severity of an attack. It is imperative that an objective measure of airflow obstruction such as FEV_1 or PEFR be obtained. These tests are safe, easy to perform, and tolerated by almost all patients. In an emergency room setting, they have been shown to accurately predict the need for hospital admission: Patients with an FEV_1 or PEFR less than 40% of predicted after 1 hour of intensive therapy require admission. In contrast, PaO_2 correlates poorly with the severity of airway obstruction. Measurement of $PaCO_2$ is more useful in assessing the severity of an attack.

430 What are the major abnormalities in pulmonary function observed with severe asthma? Is hypoxemia promptly reversed with supplemental oxygen? Does the presence of a normal or high $PaCO_2$ mandate initiation of mechanical ventilation?

❑ Airway obstruction, hyperinflation, abnormal gas exchange, and altered cardiovascular function are the four major abnormalities observed with severe asthma. Airway obstruction is caused by severe contraction of the bronchial wall, mucosal inflammation, and plugging of the lumen with mucus and debris. The hyperinflation and gas trapping lead to a marked increase in the work of breathing because tidal volume occurs on a flatter portion of the pressure-volume curve, where a given change in lung volume requires greater swings in pleural pressure. In addition, hyperinflation causes an increase in the elastic work of breathing. Furthermore, hyperinflation causes shortening of the diaphragm and other inspiratory muscles, decreasing muscle tension and leading to a marked impairment of the ventilatory muscle pump. The deranged gas exchange is caused by abnormal ventilation-perfusion ratios, whereas shunting and increased dead space are very uncommon. Consequently, hypoxemia in patients with asthma is easily reversed with supplemental oxygen therapy. Patients typically have hypoxemia and hypocapnia but PaO_2 rarely falls below 50 mm Hg. As airway obstruction worsens and FEV_1 decreases to about 15% of the predicted value, $PaCO_2$ increases. In a retrospective study, 27% of patients with acute asthma had a $PaCO_2$ higher than 38 mm Hg and only 8% of this hypercapnic group required mechanical ventilation. The major alteration in cardiovascular function in patients with acute asthma is the development of pulsus paradoxus, which is defined as an inspiratory decline in systolic arterial pressure of at least 10 mm Hg.

431 What abnormalities in $PaCO_2$ are observed in acute severe asthma?

❑ During an asthmatic attack $PaCO_2$ is typically decreased but returns to normal or becomes elevated as the severity of the attack increases. However, virtually all patients with significant hypercapnia ($PaCO_2$ >45 mm Hg) have an FEV_1 or PEFR less than 25% of predicted. Multifactorial predictive indices based on clinical features and PEFR at the time of presentation are inaccurate in predicting the course of emergency room therapy, presumably because some patients with very severe airway obstruction have a dramatic response to bronchodilator therapy. Instead, measurement of lung function following initial intensive therapy is more accurate in predicting the patient's course.

432 What is the mechanism of pulsus paradoxus in acute asthma? Is the function of the right and left cardiac ventricles abnormal in acute asthma?

❑ Patients with acute asthma have markedly negative swings in pleural pressure (about -30 cm H_2O at peak inspiration during tidal breathing as opposed to -7 cm H_2O in healthy subjects), which lead to increased venous return. However, hyperinflation associated with alveolar distention increases the resistance to flow in the pulmonary vasculature, and the net effect is a decrease in right ventricular stroke volume. The decrease in right ventricular output, combined with increased venous return, leads to right ventricular overdistention, which in turn causes a leftward shift in the interventricular septum. The decreased right ventricular output produces a decrease in left ventricular preload. In addition, left ventricular compliance is decreased because of the septal shift and the increased left ventricular afterload caused by the abnormal intrathoracic pressure. Consequently, the left ventricular dysfunction leads to a decrease in left ventricular stroke volume and a fall in systemic arterial pressure. While pulsus paradoxus is generally more common with increasing airway obstruction, it is absent in some patients with severe obstruction whereas it is present in other patients with only mild obstruction.

433 How can severe bronchial asthma (ie, acute asthma attack) be differentiated from cardiac asthma on first encounter by the clinician?

❑ Patients with severe bronchial asthma frequently have a history of similar episodes, allergic rhinitis or sinusitis, or other evidence of atopic reactions. Sweating and cyanosis are observed less often in bronchial asthma than in cardiac asthma. The chest in patients with severe bronchial asthma is generally overexpanded and hyperresonant. Furthermore, use of accessory respiratory muscles is more prominent, wheezes are high pitched and musical, and crackles (crepitations) are less evident in bronchial than in cardiac asthma. In the latter condition, the chest is often dull to percussion, and on auscultation, crackles and rhonchi are characteristically present. The chest x-ray findings of pulmonary edema (described in the answer to another question) are usually absent in severe bronchial asthma in which pulmonary hyperinflation is the most prominent abnormality.

CHRONIC OBSTRUCTIVE PULMONARY DISEASE

434 Compare the most salient clinical features of chronic bronchitis and emphysema, collectively known as *COPD.*

❑ Increased resistance to airflow during expiration is a characteristic feature of COPD independent of the underlying disease. Chronic bronchitis and emphysema are distinct disorders, with the former damaging the conducting airways and the latter involving primarily the alveolar and capillary structures (pulmonary parenchyma). The two diseases often coexist in the same individual and may be associated with reversible airway obstruction, commonly referred to as a component of "reactive airway disease" that can be demonstrated with pulmonary function testing (ie, response to bronchodilators). The diagnosis of chronic bronchitis is based on the presence of a productive cough persisting for most days of at least 3 months in a year and for at least 2 or more consecutive years. The diagnosis of chronic bronchitis requires that other infectious disorders (eg, tuberculosis) be excluded. Clinical manifestations of emphysema include progressive dyspnea and variable cough. The hallmark of emphysema is hyperinflation, airflow limitation, and reduced gas diffusing capacity (evaluated with carbon monoxide). The loss of pulmonary elastic recoil in emphysema limits airflow, facilitates dynamic airway collapse, and enlarges lung volume in the presence of a relatively unaltered chest wall recoil. Destruction of the alveolar-capillary interface results in a low diffusing capacity that is characteristic of emphysema.

Early in the course of emphysema, ventilation-perfusion relationships remain unaltered, explaining the preservation of gas exchange.

---

435 Is COPD a frequently encountered illness and a common cause of death?

❑ Yes. COPD has assumed epidemic proportions in industrialized countries and is a common cause of death (eg, it ranks fifth in the United States). Fortunately, a variety of therapeutic options are now available to manage acute respiratory failure in COPD patients, and these interventions have led to a decrease in COPD-related mortality.

---

436 What is the natural history of COPD?

❑ COPD is a progressive and disabling condition with a natural history characterized by a reduction of pulmonary function that greatly exceeds that found in normal subjects in response to aging. Discontinuation of exposure to the specific pathogenetic factors (eg, cigarette smoking, occupational environment) may slow the overall progression of COPD. Yet, episodic worsening of the disease is commonly encountered and can lead to respiratory failure (frequently associated with circulatory failure) and premature death. Measures aimed at preventing COPD may have the largest impact in the control of this disease.

---

437 What is the prognosis of advanced COPD? Does the presence of cor pulmonale increase the risk of death?

❑ The prognosis of advanced COPD is poor in spite of optimal medical management. The mortality rate of patients with an FEV_1 less than 0.75 L is 30% and 95% at 1 year and 10 years, respectively. The presence of cor pulmonale worsens the prognosis of patients with COPD.

438 What elements supporting the diagnosis of COPD can be found on physical examination of patients with this condition?

❑ Patients with advanced stages of COPD generally exhibit one or more of the following physical findings: (1) barrel-shaped chest having increased anteroposterior diameter on inspection, decreased vocal fremitus on palpation, and hyperresonance to percussion; (2) use of accessory muscles of ventilation; (3) prolonged expiratory phase; (4) diffusely diminished breath sounds and scattered wheezes during forced expiration, on auscultation; (5) tracheal tug (ie, downward movement of cricoid with each inspiration); (6) decreased cricoid-sternal distance (ie, <2 finger widths); (7) Hoover's sign (ie, paradoxical inward motion of lateral aspect of the rib cage on inspiration); and (8) inspiratory fall in arterial pressure (up to 20 mm Hg), known as *pulsus paradoxus,* and expiratory engorgement of the neck veins secondary to the associated changes in intrathoracic pressure.

439 What elements that support the diagnosis of COPD can be found on routine radiologic examination of patients with this condition?

❑ The diffuse lung hyperinflation associated with COPD may be recognized on routine chest x-ray examination (posteroanterior and lateral views) by the presence of low and flat diaphragms, elongated and narrow cardiac silhouette, increased retrosternal airspace (on lateral view), and bullae. The latter lesions consist of rounded radiolucent areas with a diameter larger than 1 cm, corresponding to lung areas affected with emphysema. The most specific sign for emphysema is an attenuation (diminution) of pulmonary vasculature on radiologic examination, but unfortunately, it has limited sensitivity.

440 What are the characteristic features of emphysema detected with radiologic evaluation of the chest? Compare the radiologic abnormalities of emphysema and those of chronic bronchitis.

❑ Typical features of emphysema detected by chest x-ray studies are increased radiolucency of the lung parenchyma and attenuation of pulmonary vascular shadows; these abnormalities are usually accompanied by hyperinflation manifested by diaphragmatic flattening and increased retrosternal airspace, best observed on the lateral projection. High-resolution chest computed tomography (CT) is more sensitive than chest x-ray studies for demonstrating emphysematous changes but is rarely needed for this purpose. Patients with chronic bronchitis have chest radiographs that either appear normal or show thickening of bronchial walls (so-called ring shadows) and tram lines, which may also be seen in bronchiectasis. The typical radiologic features of emphysema are not observed in pure chronic bronchitis.

441 How do pulmonary function tests diagnose the obstructive ventilatory defect observed in patients with COPD?

❑ Patients exhibiting an obstructive ventilatory defect caused by COPD characteristically have low values for the FEV_1 and the FEV_1/FVC ratio. The low expiratory flow rates are associated with hyperinflation of the lungs (air trapping) as demonstrated by abnormally high values of residual volume (RV), functional residual capacity (FRC), and total lung capacity (TLC). This condition is often labeled as *irreversible lung disease,* but in fact the diminished expiratory flow rates can improve by about 20% in response to bronchodilator drugs.

442 What changes in ABGs are observed during sleep in patients with COPD? What are the clinical consequences of these abnormalities?

❑ The decreased respiratory drive and hypotonia of respiratory muscles that accompany sleep may be associated with carbon dioxide retention in COPD patients. This process is independent of the presence or absence of obstructive sleep apnea. A fall in PaO_2 and saturation of arterial oxygen (SaO_2) occurs during sleep in COPD, but the long-term effect of these alterations, if any, is unknown. The lowest PaO_2 and SaO_2 values during sleep are observed in COPD patients with the highest daytime hypoxemia.

443 Is bacterial infection responsible for most acute exacerbations of COPD? What are the commonly observed precipitating factors of this condition?

❑ Although it has been assumed that bacterial infection is solely responsible for acute exacerbations of COPD, many experts dispute this view. In a recent report on patients with COPD and acute respiratory failure who required mechanical ventilation, only 50% had evidence of bacterial infection (diagnosed by bronchoscopy using the protected specimen brush technique). Therefore, it is important to exclude other factors that might precipitate acute respiratory failure, such as sedative or narcotic analgesics, pneumothorax, rib fracture, pulmonary embolism, or congestive heart failure, before attributing an acute exacerbation of COPD to bacterial infection.

444 What factors are responsible for the exacerbations frequently observed in COPD? Enumerate common causes of acute respiratory failure in COPD.

❑ The episodic worsening of pulmonary function, commonly referred to as *exacerbations,* that is observed in patients with COPD is caused by (1) respiratory tract infections (eg, acute bronchitis and bronchiolitis, pneumonia), (2) environmental exposure (eg, allergens, irritants, cold weather), (3) noncompliance to medical treatment (eg, discontinuation of bronchodilators), and (4) other complications (eg, pneumothorax, enlargement of lung bullae, trauma, abdominal distention).

445 What precipitating causes of acute respiratory failure other than infections account for the exacerbations of COPD?

❑ Precipitating causes of acute respiratory failure such as oversedation, pulmonary embolism, and congestive heart failure should be sought for in the presence of exacerbations of COPD, and appropriate therapy rapidly instituted.

446 What are the manifestations of the precipitating illness responsible for the development of acute respiratory failure in COPD?

❑ Symptoms of the precipitating illness responsible for the development of acute respiratory failure in COPD may be similar to those seen with any respiratory tract infection. The patient may be febrile, complain of back pain, and may have increased production of purulent sputum, leukocytosis, evidence of consolidation on physical examination, or an infiltrate as demonstrated on the chest x-ray film.

447 What are the manifestations of an acute exacerbation of COPD? What is the role of muscle fatigue in the development of acute respiratory failure during a COPD exacerbation?

❑ An acute exacerbation of COPD leads to multiple clinical manifestations including intensification of dyspnea, increased sputum production, difficulty in expectorating the bronchial secretions, tachypnea, wheezing, accessory muscle recruitment, intercostal and supraclavicular space recession, tracheal tug, paradoxical movement of the rib cage and abdomen, and paradoxical pulse. Worsening of the obstructive lung disease places the patient at particular risk for respiratory muscle fatigue. Many investigators believe that such fatigue plays an important role in the development of acute respiratory failure. Others believe that this fatigue is of secondary importance and that abnormalities in the mechanics of breathing are the primary determinants of ventilatory failure. The lack of a satisfactory technique for diagnosing respiratory muscle fatigue in this setting is a major problem in resolving this issue.

448 What is a "pink puffer" and a "blue bloater"?

❑ The terms *pink puffer* and *blue bloater* refer to two distinct clinical presentations of patients with advanced COPD. The absence of cyanosis in association with constant and disabling dyspnea is responsible for selecting the label *pink puffers* to describe a group of COPD patients. The presence of central and peripheral cyanosis in association with venous congestion and peripheral edema (caused by right-sided heart failure) accounts for the label *blue bloaters* to describe the other group of COPD patients. These two clinical presentations have additional characteristics that are described in the answers to pertinent questions. It must be recognized, however, that most patients with COPD have some features that are present in pink puffers (COPD, type A) and in blue bloaters (COPD, type B); consequently, the clinical pattern in patients displaying a mixed form has been called *type C*. It must be recognized that there is not a clear-cut relationship between these clinical presentations (ie, pink puffer, blue bloater) and the underlying disease. Consequently, the significance of these labels is limited.

449 Compare the main symptoms, general appearance, and cardiovascular features of patients with COPD types A and B.

❑ Type A COPD patients' (pink puffers) main complaint concerns the presence of dyspnea but cough is absent or of minor importance. These patients do not exhibit cyanosis. They are generally thin and may exhibit weight loss. Signs of lung hyperinflation are found on physical examination but cardiovascular features consistent with cor pulmonale are absent. Type B COPD patients (blue bloaters) have cough and sputum production with frequent respiratory tract infections as main manifestations. Cyanosis, central and peripheral, is generally evident. Weight loss is uncommon in blue bloaters and they tend to have a stocky body build. Cor pulmonale is typically found in patients with advanced stages of type B COPD.

---

450 Compare the chest x-ray findings, hematocrit, and ABG values of patients with COPD types A and B.

❑ Lung hyperinflation and decreased vascular markings are typical chest x-ray findings detected in pink puffers (type A); on the other hand, blue bloaters (type B) do not generally exhibit these features but have instead normal or increased markings at the lung bases (so-called dirty chest x-ray appearance). The hematocrit is normal in pink puffers and increased in blue bloaters, a finding that correlates with the PaO_2 (see below). ABG analysis demonstrates only mild abnormalities in pink buffers (small reduction in PaO_2 and normal or decreased $PaCO_2$), but more severe alterations in blue bloaters (marked reduction in PaO_2 and increased $PaCO_2$). The differences with respect to the chest x-ray films, hematocrit, and ABGs between types A and B are of very limited value because they are evident in a small fraction of COPD patients.

17. Infections and Other Conditions

BRONCHIOLITIS, BRONCHIECTASIS, ALVEOLAR PROTEINOSIS

451 What is bronchiolitis? Explain the clinical forms and main causes of this disease.

❑ *Bronchiolitis* is defined as an inflammatory process of the small airways (eg, bronchioles) that may be accompanied by fibrosis. There are two main forms of the disease: constrictive bronchiolitis (characterized by luminal narrowing caused by bronchiolar inflammation with peribronchial and submucosal scarring producing airflow obstruction) and bronchiolitis obliterans with organizing pneumonia (BOOP) (characterized by an inflammatory process of the small airways that are occluded by intraluminal fibrous plugs, and often associated with parenchymal infiltrates as seen on chest radiographs, and a restrictive pattern on pulmonary function testing). The causes of bronchiolitis include (1) cigarette smoking, which commonly leads to a form of bronchiolitis that resembles interstitial lung disease and improves after cessation of exposure; (2) viral infections (eg, measles); (3) toxic inhalation (eg, nitrogen dioxide); (4) connective-tissue disease (eg, rheumatoid arthritis); (5) inherited disorders (eg, cystic fibrosis); (6) drugs (eg, penicillamine); and (7) chronic rejection (eg, lung and heart-lung transplants).

452 How is *bronchiectasis* defined and what are the symptoms of this condition?

❑ Bronchiectasis consists of an abnormal and permanent dilation of airways caused by destructive and inflammatory changes in their walls. The dilated airways facilitate the accumulation of secretions and bacterial colonization (eg, *Streptococcus pneumoniae, Haemophilus influenzae, Pseudomonas aeruginosa, Staphylococcus aureus,* and nontuberculous atypical mycobacteria).

Consequently, the symptoms of the disease consist of chronic cough, purulent sputum production, blood streaking of sputum, and hemoptysis.

453 What are the causes and predisposing conditions for the development of bronchiectasis?

- ❑ Airway infection, either as a single severe episode or as multiple mild bouts, is usually responsible for the development of bronchiectasis. Predisposing factors for the development of recurrent bronchial infections that can initiate bronchiectasis include impaired pulmonary defense mechanisms (either secondary to local airway obstruction or because of immunoglobulin deficiency), primary ciliary disorders, and cystic fibrosis.

454 What is pulmonary alveolar proteinosis? How is the diagnosis established? What is the treatment for this condition?

- ❑ Pulmonary alveolar proteinosis, a disease of unknown etiology, has many features that resemble an interstitial lung disease including symptoms (progressive dyspnea, nonproductive cough) and data from pulmonary function tests (ie, restrictive ventilatory pattern). Yet, pulmonary alveolar proteinosis is not an interstitial lung disease because it represents an intra-alveolar process. The chest x-ray film of pulmonary alveolar proteinosis reveals diffuse alveolar consolidation and nodular shadows typically radiating from the hilar regions that resemble pulmonary edema. The alveoli of patients with this disease are filled with granular material that stains positive with periodic acid–Schiff (PAS) reagent but there is no evidence of alveolar inflammation. Diagnosis is established by demonstration of PAS-positive granular material obtained by bronchoscopic biopsy or bronchoalveolar lavage. Whole lung lavage(s) may provide relief of dyspnea, improvement of hypoxemia, and long-term benefit.

455 What conditions can closely resemble pulmonary alveolar proteinosis?

❑ Patients having chronic pulmonary infection, malignancy, or inhaled dust exposure to silica and aluminum may develop a proteinaceous alveolar response that closely resembles that found in patients with pulmonary alveolar proteinosis. The syndrome is known as *secondary pulmonary alveolar proteinosis,* and its differential diagnosis from the primary form may require a lung biopsy.

PNEUMONIA

456 What are the microorganisms responsible for the development of community-acquired pneumonia?

❑ A specific pathogen is not identified in 33% to 50% of patients with community-acquired pneumonia. The microorganisms responsible for all other cases are *S. pneumoniae* (about 50% of patients), mycoplasma organisms, *Legionella* species, and viral agents. *H. influenzae, Moraxella catarrhalis,* and *S. aureus* are less common causes but may be important in patients with mildly to moderately impaired host defenses, such as diabetics, smokers, alcoholics, and patients with COPD. Anaerobic infections may be responsible for pneumonia when loss of consciousness and aspiration have occurred, and *Klebsiella* species may play a more significant role in pneumonia observed in alcoholics.

457 What microorganisms are responsible for the development of nosocomial pneumonia? How does it develop and how common is this disease?

❑ Mixed infections with two or more microorganisms are common in nosocomial pneumonia. Gram-negative bacilli, anaerobes, and *S. aureus* (about 60%, 35%, and 15% of cases, respectively), and in some areas *Legionella pneumophila,* are the most important causes of this disease. The institutional origin of the bacteria becomes evident by examining the change in oropharyngeal flora within 72 hours after the patient's admission to a hospital or nursing home. The new flora of the oropharyngeal cavity leads to the development of nosocomial pneumonia, which occurs in 1.0% to 5.0% of hospitalized patients and in up to 60% of critically ill patients.

458 What are the most important risk factors for nosocomial pneumonia?

❑ The major risk factors for nosocomial pneumonia might be grouped as dependent on the (1) instrumentation (eg, intubation, too frequent changes of ventilator tubing, intracranial pressure monitors), (2) current ailments (eg, depressed sensorium, aspiration of gastric content, chest surgery), (3) previous illness (eg, chronic lung disease), (4) host (ie, elderly subjects), and (5) season (ie, fall, winter).

459 Enumerate the available methods that may allow a precise etiologic diagnosis of bronchopulmonary infections.

❑ The methods that assist in the diagnosis of bronchopulmonary infections (eg, pneumonia) include (1) clinical diagnosis, (2) examination of the tracheobronchial secretions, (3) blood cultures, (4) transtracheal aspiration, (5) transthoracic aspiration, (6) bronchoscopic specimen evaluations (eg, bronchial washes, plugged telescoping catheter brush, quantitative culture, antibody coating of bacteria, transbronchial needle aspiration, bronchoalveolar lavage, and transbronchial biopsy), (7) open lung biopsy, and (8) immunologic methods.

460 What is the role of examination of sputum and bronchial secretions in the treatment of both community-acquired and nosocomial pneumonia? How useful are bronchoscopy-obtained specimens and thoracentesis in the management of pneumonias?

❑ Expectorated sputum is of value if it represents a sample of lower respiratory tract secretions (ie, <10 squamous epithelial cells and >25 polymorphonuclear cells/low-power field). Cultures of such specimens have variable concordance with specimens obtained by invasive techniques (eg, bronchoscopy, bronchoalveolar lavage). In patients suspected of nosocomial pneumonia, findings by examination of sputum are likely to be very misleading due to contamination with organisms that colonize the respiratory tract. Bronchoscopy-obtained specimens may be useful in patients who are seriously ill or mechanically ventilated, especially if antibiotics have not been administered. Bronchoalveolar lavage is of significant value in the search for opportunistic pathogens from immunosuppressed patients. Pleural effusions should be sampled by thoracentesis to aid diagnosis and establish the need of drainage.

---

461 A 71-year-old woman with end-stage renal disease on chronic hemodialysis consults after 3 days of chills, fever, and nonproductive cough. Her history is negative for smoking or alcohol abuse. Vital signs include rectal temperature of 39.5°C, respiration rate of 32 breaths/min, and blood pressure of 172/82 mm Hg. Physical examination reveals dullness and decreased breath sounds over the right lower posterior and lateral aspects of the hemithorax. A chest x-ray study confirms the presence of a right lower lobe pneumonia and possible right pleural effusion. Laboratory data include a leukocyte count of 12,800/µL with 86% polymorphonuclear cells and 15% band forms.

What are the most likely microorganisms responsible for the patient's pneumonia?

❑ The patient presents with a community-acquired pneumonia that had developed in a host with a chronic extrapulmonary illness (ie, end-stage renal disease on chronic dialysis). Organisms commonly found in this condition include *S. pneumoniae, Legionella* species, *S. aureus,* and enteric gram-negative bacilli. In the absence of neutropenia or bronchiectasis, patients with chronic extrapulmonary disease do not generally grow *Pseudomonas aeruginosa* in the airway.

462 Explain the pneumonia secondary to aspiration of oropharyngeal bacteria (as opposed to pneumonia secondary to aspiration of gastric contents).

❑ Pneumonia secondary to aspiration of oropharyngeal bacteria is considered to be present to account for the development of pneumonia in a patient with a condition that predisposes to aspiration or in a patient with dental disease who did not aspirate the gastric contents. More than 200 microbial species are found in the healthy human mouth, and the concentration and bacterial type vary throughout the oral cavity. Aspiration of oropharyngeal contents is more likely to cause pneumonia in patients with gingivitis and periodontal disease. The organisms predominantly responsible for this form of aspiration pneumonia are *Peptostreptococcus* species (anaerobic streptococci), *Bacteroides melaninogenicus,* and *Fusobacterium nucleatum.* Infection is rarely due to a single organism and most infections are polymicrobial in nature.

463 What are the main characteristics of pneumonia secondary to aspiration of oropharyngeal bacteria?

❑ Many patients have an impaired level of consciousness, dysphagia, periodontal disease, or gingivitis. Microbial identification, taking care to avoid upper-airway contamination and employing the proper transport and processing precautions, usually reveals anaerobes. About 90% of these pneumonias are localized to regions of the lung that are favored by gravitational flow. This contrasts with aspiration of gastric contents, which does not have a distinctive radiologic picture. If the patient was supine at the time of aspiration, the posterior segments of the upper lobes and the superior segments of the lower lobes are most frequently affected. In the erect posture, the basilar segments of the lower lobes are most frequently involved. The right lung is involved twice as frequently as the left because the right main-stem bronchus has a more direct takeoff. More than one segment is commonly involved. Finally, the putrid discharge typical of anaerobic pneumonia may be observed if 1 to 2 weeks have elapsed after the acute event, at which time tissue necrosis and cavity formation may occur. Later in the course of the disease, the clinical picture is characterized by complications such as lung abscess formation, necrotizing pneumonia, or empyema.

18. Cardiorespiratory Failure

EMBOLISM AND PULMONARY HYPERTENSION

464 What are the major predisposing factors and conditions for the development of deep vein thrombosis (DVT) and pulmonary embolism?

❑ Predisposing factors and conditions for the development of pulmonary embolism arising from DVT include (1) venous stasis (eg, low cardiac output, recent surgery, prolonged bed rest, immobility, extended travel), (2) local damage to vascular intima (eg, trauma, varicosities, thrombophlebitis), and (3) hypercoagulable state (eg, birth control pills, pregnancy, cancer, sickle cell disease, erythrocytosis, abnormalities in clotting factors).

465 Explain further the risk factors for the development of pulmonary thromboembolism.

❑ An augmented risk for the development of pulmonary emboli is observed with (1) advanced age, (2) obesity, (3) prolonged immobilization, (4) pregnancy and postpartum period, (5) pelvic and lower-extremity injury and surgery, (6) burns, (7) history of DVT, (8) coagulation disorders (eg, deficiency of antithrombin C), (9) malignancies, (10) right-sided heart failure, (11) estrogen-containing medication, and (12) prolonged general anesthesia.

466 How common is the development of pulmonary embolism in patients with DVT? How effective is the treatment of these two conditions?

❑ Pulmonary embolism develops in 10% of patients with DVT and 10% of these patients have a fatal outcome. Pulmonary embolism is more common when DVT occurs in the popliteal or more proximal veins in comparison to the more distal veins of the lower extremities. Because only 25% of pulmonary embolisms are diagnosed, this disease must be carefully considered in patients having predisposing conditions for DVT (see pertinent question). Patients with pulmonary embolism and DVT generally respond well to treatment (see pertinent question).

467 What signs and symptoms are associated with pulmonary infarction?

❑ Manifestations of pulmonary infarction can include low-grade fever, hemoptysis, and pleuritic chest pain. Chest x-ray films can reveal a wedged-shaped consolidation accompanied with a small pleural effusion (ie, exudate that not unusually is hemorrhagic). Pulmonary infarction develops in approximately 10% of patients with pulmonary thromboembolism.

468 What are the chest x-ray findings of patients with pulmonary emboli?

❑ A normal-appearing chest x-ray film is commonly obtained in patients with acute pulmonary emboli. In a small fraction of patients, characteristic changes, such as increased radiolucency in some areas (due to absent blood perfusion), abrupt ending of a vessel, and differences in diameter of vessels within the same ipsilateral or contralateral region, can be detected. These abnormalities, if present, need to be closely searched for by the astute clinician; otherwise, they remain undetected.

469 How is the diagnosis of pulmonary embolism established?

❑ Demonstration of segmental perfusion defects in the lung leading to mismatched ventilation-perfusion ($\dot{V}_A/\dot{Q}$) scans with radioisotope techniques are highly suggestive of pulmonary embolism in a patient with DVT. Other findings that lead to a suspicion of pulmonary embolism include an abnormally high alveolar-arterial gradient for oxygen ($P_A\text{-}aO_2$), hypocapnia, and hypoxemia (not constant). If the previously mentioned evaluation is nondiagnostic of embolism, pulmonary angiography may be required. The latter technique, performed with selected dye injection guided by lung scan defects, is generally safe even when pulmonary hypertension is present.

470 What procedures can be used to establish the diagnosis of pulmonary emboli?

❑ The ventilation-perfusion ($\dot{V}/\dot{Q}$) lung scan can be useful for the diagnosis of acute pulmonary emboli. This noninvasive test is highly sensitive but not specific; furthermore, interpretation of results is difficult in patients having underlying pulmonary disease. The most reliable test for the diagnosis of pulmonary emboli consists of pulmonary angiography, an invasive procedure that is not risk free. Consequently, the procedure selected for the diagnosis of pulmonary emboli depends on the clinician's assessment of the risk-benefit ratio of these tests in a given patient.

471 What clinical forms of pulmonary embolism other than those arising from blood thrombi can be observed?

❑ Fat emboli and amniotic fluid emboli are the most commonly observed clinical forms of nonthrombotic pulmonary embolism. Fat emboli are observed within the first 48 hours after major trauma and bone fractures have occurred. Signs and symptoms include dyspnea, hypoxemia, low platelet count, and petechiae. Amniotic fluid embolism is a serious complication of pregnancy caused by the entrance of amniotic fluid into the systemic circulation. The latter condition can lead to DIC and circulatory collapse. All forms of pulmonary emboli, thrombotic and nonthrombotic, are serious and life-threatening conditions.

472 What are the diagnostic tests for DVT?

❑ Useful noninvasive tests for DVT are Doppler techniques (ultrasound based) and impedance plethysmography. However, the gold standard for the diagnosis of DVT is an invasive radiographic test that requires administration of contrast medium (ie, contrast venography). The latter method has the additional disadvantage of technical difficulties for its application in some patients.

473 What are the most common causes of venous air embolism?

❑ Venous air embolism is most commonly reported in surgical patients, especially during craniotomy performed in the sitting (Fowler's) position. Prospective studies have reported an incidence of venous air embolism of 20% to 40% during craniotomy. Accidental intravenous injections of 100 to 300 mL of air have been reported to be fatal in humans. This is a particular risk if the site of infusion is above the heart (internal jugular or subclavian cannulation) and the patient generates large negative intrathoracic pressure swings. It is estimated that during 1 second, 100 mL of air can flow through a 14-gauge needle with a 5 cm H_2O pressure drop across it. Other reported causes of venous air embolism include penetrating lung injury, positive-pressure mechanical ventilation, pneumothorax, insufflation of the genitourinary tract, and obstructed obstetric delivery.

474 What are the signs and symptoms of venous air embolism?

❑ The clinical presentation of venous air embolism is nonspecific. Cardiac arrest can occur if the volume of infused air is sufficient to obstruct the right ventricular outflow tract. A mill wheel murmur, although specific for air embolism, is infrequently heard. Large emboli cause elevation of right-sided heart pressures and systemic hypotension. Obstruction of the pulmonary vascular bed leads to severe hypoxemia. The increase in right-sided heart pressures associated with large air emboli facilitates the opening of the foramen ovale and leads to systemic embolization (paradoxical emboli). Pulmonary edema due to increased microvascular permeability (ARDS) may develop. This is usually self-limiting, provided that air is not infused in very large amounts or over a long period.

475 What measures help prevent venous air embolism?

❑ Measures that prevent the development of air embolism during central venous cannulation include placing the patient in the

Trendelenburg position, having the patient breath-hold or perform Valsalva's maneuver when the catheter is being inserted into the needle or introducer, and occluding the hub as much as possible with the operator's finger. During high-risk surgical procedures, placing a Doppler probe over the right side of the heart can alert the physician to air bubbling into the circulation.

476 What are the causes of pulmonary hypertension?

❑ Pulmonary hypertension (ie, mean pulmonary artery pressure >20 mm Hg) can be caused by precapillary and postcapillary abnormalities. Precapillary causes include (1) obstruction of the pulmonary arteries (eg, embolism, vasculitis, intravenous drug use, COPD, interstitial lung disease, primary pulmonary hypertension), (2) hypoxemia (eg, sleep apnea syndrome, altitude, chronic bronchitis), (3) overperfusion of the pulmonary circulation (eg, left-to-right shunt), and (4) mechanical compression (eg, kyphoscoliosis, positive-pressure ventilation). Postcapillary causes include (1) cardiac conditions (eg, left ventricular failure, mitral valve disease, left atrial myoma) and (2) pulmonary venous abnormalities (eg, mediastinal neoplasm or fibrosis, veno-occlusive disease, anomalous venous return).

477 How is the diagnosis of pulmonary hypertension suspected and established?

❑ The presence of pulmonary hypertension should be suspected in patients developing syncope, dyspnea, or exercise intolerance of uncertain cause. The physician must confirm the diagnosis, establish the cause, and determine the severity of pulmonary hypertension. Right-sided heart catheterization is the definitive method for measuring pulmonary vascular pressures (ie, mean pulmonary artery pressure >20 mm Hg in pulmonary hypertension). In addition, this procedure facilitates pulmonary angiography, allows detection of left-to-right shunts (presence of a step-up in oxygen saturation), and helps to determine the efficacy of therapy. Complementary diagnostic methods for pulmonary hypertension include echocardiography, pulmonary function testing, ABG measurement, and other procedures.

COR PULMONALE

478 What is cor pulmonale?

❑ *Cor pulmonale* is a syndrome characterized by right ventricular overload that can include hypertrophy, dilatation, and sometimes failure of this cardiac chamber, caused by pulmonary hypertension.

479 What are the causes of cor pulmonale?

❑ Any condition leading to pulmonary hypertension can cause cor pulmonale. The most relevant causes of cor pulmonale are (1) diseases of the airways and lungs (eg, COPD, restrictive lung diseases, pneumoconiosis, sarcoidosis), (2) diseases of the pulmonary circulation (eg, recurrent lung embolism, primary pulmonary hypertension), and (3) diseases of the left side of the circulation that lead to pulmonary hypertension (eg, mitral valve disease, left ventricular failure).

480 What are the major causes of right-sided heart failure?

❑ The major causes of right-sided heart failure are (1) chronic left-sided congestive heart failure such as that due to ischemic or valvular heart disease; (2) mitral stenosis with pulmonary hypertension; (3) cor pulmonale due to COPD; (4) pulmonary hypertension due to either an unknown cause (primary form), congenital heart abnormalities, or collagen vascular diseases; (5) valvular diseases of the right ventricle including pulmonic stenosis, tricuspid stenosis, and regurgitation; and (6) myocardial diseases of the right ventricle such as infarction and dysplasia involving this chamber.

481 Describe the signs and symptoms of right-sided heart failure.

❑ The signs and symptoms of right-sided heart failure are those of venous congestion in the systemic circulation. Distention of jugular veins, hepatojugular reflux, hepatomegaly, ascites, and lower-extremity edema are commonly observed. Patients might complain of right upper quadrant pain caused by stretching of the hepatic capsule from liver congestion. In addition, anorexia, nausea, and abdominal bloating from venous congestion of abdominal viscera including the liver, mesentery, and spleen might be present. In the absence of left-sided heart failure, pulmonary symptoms are uncommon but fatigue is a frequent complaint. Examination of the heart in patients with right-sided cardiac failure might reveal additional signs (described in the answers to subsequent questions), especially if enlargement of the right chambers is present.

482 How is the clinical evaluation of systemic venous hypertension performed?

❑ When patients are examined in a semirecumbent position (ie, at a 45-degree angle), the jugular vein might be distended as much as 4 cm above the sternal angle in the normal state. Higher values are observed with systemic venous hypertension (eg, right-sided heart failure, cor pulmonale). Exertion decreases jugular venous pressure in normal individuals but it increases this parameter in patients with heart failure. This physical finding is known as *Kussmaul's sign.* Prominence of the veins in the back of the hands is a valuable sign of systemic venous congestion in infants whose short necks make detection of jugular vein distention difficult.

483 What are the mechanisms of salt and water retention commonly observed in chronic hypercapnia, especially in the presence of cor pulmonale?

❑ The mechanisms of salt and water retention in these patients include the renal effects of heart failure, the prevailing stimulation of the renin-angiotensin-aldosterone axis and of the sympathetic nervous system, elevated levels of cortisol and antidiuretic hormone (ADH), and increased renal vascular resistance.

484 What chest x-ray abnormalities in the systemic veins might be recognized in patients with right-sided heart failure?

❑ Dilation of the superior vena cava and azygos veins might be present in patients with right-sided congestive heart failure. These abnormalities are caused by backward failure of the right cardiac chambers, increased blood volume, and constriction of arteries and veins of the systemic circulation.

485 What physical findings might be detected on cardiac examination of patients with cor pulmonale or right-sided heart failure? What are the physical findings indicative of right ventricular hypertrophy?

❑ Physical findings that might be detected in patients with cor pulmonale or right-sided heart failure include signs of right ventricular enlargement or pulmonary hypertension as well as ''gallop'' sounds or murmurs of tricuspid regurgitation. When right ventricular enlargement is present, a right ventricular heave may be recognized on inspection and palpation of the precordium as a diffuse lift over the lower portion of the sternum (the right ventricle is positioned behind the lower portion of the sternum). Accentuation of the pulmonary component of the second heart sound is generally evident with pulmonary hypertension. A right ventricular gallop due to a third heart sound (commonly called S_3) might be evident on cardiac auscultation. This S_3 sound is due to a rapid deceleration of blood entering a right ventricle with reduced distensibility in the filling phase of the cardiac cycle. A fourth heart sound (commonly called S_4) might also be detected immediately preceding the first heart sound (S_1) and is due to a forceful contraction of the right atrium expelling blood into a noncompliant and thickened right ventricle (hypertrophy of this chamber). Because S_3 and S_4 occur during ventricular diastole (ie, after S_2 and before S_1), their presence along with the normal S_1 and S_2 produces a characteristic pattern of sounds that resembles a galloping horse. Thus, these extra sounds are commonly known as *S_3 gallop* and *S_4 gallop.* The gallop sounds are better auscultated with the bell (due to their low frequency) rather than the diaphragm of the stethoscope. Gallops that originate in the right ventricle are best heard at the lower sternal border and increase with inspiration. Tricuspid regurgitation due to right ventricular enlargement is present in some patients with right-sided heart failure and produces a characteristic holosystolic murmur with a systolic distention or "v" wave that may be seen and palpated in the jugular veins at the neck.

486 How common is the development of cardiac arrhythmias in respiratory acidosis? What is their management?

❑ Cardiac arrhythmias occur frequently in patients with carbon dioxide retention, both acute and chronic, especially those with cor pulmonale and receiving digitalis therapy. Supraventricular tachyarrhythmias with ventricular rates of 120 to 160 beats/min are particularly common; they are usually not associated with major hemodynamic compromise and respond poorly to antiarrhythmic medication. The use of digitalis in the treatment of these arrhythmias is frequently more harmful than the arrhythmias per se. Because remarkably little, if any, augmentation in cardiac irritability occurs with hypercapnia, development of the arrhythmias is the result of the associated hypoxemia, sympathetic discharge, concomitant medication (eg, xanthines, beta-adrenergic agonists, digitalis), electrolyte abnormalities, and underlying heart disease. Cardiac arrhythmias, including those of ventricular origin, frequently develop with rapid restoration of normal $PaCO_2$ from very high levels by means of mechanical ventilation; similarly, generalized convulsions might be observed, and the pathogenesis of the brain and heart hyperexcitability is probably related to the associated rapid decrease in acidity of body fluids (ie, increase in blood pH).

487 What is the role of echocardiography in the evaluation of heart function? Does the presence of COPD have any effect on this evaluation?

❑ Echocardiography helps to establish whether a valvular disease (which is potentially correctable) is present, whether wall motion abnormalities exist, and whether they are regional or diffuse. While diffuse or global left ventricular dysfunction suggests a cardiomyopathy, regional wall motion abnormalities are more consistent with coronary artery disease. Doppler echocardiography permits measurements of blood flow. However, suboptimal sound penetration prevents optimal evaluation in some elderly patients, as well as others having COPD or obesity.

CIRCULATORY FAILURE

488 Contrast the conceptual meaning of circulatory failure, heart failure, and myocardial failure, conditions that might be observed in patients with respiratory failure.

❑ Circulatory failure denotes an abnormal blood flow through the cardiovascular circuitry that compromises tissue function with or without the presence of abnormal heart function. Examples of circulatory failure in which heart function might be normal include volume overload and tissue congestion due to renal failure, sepsis-induced vasodilation, and polycythemia-induced hyperviscosity, all causing reduced tissue perfusion. Heart failure refers to abnormal cardiac pumping of blood with or without an abnormal heart muscle (ie, presence or absence of myocardial failure). An example of heart failure without myocardial failure is valvular heart disease. Myocardial failure denotes abnormal cardiac pumping of blood due to a defective heart muscle. It should be apparent that myocardial failure is a subset of heart failure, which is in turn a subset of circulatory failure. Furthermore, some patients have only one of these abnormalities at a given time or, on the contrary, might have all of them. Circulatory failure without heart failure or myocardial failure is typically present in the early phase of a severe bleeding episode (eg, major blood loss caused by a gastrointestinal hemorrhage) leading to shock secondary to hypovolemia. All three disorders are present in patients with congestive heart failure caused by ischemic heart disease because myocardial failure due to reduced coronary blood flow is responsible for the heart failure and tissue underperfusion.

489 Do the terms *heart failure* and *circulatory failure* describe the same process?

❑ No. *Circulatory failure* describes a broader concept than *heart failure* because the former term refers to the inability of the cardiovascular system to perform its basic function to provide nutrition to and remove wastes from tissues. An abnormality in any component of the circulatory system including the heart (ie, heart failure), vessels (eg, decreased venous return, vasodilation), and blood (eg, decreased blood volume) might produce circulatory failure. Other conditions such as severe hypoxemia might also cause circulatory failure. The term *shock* is commonly used to refer to a state of severe circulatory failure.

490 Explain further the concept of heart failure. Is the presence of dyspnea, jugular vein distention, and peripheral edema diagnostic of heart failure?

❑ Heart failure is the condition in which, in the presence of adequate venous return, a cardiac abnormality makes this organ unable to pump blood at a rate that satisfies the metabolic needs of tissues. Heart failure is also present if an adequate rate of blood pumping can be accomplished only with abnormally elevated filling pressure. It is also called *cardiac failure.* The presence of dyspnea, jugular vein distention, and peripheral edema is not diagnostic of heart failure because these manifestations (ie, signs and symptoms) can be observed in states of fluid overload in the absence of heart failure (eg, renal failure).

491 Describe left-sided and right-sided heart failure. Explain acute and chronic heart failure.

❑ *Left-sided heart failure* refers to abnormal function of the left cardiac chambers. Likewise, *right-sided heart failure* refers to abnormal function of the right cardiac chambers. Left- and right-sided heart failure can manifest signs and symptoms of forward or backward failure of their respective chambers. Most commonly, the initial manifestations of heart failure (eg, due to hypertension, ischemic heart disease, aortic and mitral valve defects) are those of left-sided heart failure such as shortness of breath and weakness. Thereafter, right-sided heart failure leading to hepatic congestion and effusion in body cavities commonly ensues. *Acute heart failure* is the unfolding of cardiac failure in minutes, hours, or only a few days; its time of onset is usually detectable with precision. By contrast, *chronic heart failure* gradually evolves over months to years such that establishing its time of onset is more difficult.

492 What are the most relevant chest x-ray findings of patients with heart failure?

❑ Examination of the chest x-ray film of patients with heart failure might reveal (1) prominence of the superior pulmonary veins—generalized dilatation of these vessels on an upright chest x-ray film indicates pulmonary venous hypertension, (2) enlarged systemic veins (superior vena cava, azygos veins), (3) lung field shadows indicative of interstitial or alveolar edema, (4) fluid accumulation in the pleural space (eg, subpleural location, free pleural fluid effusion, interlobar fissure "thickening," pseudotumor), and (5) an enlarged cardiac silhouette (ie, cardiothoracic ratio >0.5) with possible changes in the shape and size of one or more heart chambers.

493 What are the major elements of the hemodynamic profile that accompanies common forms of shock of cardiac and noncardiac pathogenesis?

❑ Clinical forms of shock that are commonly observed in patients with actual or impending respiratory failure include (1) cardiogenic shock, (2) cardiac tamponade, (3) recurrent pulmonary embolism, (4) hypovolemic shock, and (5) septic shock. Cardiogenic shock is characterized by a low cardiac output accompanied with elevated pulmonary artery wedge pressure and right atrial pressure. Cardiac tamponade has typical features that include pulsus paradoxus (fall in systolic pressure >10 mm Hg with inspiration) and an equally elevated (eg, 15 to 30 mm Hg) diastolic pressure in all cardiac chambers assessed with right-side catheterization (ie, right atrial pressure, right ventricular end-diastolic pressure, pulmonary artery diastolic pressure, and pulmonary artery wedge pressure). Recurrent pulmonary embolism is characterized by a low or normal pulmonary artery wedge pressure and increased pulmonary vascular resistance (ie, high systolic and diastolic pulmonary artery pressures with more than 5 mm Hg of gradient between the diastolic and wedge pressures, and elevated right atrial pressure). Hypovolemic shock presents with a decreased cardiac output, low right atrial pressure, and low pulmonary artery wedge pressure (ie, low filling or diastolic pressures in left and right ventricles). Finally, septic shock presents with a very low diastolic pressure caused by arteriolar dilation, and increased pulse pressure accompanied with augmented stroke volume and cardiac output.

494 What is the role of radionuclide ventriculography, coronary angiography, and cardiac catheterization in the evaluation and management of patients with circulatory failure?

❑ Radionuclide ventriculography is a noninvasive technique that can assess ventricular function at rest and during exercise.

Coronary angiography allows recognition of coronary artery disease and it guides subsequent treatment with angioplasty or coronary artery bypass surgery. Cardiac catheterization is of special value in assessing the effect of drugs (eg, vasodilators, inotropic agents) in patients with circulatory failure refractory to standard medical therapy. In addition, cardiac catheterization might help to establish the cause of circulatory failure.

---

495 Compare the information obtained with radionuclide ventriculography, echocardiography, and Doppler studies in the evaluation of patients with circulatory failure.

❑ Radionuclide ventriculography can measure ejection fraction of the left and right ventricles, thereby helping to establish what cardiac chamber is primarily or more severely affected. The echocardiogram and Doppler studies can assess cardiac function and identify valvular and congenital defects. Regional wall motion abnormalities caused by myocardial infarction can be recognized with all three techniques.

19. Abnormal Control of Breathing

PERIODIC BREATHING

496 Explain apnea, hypopnea, and hyperpnea.

❑ *Apnea* is the cessation of airflow in the respiratory system lasting at least 10 seconds. *Hypopnea* indicates a reduction of tidal volume and *hyperpnea* (opposite process) indicates an increase of tidal volume.

497 What is Cheyne-Stokes respiration?

❑ *Cheyne-Stokes respiration* is a form of periodic breathing characterized by regular cycles of crescendo-decrescendo tidal volume breathing separated by central apneas or hypopneas.

498 Describe the Cheyne-Stokes ventilatory pattern.

❑ Cheyne-Stokes respiration, with its characteristic waxing-waning ventilatory pattern, in which hyperventilation alternates with apnea, is exhibited by patients with bifrontal or massive cerebral lesions, obesity associated with diffuse brain disease, and cardiac failure.

499 Explain further the relevant feature of Cheyne-Stokes respiration and methods that may help its diagnosis. Is the presence of Cheyne-Stokes respiration always indicative of a disease?

❑ Cheyne-Stokes respiration consists of regularly recurring cycles composed of a crescendo increase of tidal volume followed by a decrescendo decrease of tidal volume that are separated by periods of apnea or hypopnea. Intraesophageal pressure recordings help to differentiate whether the hypopneic period is central or obstructive, particularly when the hyperpneic period is brief. Cheyne-Stokes respiration is observed most commonly in patients with combined cardiac and neurologic disease and the mechanisms appear to be a delayed circulation time and abnormal function of the respiratory control centers. This pattern also appears to occur frequently in elderly subjects with apparently normal cardiovascular and neurologic systems and in normal young subjects ascending to high altitude.

500 What cardiovascular and neurologic abnormalities participate in the pathogenesis of Cheyne-Stokes respiration?

❑ Prolongation of the circulation time and greater dependency on oxygen than on carbon dioxide of the respiratory control system are the dominant cardiovascular and neurologic abnormalities responsible for the development of Cheyne-Stokes respiration. This pathogenesis explains the common presence of disease of the heart and brain in association with Cheyne-Stokes respiration.

501 What cardiac and neurologic diseases are associated with Cheyne-Stokes respiration?

❑ Most patients with Cheyne-Stokes respiration have both cardiac and neurologic disease, although the underlying illness may be limited to only one system. A prolonged circulation time is considered the major factor responsible for Cheyne-Stokes respiration in patients with cardiac failure but the associated pulmonary congestion further increases the likelihood of this periodic breathing. Hypoxemia augments the sensitivity and the instability of the respiratory control center. The sensitivity of the respiratory control center may also be heightened by increased reflex activity of mechanoreceptors in the presence of pulmonary congestion. Cheyne-Stokes respiration is also observed in a variety of neurologic disorders including cerebrovascular accident caused by hemorrhage, infarct, or embolism; tumors; meningitis; encephalitis; trauma; or intracranial tumor.

SLEEP APNEA

502 What is apnea? What types of apnea are most commonly observed in clinical practice?

❑ Apnea is an interruption of respiration lasting more than 10 seconds. Among the clinical presentations of apnea, obstructive sleep apnea is probably the most frequently observed and consists of cessation of airflow in association with persistence of respiratory effort. Conversely, absence of respiratory effort accompanies cessation of airflow in patients with central apnea (other important clinical form of apnea).

503 What is the overall effect on blood gases of a respiratory arrest?

❑ Abrupt cessation of ventilation in any clinical setting leads to death from hypoxia in approximately 4 minutes or less. The degree of the associated carbon dioxide retention in this period is modest, for $PaCO_2$ rises at an average rate of 3 to 5 mm Hg per min; thus, 10 to 15 minutes is required before extreme hypercapnia develops if the patient previously had hypocapnia or eucapnia. Patients with circulatory shock or cardiac arrest might display an unusual pattern of blood gas composition; the respiratory acidosis can be confined to the tissues and the venous circulation, whereas the arterial blood might evidence eucapnia or even hypocapnia, because of the prevailing high $\dot{V}_A/\dot{Q}$ in the lungs.

504 How important is detection of breathing abnormalities during sleep?

❑ Sleep apnea syndrome can no longer be regarded as a curiosity linked with fictitious characters in the writings of Charles Dickens (Joe, the fat boy in *Pickwick Papers*) and Jean Giraudoux

(Ondine's curse). Instead, it is a potentially lethal condition that is much more prevalent than commonly suspected. Because of the wide variety of conditions that predispose to the sleep apnea syndrome and other abnormal patterns of breathing during sleep, physicians of almost every specialty should be aware of the clinical features and methods available for diagnosis of these disorders.

505 What conditions are associated with the sleep apnea syndromes?

❑ Sleep apnea syndromes are observed in association with (1) neurologic conditions (eg, bilateral cervical cordotomy, myotonic dystrophy, bulbar poliomyelitis, brain stem infarction, Shy-Drager syndrome, encephalitis, Guillain-Barré syndrome, and Cheyne-Stokes respiration); (2) upper-airway obstruction (eg, micrognathia, enlarged tonsils and adenoids, enlarged uvula and posterior oronasopharyngeal tissue, obesity, acromegaly, myxedema, Down syndrome, Scheie's syndrome, platybasia, neck infiltration with lymphoma, atlantoaxial dislocation, Prader-Willi syndrome, and posterior nasal packing); and (3) alveolar hypoventilation (eg, Ondine's curse, pickwickian syndrome, and kyphoscoliosis).

506 Compare the episodes of sleep apnea observed in normal subjects with those found in patients with breathing abnormalities.

❑ Normal men have an average of seven episodes (range, 1 to 25 episodes) of central apnea per night and women have only about two episodes (range, 0 to 5). In normal persons, the apnea index that represents the number of apneas per sleep hour is less than 5 and is of a central origin. The central apneic episodes observed in normal subjects are rarely longer than 30 seconds in duration, whereas episodes longer than 60 seconds frequently occur in patients with the obstructive or mixed sleep apnea syndrome.

507 What features can be detected by physical examination of patients with sleep apnea?

❑ On physical examination, the patient with sleep apnea syndrome is often obese and may have a short, thick neck and large jowls. A narrowed posterior pharyngeal aperture, hypertrophied or long uvula, and prominent tonsils may be present. Nasal obstruction manifested by collapse of the nares with forced inspiration through the nose is often detected. In addition, there is an increased frequency of daytime systemic hypertension in patients with sleep apnea.

508 Is the prevalence of sleep apnea similar in men and women? Is there a genetic predisposition to sleep apnea?

❑ Like snoring, sleep apnea is less common among women, but the prevalence increases after the menopause. Hormonal factors are probably involved and administration of medroxyprogesterone acetate to patients with sleep apnea may improve the disorder. The gender difference may be caused by the stimulant effect of progesterone on ventilation as well as the pharyngeal fat deposition promoted by male sex hormones. Genetic predisposition has been implicated for the development of the syndrome of obstructive sleep apnea.

509 What is the risk, if any, of sedatives and alcohol intake in patients with sleep apnea syndrome?

❑ Patients with obstructive sleep apnea are particularly vulnerable to more severe hypoxia and life-threatening arrhythmias after sedation with alcohol and drugs. Consequently, intake of alcoholic beverages before retiring (''nightcaps'') should be avoided in patients with sleep apnea syndrome as apneas and oxygen desaturation are more frequent and of longer duration with the use of this substance. Alcoholic beverages may also precipitate obstructive apneas in asymptomatic men.

510 What daytime symptoms may be observed in patients with sleep apnea?

☐ Morning headaches are common in patients with sleep apnea and gradually disappear over several hours. The patient's headaches in association with nausea and mental confusion may lead physicians to erroneously suspect the presence of an intracranial lesion. Personality changes, such as paranoia, agitated depression, and hostility, often occur. Problems at work arise because of intellectual deterioration and difficulty in mental concentration caused by the chronic sleep deprivation. Reduced libido and impotence are also frequently present in patients with sleep apnea.

511 Explain the daytime hypersomnolence of patients with sleep apnea.

☐ Disturbance of normal nocturnal sleep in patients with sleep apnea is caused by frequent arousals at the termination of apneic periods. Consequently, deep sleep is rarely achieved and this sleep deprivation causes varying degrees of daytime hypersomnolence. In mild cases, it may be limited to certain times such as the postprandial period or while viewing television. In severe cases, the irresistible urge to sleep may lead to virtual incapacitation and endanger the life of the patient and those of others. For example, inappropriate onset of sleep during driving may be associated with automobile accidents. In advanced stages of the disorder, it may be difficult to differentiate severe somnolence from the semicomatose state.

512 What cardiovascular abnormalities are commonly observed in the sleep apnea syndrome? What is the role of hypercapnia in the development of these abnormalities?

☐ Sinus bradycardia caused by increased parasympathetic activity develops during episodes of apnea and its development does not correlate with any abnormality in ABGs. Sudden death caused by hypoxemic-induced ventricular arrhythmias is fortunately rare in patients with the sleep apnea syndrome. It should be recognized that hypercapnia does not play any role in the disturbances of heart rhythm in these patients because carbon dioxide retention does not occur in the course of the short episodes of apnea (eg, it takes 1 minute of apnea to increase PCO_2 by approximately 4 mm Hg). Hypertension is more prevalent in individuals with sleep apnea syndrome than in the general population but its pathogenesis remains unclear.

---

513 Provide more information on the cardiovascular and hematologic disturbances that might develop in patients with sleep apnea.

❑ Abnormalities of cardiac rhythm, such as sinus arrhythmia, sinus arrest, paroxysmal atrial tachycardia, atrial fibrillation, atrioventricular block, and ventricular tachycardia, can occur in patients with sleep apnea, but life-threatening arrhythmias are uncommon. Elevations of pulmonary and systemic blood pressures are observed during the apneic episodes. Marked hypoxia during the obstructive apneas plays a role in the development of these cardiovascular disturbances. In advanced sleep apnea syndrome, cardiac failure with pulmonary hypertension, right ventricular failure, cyanosis, polycythemia, and carbon dioxide retention may develop and the patient may be termed *pickwickian* if he or she is also obese. However, patients with the pickwickian syndrome do not necessarily have sleep apnea.

---

514 Explain the various forms of apnea including central, obstructive, and mixed, as well as the sleep apnea syndrome. What is the apnea index?

❑ *Central apnea* refers to the cessation of both airflow and respiratory movements and may be present in normal persons during sleep onset or during rapid eye movement (REM) periods. Conversely, *obstructive apnea* refers to the cessation of airflow caused by upper-airway obstruction accompanied with persistent respiratory movements. *Mixed apnea* is characterized by the presence of central apnea at the initiation of an episode followed by obstructive apnea at the completion of the episode. *Sleep apnea syndrome* refers to the presence of at least 30 apneas during 6 hours of nocturnal sleep in association with insomnia or daytime hypersomnolence. The *apnea index* is the number of apneas per hour of sleep and this parameter helps to ascertain the severity of a sleep apnea syndrome.

515 What are the underlying mechanism and the main features of the obstructive type of sleep apnea and hypopnea?

❑ Occlusion of the airway above the level of the glottis is caused by apposition of the tongue against the posterolateral pharyngeal wall during the apneic phase. Contraction of the diaphragm during the apneic phase produces subatmospheric pressure in the pharynx, thereby causing retraction of the tongue which facilitates obstruction of the airway. The apneic episode continues until arousal occurs, possibly triggered by hypoxic stimulation of the reticular neurons of the central nervous system (CNS). The increase in motoneuron activity observed after arousal activates the upper-airway musculature, leading to a dissipation of the obstruction and resumption of ventilation. Periods of obstructive apneas alternating with arousals can occur throughout the entire night and as many as 400 to 500 episodes can occur in some patients.

516 What are the clinical features of obstructive sleep apnea?

❑ Important clinical features associated with obstructive sleep apnea are obesity, loud snoring, repeated awakening during sleep, daytime hypersomnolence, nocturnal enuresis, sexual dysfunction, and morning headache. In patients with obstructive sleep apnea, the bed partner on direct questioning will usually describe intermittent loud sonorous snoring. These episodes of loud gasping snoring followed by silence that lasts typically from 30 to 100 seconds or longer are described by the witness as if the patient exhibits struggling motions of the thorax and abdomen. The silent period is terminated by a loud snore, and airflow resumes with a few additional snores. As many as 500 such episodes are often documented through the night. Thrashing of the upper and lower limbs is common, as are talking and walking during sleep. These features combined with the noisy loud snoring frequently lead the bed partner to seek refuge in another room. The prevalence of multiple divorces is quite high in patients with obstructive sleep apnea because the bed partner becomes emotionally disturbed by the loud snoring. The history of snoring is frequently lifelong, extending from childhood or the adolescent period, but it is not a sine qua non for diagnosis. Patients with associated neuromuscular disease or kyphoscoliosis may have respiratory efforts so feeble that snoring is not heard.

---

517 Is the specific cause of upper-airway obstruction similar in the various diseases associated with breathing abnormalities?

❑ No. In acromegaly, the obstructive sleep apnea syndrome may have as a specific cause the associated prognathism, overgrowth of pharyngeal soft tissue, and macroglossia. Macroglossia, often present in Down syndrome and hypothyroidism, may predispose to the development of sleep apnea. Accentuation of the breathing abnormality in hypothyroidism and thyroid diseases may occur as a result of goiter producing upper-airway narrowing, and myxedema, diminishing respiratory center drive. Similar to airway narrowing associated with anatomic abnormalities, increased deposition of fat in the pharyngeal space in obese subjects may predispose them to the obstructive sleep apnea syndrome. Computed tomography in patients with obstructive sleep apnea syndrome may reveal upper-airway narrowing in the posterior nasal, oral, or hypopharyngeal region.

518 What are the underlying mechanism and the main features of the central type of sleep apnea and hypopnea?

❑ Features associated with central sleep apnea include insomnia, frequent awakening during sleep, depression, and absence of loud snoring during sleep as well as obesity. This form of sleep apnea syndrome is the least common, and is caused by decreased respiratory center output. It must be recognized that a few brief central apneas may occur in normal persons, especially at sleep onset and during REM sleep. Diminished respiratory center output may be found in patients with CNS lesions and is manifested either by complete cessation or by reduced excursions of both rib cage and abdominal compartments. This syndrome is distinguished from Cheyne-Stokes respiration in that apneas or hypopneas do not occur on a periodic basis. In addition, the breaths following the intermittent central apneas or hyperpneas rarely are of equal magnitude; instead, crescendo-decrescendo or a single deep breath followed by decrescendo tidal volumes are observed before regular tidal breathing is established.

519 What are the main features of the mixed type of sleep apnea and hypopnea?

❑ The mixed type of sleep apnea starts as a central apnea but is immediately followed by paradoxical thoracoabdominal movements with upper-airway obstruction as in the obstructive type of apnea. The reverse sequence rarely occurs. A similar pattern is observed with the mixed type of sleep hypopnea. Mixed apneas and hypopneas are less common than the obstructive type but are far more frequently observed than the central type.

520 What diagnostic methods are used to establish with certainty the specific sleep-breathing abnormality observed in a patient?

❑ The definitive diagnosis of breathing abnormalities during sleep rests on the analysis of nocturnal sleep stages (with the use of electroencephalography, electro-oculography, and chin-digastric electromyography), breathing pattern (respiratory inductive plethysmography) and pleural pressure swings (esophageal balloon catheter), and oxygen saturation (ear oximetry). Electrocardiographic and leg electromyographic monitoring are complementary procedures for the diagnosis of cardiac arrhythmias and nocturnal myoclonus, respectively. Patients with central apnea exhibit absence of all ventilatory movements in the abdomen and rib cage as well as a small decrease in SaO_2 measured via ear oximetry. In contrast, in obstructive sleep apnea there is paradoxical movement of the rib cage (movement downward) and abdominal (movement upward) compartments that is associated with the marked decrease in SaO_2.

521 How can the oxygen desaturation observed with breathing abnormalities be evaluated?

❑ The oxygen saturation can be measured noninvasively and continuously with ear oximetry. Values lower than 50% may be observed during prolonged obstructive or mixed apneas as a result of the prolonged breath-hold and the shrinking lung volume with increasing ventilation-perfusion inequalities. During central apneas or partial obstructions of the upper airway, oxygen saturation rarely falls below 80% because lung volume does not decrease owing to persistent uptake of fresh air. There is not an accepted definition of significant hypoxemia or oxygen desaturation, although values of 4% to 10% below the baseline saturation levels are generally considered significant.

522 What is the pickwickian syndrome?

❑ *Pickwickian syndrome* refers to a clinical entity that includes alveolar hypoventilation during sleep with or without apneas, obesity, hypersomnolence, periodic breathing, cor pulmonale, and polycythemia.

523 Explain the breathing abnormalities observed in association with Ondine's curse and pickwickian syndrome.

❑ *Ondine's curse* refers to a rare condition in which the patient breathes inadequately or not at all unless commanded to ventilate. The term is derived from a French play by Giraudoux where the jilter of a mermaid, Ondine, found that his bodily functions no longer operated automatically. Fortunately, this condition is a very rare cause of central apneas and hypopneas during sleep. A variant of this syndrome that occurs after bilateral cervical cordotomy for palliation of pain usually lasts 24 to 48 hours after surgery. Pickwickian patients (obesity is a constant feature of this syndrome) have central alveolar hypoventilation and some afflicted patients have obstructive sleep apneas.

524 Elaborate on the causes and importance of nocturnal disturbances in ventilation and gas exchange in the absence of obstructive sleep apnea. What forms of ventilatory support might be used?

❑ Worsening hypoxemia and hypercapnia at night are commonly observed in patients with significant respiratory impairment from chest wall or neuromuscular disease. Transient or sustained hypoventilation (caused by decreased respiratory drive and hypotonia of respiratory muscles) and decreased ventilation-perfusion ratio in some regions of the lung (caused by smaller tidal volumes and decreased functional residual capacity [FRC] in the supine position) during nocturnal sleep may increase PCO_2 and decrease PaO_2 and SaO_2. Therapy usually involves nocturnal mechanical ventilator support, ideally noninvasive, in the form of either positive-pressure mask ventilation or negative-pressure ventilation with a cuirass (rigid shell) or poncho ventilator around the chest wall. In COPD, patients with the lowest daytime SaO_2 are most likely to have the lowest SaO_2 during sleep. Transient increases in pulmonary artery pressure accompany these nocturnal falls in SaO_2, but important long-term clinical consequences of nocturnal falls in oxygen saturation have not been demonstrated in the absence of daytime desaturation.

525 A 42-year-old obese man presents to the physician's office at the request of his wife who claims that he had been snoring loudly for the past 6 months. He has a history of untreated hypertension and smoking 1 pack of cigarettes per day for 25 years. The patient complains of feeling sleepy during the daytime but capable of performing his daily work. Physical examination reveals a height and weight of 162 cm and 96 kg, respectively. Blood pressure is 152/92 mm Hg. The rest of the examination including evaluation of the oropharynx revealed normal findings.

What is the most appropriate test to be performed at this time to evaluate the patient's condition? What is the role of ABG measurements?

❑ The daytime hypersomnolence and loud snoring that led the patient to consult a physician are suggestive of the presence of obstructive sleep apnea. The most appropriate test to evaluate the patient's condition and reach a diagnosis is overnight polysomnography. Other tests might have some value but will not establish the diagnosis with certainty. ABG measurements should not be requested because the values are usually normal while the patient is awake. Radiographs of the sinuses are not appropriate in this obese patient who does not have symptoms of congestion of upper airways.

20. Miscellaneous Disorders

UPPER-AIRWAY OBSTRUCTION

526 Compare the effects of inspiration and expiration on the extrathoracic and intrathoracic airways.

❑ The upper airway undergoes dynamic alterations in its caliber during the respiratory cycle. These alterations differ for the extrathoracic and intrathoracic airways. For the extrathoracic airway, intraluminal pressure is negative when compared with the surrounding atmospheric pressure during inspiration, and the extrathoracic airway tends to collapse. During expiration, the intraluminal pressure is positive, which causes the lumen to distend. For the intrathoracic airway, pleural pressure is more negative than the intraluminal pressure is during inspiration, which causes the lumen to expand. During expiration, pleural pressure is higher than intraluminal pressure, and the intrathoracic airway tends to collapse. During quiet breathing, the airway caliber changes by less than 15%, whereas during increased respiratory effort in patients with airway obstruction, a more than 50% change in caliber may occur. On the basis of these principles and by employing flow-volume loops, upper-airway obstruction can be divided into three types: fixed obstruction, variable extrathoracic obstruction, and variable intrathoracic obstruction. Characteristic flow-volume loop patterns are observed with each type of obstruction.

527 What spirometric indices suggest the existence of upper-airway obstruction?

❑ Four spirometric indices help to establish the presence of upper-airway obstruction, as follows: (1) forced inspiratory flow at 50% of vital capacity (FIF 50%) less than 100 L/min; (2) the ratio of forced expiratory flow at 50% of vital capacity to FIF 50% (mid–vital capacity ratio) equal or greater than 1.0; (3) FEV_1/PEFR equal or greater than 10 mL/L/min because the reduction in PEFR with upper-airway obstruction is greater than the reduction in FEV_1; and (4) forced expiratory volume in 0.5 second ($FEV_{0.5}$) more severely affected by upper-airway obstruction than is FEV_1, with the result that the $FEV_1/FEV_{0.5}$ ratio is equal or greater than 1.5.

528 What are the main features of an upper-airway obstruction?

❑ Upper-airway obstruction is a relatively uncommon cause of obstruction to airflow, and it is frequently unrecognized or misdiagnosed. Presenting symptoms include dyspnea, stridor, wheezing (leading to a misdiagnosis of asthma), hoarseness, dysphonia, and an unusual cough. Some patients may have features of the sleep apnea syndrome. Initially, symptoms might occur only with exercise, but later they might occur at rest. Symptoms can be related to variations in posture, and stridor varying with the position of the head suggests the presence of a thoracic inlet lesion. The loudness of stridor bears no relationship to the severity of obstruction.

529 What are the causes and main features of a fixed upper-airway obstruction?

❑ Causes of fixed upper-airway obstruction include tumor or stricture secondary to previous intubation. Upper-airway obstruction of the fixed type (whether intrathoracic or extrathoracic) is not influenced by dynamic changes in the tracheal cross-sectional airway, and airflow is equally reduced during inspiration and expiration. The appearance of the flow-volume loop is most helpful in making the diagnosis. The ratio of expired to inspired flow at 50% of vital capacity, the mid–vital capacity ratio, is approximately 1.0 (similar to the normal value of about 0.9).

530 What is a variable extrathoracic obstruction? What are its causes?

❑ Obstructions that vary with the phase of the respiratory cycle are termed *variable obstructions.* Causes of variable extrathoracic obstruction include vocal cord paralysis, scars, malignancy, goiter, lymphadenopathy, and fat deposits. Variable extrathoracic obstruction causes a greater reduction in inspiratory flow as compared with expiratory flow (mid–vital capacity ratio >2.0) because intraluminal pressure during inspiration is considerably lower than peritracheal pressure, with the result that dynamic narrowing of the trachea occurs.

---

531 Explain the characteristics and causes of a variable intrathoracic obstruction.

❑ A variable intrathoracic obstruction is usually due to tumor and causes a higher reduction in expiratory flow than in inspiratory flow (mid–vital capacity ratio is very low, about 0.3). During expiration, peritracheal pressure is higher than the intraluminal pressure of the intrathoracic portion of the trachea, thereby causing dynamic compression of the airway.

---

532 How is the diagnosis of upper-airway obstruction made? What is the management of this condition?

❑ Once upper-airway obstruction is suspected on the basis of pulmonary function testing, the etiology of the obstruction should be established radiologically or by endoscopic examination. In most patients, the treatment is surgical. While awaiting definitive treatment, some patients with severe obstruction may require endotracheal intubation, tracheotomy, or cricothyroidotomy.

RESTRICTIVE VENTILATORY DEFECTS. PULMONARY FIBROSIS

---

533 Name common causes of a restrictive ventilatory defect. How is this defect recognized?

❑ Intrathoracic abnormalities arising within the lungs (eg, some tumors, interstitial lung diseases including pulmonary edema, fibrosis, pneumoconiosis), pleura (eg, tumor, effusion), and chest wall (eg, kyphoscoliosis, neuromuscular disease) are prominent causes of a restrictive ventilatory defect. In addition, other common conditions leading to a restrictive ventilatory defect include obesity, ascites, and pregnancy (extrathoracic conditions). Pulmonary function tests allow clinicians to establish the presence of a restrictive ventilatory defect. Additional information obtained from the clinical history and other laboratory tests allows one to establish the specific cause of the restrictive ventilatory defect.

534 What is Hamman-Rich syndrome?

❑ Hamman-Rich syndrome is a serious condition leading to hypoxemic respiratory failure, characterized by the presence of pulmonary fibrosis of unknown cause (idiopathic pulmonary fibrosis [IPF]). This entity produces a restrictive ventilatory defect, diminished lung compliance, and decreased alveolar-capillary diffusion of carbon monoxide (DLCO). It has been proposed that these patients may actually have ARDS superimposed on the IPF, and the summation of effects may explain the severity of their condition.

535 A 59-year-old woman consults because of persistent nonproductive cough and progressive shortness of breath for 18 to 24 months. Previous history is negative for cigarette smoking and exposure to inhalants and toxic products. A chest x-ray film reveals a diffuse interstitial pattern, most evident in the lower fields.

What is the presumptive diagnosis? What is the value of pulmonary function tests in the evaluation of diffuse lung diseases?

❑ The available information suggests the presence of interstitial pulmonary fibrosis. Routine pulmonary function tests (eg, spirometry, flow-volume loops) are neither sensitive nor specific for the diagnosis of interstitial pulmonary fibrosis in patients with early disease. In addition, a reduction of total lung capacity as well as spirometric measures and flow-volume loops does not correlate with lung histology, prognosis, or survival of patients with interstitial pulmonary fibrosis. However, a reduction of vital capacity to less than 50% of the predicted value is accompanied by pulmonary hypertension and a reduced survival. As previously indicated, patients with interstitial lung disease generally have a restrictive defect that is characterized by decreased values of total lung capacity, FRC, vital capacity, and residual volume. The values of FEV_1 and forced vital capacity (FVC) are decreased because of small lung volumes but the FEV_1/FVC ratio is normal or increased. Yet, some patients with interstitial lung disease also demonstrate an obstructive ventilatory defect.

---

536 What are the expected blood gas abnormalities in this patient? Explain the role of exercise testing and the evaluation of pulmonary diffusion capacity (DLCO) in the diagnosis and follow-up of patients with interstitial lung disease.

❑ Resting hypoxemia caused by ventilation-perfusion mismatching, and respiratory alkalosis are commonly observed in patients with interstitial lung disease. Exercise testing is more sensitive than evaluations at rest to detect an abnormal oxygen transfer in patients with this condition. Furthermore, the increase in the alveolar-arterial oxygen gradient (P_A-aO_2) with exercise is a sensitive measure to evaluate the clinical course of the disease and the response to treatment. Measurement of pulmonary diffusion capacity (DLCO) has a limited value to evaluate the course of the disease and does not correlate with lung histology. However, a normal DLCO may be observed in patients with early disease and relatively normal gas exchange, whereas a marked reduction of DLCO correlates with the presence of pulmonary hypertension and decreased survival.

---

537 What connective-tissue disorders can lead to the development of chronic interstitial lung diseases (diffuse interstitial fibrosis)?

❑ Connective-tissue disorders possibly leading to the development of chronic interstitial lung diseases include rheumatoid arthritis, systemic lupus erythematosus, systemic sclerosis, polymyositis, dermatomyositis, and Sjögren's syndrome. The clinical form of chronic interstitial lung disease most commonly encountered is caused by rheumatoid arthritis and is observed in men having other manifestations of this connective-tissue disorder including joint involvement and subcutaneous nodules. The association of rheumatoid arthritis and pneumoconiosis in a patient with diffuse interstitial fibrosis is known as *Caplan's syndrome.*

NEUROMUSCULAR IMPAIRMENT

538 What conditions can lead to respiratory muscle dysfunction caused by decreased neuromuscular capacity?

❑ Decreased neuromuscular capacity can occur as a result of (1) depression of respiratory center output (eg, sedatives, structural neurologic damage secondary to vascular disease or trauma, sleep deprivation, starvation, hypothyroidism, metabolic alkalosis), (2) phrenic nerve dysfunction (eg, bilateral diaphragmatic paralysis of idiopathic origin or secondary to trauma or diffuse neuropathies and myopathies), (3) neuromuscular disorders (eg, spinal cord injuries, myasthenia gravis, amyotrophic lateral sclerosis, poliomyelitis, Guillain-Barré syndrome, and muscular dystrophies), (4) thoracic cage deformity (eg, scoliosis, ankylosing spondylitis, and fibrothorax), (5) hyperinflation (one of the most common and important causes of respiratory muscle dysfunction in an acute care setting that is observed with COPD and asthma), (6) respiratory muscle fatigue, (7) drug-induced disorders (eg, pancuronium, succinylcholine, aminoglycoside antibiotics), (8) malnutrition, and (9) decreased oxygen supply (eg, anemia, circulatory failure, hypoxemia, sepsis) to peripheral tissues.

539 Explain the causes and importance of diseases of the anterior horn cells (motoneurons of the spinal cord) in the development of respiratory failure. What abnormalities in pulmonary function tests and ABGs are observed?

❑ In the first half of the century, poliomyelitis was the major neuromuscular disease affecting respiration, and some patients with poliomyelitis are still being treated for respiratory failure. Currently, amyotrophic lateral sclerosis is the most important entity within this group of diseases and the most common cause of death is respiratory failure. Patients display a restrictive ventilatory pattern, decreased respiratory muscle strength, and rapid shallow breathing. The ventilatory response to hypercapnia is also mildly decreased, and correlates with the level of respiratory muscle strength and vital capacity. Hypercapnia is uncommon until the terminal stages of the disease.

540 What is the most common peripheral neuropathy leading to acute respiratory failure?

❑ Guillain-Barré syndrome is the most common peripheral neuropathy leading to acute respiratory failure and accounts for more than half the patients with neuromuscular disease who are admitted to intensive care units. Early detection of ventilatory failure is essential because approximately 20% to 45% of afflicted patients require mechanical ventilation.

541 What are the causes and consequences of *unilateral* diaphragmatic paralysis? How is this diagnosis made?

❑ *Unilateral* diaphragmatic paralysis may result from malignancy, trauma, pneumonia, or herpes zoster or may be idiopathic in origin. It usually presents as an elevated hemidiaphragm that needs to be differentiated from a pleural or subpulmonic effusion. Pulmonary function is slightly impaired: Vital capacity and TLC are decreased by 26% and 13%, respectively, in the sitting position, while FRC remains normal. Fluoroscopy is the method most commonly employed to make the diagnosis. Normally, the diaphragm descends during "sniffing," whereas the entire leaf of a paralyzed diaphragm may show at least 2 cm of paradoxical motion, provided the abdominal muscles are relaxed. Unfortunately, paradoxical motion also can be observed in 6% of healthy subjects. Demonstration of a delayed phrenic nerve conduction time is a more specific test for the diagnosis of unilateral diaphragmatic paralysis.

542 What are the causes and consequences of *bilateral* diaphragmatic paralysis? How is this diagnosis made? What abnormalities in pulmonary function tests are observed in this condition?

❑ *Bilateral* diaphragmatic paralysis can be caused by diffuse neuropathies and myopathies or trauma, or can be idiopathic. Patients display a severe restrictive ventilatory pattern; vital capacity while the patient is in the erect position is about 50% of the predicted value and pulmonary compliance is decreased. When the patient changes to the supine position, abdominal paradox develops and the vital capacity falls by 50%. This probably is caused by gravitational forces displacing the paralyzed diaphragm cephalad, causing a further reduction in FRC. In one study, 63% of the patients developed hypercapnia ($PaCO_2$ >50 mm Hg) on assuming the supine posture and 86% showed worsening of gas exchange during sleep. It is thought that inhibition of the intercostal and accessory muscles during REM sleep leads to profound hypoventilation, given that patients with paralyzed diaphragms are totally dependent on these muscles for breathing. Fluoroscopy can be a very misleading diagnostic method, since paradoxical diaphragmatic motion may be absent. This occurs because some patients with paralyzed diaphragms contract their abdominal muscles during expiration, displacing the abdomen inward and the diaphragm toward the rib cage. At the onset of inspiration, relaxation of the abdominal muscles causes outward recoil to the abdominal wall and diaphragmatic descent. Measurement of transdiaphragmatic pressure (Pdi, assessed with balloons introduced in the lumen of the stomach and esophagus) is a more reliable diagnostic approach. Healthy subjects show a pressure change of at least 25 cm H_2O during maximum inspiration, compared with a value of 0 cm H_2O in patients with total paralysis, or less than 6 cm H_2O in patients with severe weakness.

543 What method other than measurement of maximum airway pressures can reliably assess respiratory muscle dysfunction? How can the diagnosis of diaphragmatic paralysis be established?

❑ Evaluation of transdiaphragmatic pressure with balloon catheters in the esophagus and stomach represents a reliable test of respiratory muscle strength. Measurements are made during a maximal inspiratory effort against a closed airway or while the patient generates a sniff; the transdiaphragmatic pressure is then calculated by electrically subtracting esophageal from gastric pressure. This technique assesses diaphragmatic muscle strength and is useful in the diagnosis of diaphragmatic paralysis (in this condition the negative esophageal pressure generated by the other respiratory muscles during a maximal inspiratory effort pulls the flaccid diaphragm cephalad, thereby causing a decrease as opposed to the normal increase in gastric pressure). Its major drawback is the invasive nature of this procedure, as it entails passing balloon catheters into both the esophagus and the stomach.

MUSCLE DYSFUNCTION. MUSCULAR DYSTROPHY AND SCOLIOSIS

544 What are the breathing pattern abnormalities known as asynchronous breathing, abdominal paradox, and respiratory alternans?

❑ During normal breathing, the rib cage and abdomen expand and contract in unison (synchrony). Abnormal movements of the rib cage and abdomen can be categorized as *asynchronous movements* when differences in the rate of motion of the two compartments are present, and *paradox* indicates that the two compartments move in opposite directions. A third category of abnormal movement, called *respiratory alternans,* is characterized by breath-to-breath variation in the relative contribution of the rib cage and abdomen to tidal volume. There is recruitment and derecruitment of different groups of respiratory muscles in patients with respiratory alternans.

545 What are the conditions that predispose to respiratory muscle fatigue?

❑ From a clinical standpoint, conditions that predispose to respiratory muscle fatigue can be divided into two types: those that increase the respiratory load and those that cause muscle weakness. Conditions that increase the respiratory load include airway obstruction, parenchymal lung disease, and chest bellows disease. Conditions that cause muscle weakness include neuromuscular disease, hypoperfusion, hypoxemia, hypercapnia, malnutrition, electrolyte imbalance, hyperinflation, postoperative diaphragmatic dysfunction, muscle atrophy, and advanced age.

546 What conditions can lead to respiratory muscle fatigue caused by increased respiratory load? Explain the relationship between the patient's transpulmonary pressure and the maximal voluntary inspiratory pressure with respect to the development of respiratory muscle fatigue.

❑ An increased load on the respiratory muscles can result from higher ventilatory requirements (ie, augmented carbon dioxide production, increased dead space ventilation, or inappropriately elevated respiratory drive) or increased work of breathing. If carbon dioxide production is increased, a dead space to tidal volume ratio (V_D/V_T) of 0.6 or higher generally leads to the development of hypercapnia, because the associated increase in minute ventilation necessary for satisfactory gas exchange causes a marked reduction of ventilatory reserve. Although an inadequate level of respiratory drive causes hypoventilation and respiratory acidosis, an inappropriately elevated drive places unnecessary stress on the respiratory muscles and can predispose to fatigue. In the presence of augmented airway resistance (eg, status asthmaticus, chronic bronchitis) or decreased lung compliance (eg, pulmonary fibrosis), increased transpulmonary pressure is required to achieve a given tidal volume, therefore causing increased work of breathing. As the required transpulmonary pressure for ventilation increases, the reserve capacity of the respiratory muscles decreases and respiratory muscle fatigue can ensue. Fatigue is likely to occur when the mean pleural pressure of each breath is 60% or more of the maximal voluntary inspiratory pressure (PImax).

547 How easily can the cause of respiratory muscle dysfunction be identified as secondary to increased load as opposed to muscle weakness? Explain the role of respiratory muscle fatigue in COPD.

❑ The distinction between respiratory muscle dysfunction caused by either increased load or muscle weakness is not quite as neat as it appears in any given patient and there may be some overlap. For example, COPD is one of the most common conditions (other than primary neuromuscular diseases) in which respiratory muscle dysfunction plays an important role in the development of respiratory failure. In patients with COPD, increased airway resistance and hyperinflation can raise the energy cost of breathing up to 15% of total oxygen consumption; in comparison, the energy cost of breathing is 1% to 5% in healthy persons. Ventilatory reserve is also decreased in COPD patients because resting ventilation constitutes up to about 40% of maximum ventilatory capacity, compared with 5% in healthy persons. In addition, patients with COPD typically display hyperinflation, which decreases the capacity of the muscles to generate pressure, and they also might have hypoxemia, hypercapnia, and other metabolic disturbances secondary to the airway obstruction that can also adversely affect respiratory muscle function.

548 What are the most commonly observed causes of drug-induced acute respiratory failure secondary to respiratory muscle dysfunction?

❑ Interference with neuromuscular transmission is a desired action of pancuronium or succinylcholine, but it can also occur as a side effect of other agents, especially aminoglycoside antibiotics. This complication usually presents as postoperative respiratory depression in patients who received muscle relaxants and general anesthesia during a surgical procedure. In some patients, myasthenia gravis may be unmasked or aggravated by agents such as quinidine, propranolol, or lithium. Drug-induced disorders of neuromuscular transmission are uncommon, and usually occur in patients who recently received a muscle relaxant, who have subliminal myasthenia, or who have electrolyte disorders (eg, hypokalemia and potassium depletion).

---

549 Explain the development of respiratory muscle dysfunction in patients undergoing cardiothoracic surgery. What is the cause of an elevated left hemidiaphragm in these patients?

❑ Patients undergoing cardiothoracic surgery (eg, coronary artery bypass) frequently develop a raised left hemidiaphragm and considerable reduction in lung volume in the early postoperative period. This reduction in lung volume correlates well with a decrease in PImax. The elevated hemidiaphragm has generally been attributed to cold injury of the left phrenic nerve caused by the use of topical cardioplegia, for which the pericardial sac is filled with crushed ice or chilled saline solution. However, postoperative loss of lung volume only occasionally is caused by phrenic nerve paralysis. Other potential mechanisms include atelectasis because of a decreased frequency of sighing or direct injury caused by retraction of the left lower lobe during surgery.

---

550 What clinical forms of muscle dystrophy can lead to respiratory failure? Compare the development of respiratory failure in Duchenne's dystrophy with that in limb-girdle dystrophy.

❑ Respiratory failure is the cause of death in 75% of patients with Duchenne's dystrophy. Respiratory muscle weakness occurs early in the disease but the diaphragm remains relatively spared, with the result that hypercapnia is uncommon except as a terminal event. In contrast, diaphragmatic involvement occurs relatively early in patients with limb-girdle dystrophy, and these patients seem more likely to develop hypercapnia. Patients with myotonic dystrophy may have disproportionately large involvement of the respiratory muscles compared with the remaining musculature. The ventilatory response to hypercapnia, however, has been reported variably to be either normal or decreased in patients with myotonic dystrophy.

551 What abnormalities in the ventilatory function might be observed in patients with scoliosis (ie, lateral deviation of the spine)? How do they correlate with the severity of the thoracic cage deformity? What is the management of these patients?

❑ The severity of scoliosis is quantitated by measuring the degree of angulation between the upper and lower limbs of the primary spinal curve on the radiograph (ie, perpendicular lines are drawn to the superior surface of the proximal vertebra and the inferior surface of the distal vertebra involved; the intersection of these lines produces an angle that defines the severity of the scoliosis). While mild scoliosis is common (incidence, 1 in 1000), respiratory dysfunction is uncommon in these patients and becomes detectable only when the angle is more than 70 degrees (incidence, 1 in 10,000); early cardiopulmonary failure is expected when the angle is more than 120 degrees. Scoliosis is associated with a number of abnormalities in pulmonary function. In patients with a mean angle of 80 degrees and a mean age of 25 years, TLC was 70% of predicted, vital capacity was 61% of predicted, and FRC was 79% of predicted, while RV was normal. Reductions in chest wall compliance and the ventilatory response to hypercapnia are also observed with severe scoliosis. The risk of cardiopulmonary complications appears to be higher in patients whose scoliosis is apparent before the age of 5 years compared with those developing it after the age of 11. In severe cases, the V_D/V_T ratio and $PaCO_2$ increase because of a reduction in tidal volume. Severe oxygen desaturation can occur at night, especially during REM sleep. Pulmonary hypertension and cor pulmonale are well-recognized complications but usually are observed only when the spinal angle is more than 80 degrees. Kinking or compression of the great vessels by the deformed chest wall does not play a role, but the pulmonary hypertension is related to the decreased lung volumes. Hypoxic vasoconstriction is important and lung deflation, causing compression of the pulmonary vascular bed, also may play a role. Controversy exists regarding the value of surgical correction of the scoliosis. Despite the development of fulminant cardiorespiratory failure, medical management, especially employing nighttime mechanical ventilation, can result in remarkable clinical improvement and increased longevity.

ELECTROLYTES AND RESPIRATORY MUSCLE DYSFUNCTION. HYPERKALEMIA AND HYPOKALEMIA

552 What are the electrolyte disturbances responsible for muscle weakness and those that can result in paralysis possibly involving the respiratory muscles?

❑ Multiple electrolyte abnormalities (abnormally high and low levels of K^+, Na^+, Ca^{++}, and Mg^{++} and low phosphate levels) can cause weakness. However, they are more severe with hypokalemia, hypophosphatemia, and hypercalcemia. On the other hand, few electrolyte disturbances cause paralysis that might involve the respiratory muscles, namely, hypokalemia, hyperkalemia, and hypomagnesemia.

553 What are the clinical forms of hyperkalemic skeletal muscle paralysis that might involve the respiratory muscles?

❑ The most common clinical form of hyperkalemic paralysis is the so-called secondary hyperkalemic paralysis, which is a consequence of hyperkalemia of any cause (ie, renal insufficiency, adrenal insufficiency, etc). The other clinical presentation of hyperkalemic paralysis is known as *primary hyperkalemic periodic paralysis.* The primary form is an extremely rare familial disease in which attacks of paresis or paralysis occur in association with potassium efflux from skeletal muscle. Thus, hyperkalemia is induced by an abnormal internal K^+ balance of unknown cause since abnormalities in insulin secretion, glucagon, catecholamines, mineralocorticosteroids, or glucocorticosteroids are not present in this condition; furthermore, during attacks of paralysis, external K^+ balance remains unchanged or even becomes negative.

554 At what elevated level might serum $[K^+]$ lead to paresis or paralysis of respiratory muscles? Provide a practical classification of the severity of hyperkalemia that can be used in patient management.

❑ The following is a clinically useful classification: (1) *mild* hyperkalemia, which includes patients with $[K^+]_p$ between 5.0 and 6.0 mEq/L, and absent or equivocal electrocardiographic (ECG) changes; (2) *moderate* hyperkalemia, which includes patients with $[K^+]_p$ between 6.0 and 7.0 mEq/L and/or definite ECG changes in ventricular repolarization (narrow and tall T waves, also referred to as *peaked T waves*); and (3) *severe* hyperkalemia, which includes patients with $[K^+]_p$ above 7.0 mEq/L and/or severe ECG abnormalities including atrial standstill, advanced atrioventricular heart block, intraventricular block (QRS widening), or ventricular arrhythmias, and/or profound weakness or paralysis of skeletal muscle. Thus, severe hyperkalemia represents a significant risk factor for the development of paresis or paralysis of respiratory muscles that might lead to respiratory failure.

555 Explain the hyperkalemic effects of skeletal muscle relaxants (eg, succinylcholine, suxamethonium).

❑ Because succinylcholine is a muscle relaxant that depolarizes skeletal muscle, increasing potassium permeability of its cells, a modest increment in $[K^+]_p$ occurs in most patients receiving this drug. However, severe hyperkalemia is found in some patients with neuromuscular diseases and those with increased total body potassium stores. Hyperkalemia, occasionally very severe, can occur with the use of skeletal muscle relaxants (depolarizing agents), and is caused by the exit of potassium from skeletal muscle. These agents are administered most frequently in the course of general anesthesia. In most patients, the rise in $[K^+]_p$, when present, is mild and short-lasting.

---

556 Are the neuromuscular effects of potassium depletion and hypokalemia a possible cause of respiratory failure?

❑ Hypokalemia impairs skeletal muscle function, resulting in weakness, cramps, myalgias, myolysis, paresis, and paralysis that might lead to respiratory failure. The skeletal muscle dysfunction can involve the extremities and the torso, including the respiratory muscles. Most commonly, potassium depletion is not the exclusive primary cause of respiratory failure but a cofactor that aggravates this condition in patients with other diseases (eg, myasthenia gravis). Hypokalemia also impairs the function of smooth muscle in the gastrointestinal (eg, gastric atony, ileus) and urinary (bladder atony, urinary retention) systems.

---

557 At what depressed level might serum $[K^+]$ lead to paresis or paralysis of respiratory muscles? Provide a practical classification of the severity of hypokalemia that can be used in patient management.

❑ The following is a clinically useful classification of hypokalemia: (1) *mild* hypokalemia, which includes patients with $[K^+]_p$ between 3.0 and 3.5 mEq/L and absent or equivocal ECG changes; (2) *moderate* hypokalemia, which includes patients with $[K^+]_p$ between 2.0 and 3.0 mEq/L and/or definite ECG changes indicative of hypokalemia; and (3) *severe* hypokalemia, which includes patients with $[K^+]_p$ below 2.0 mEq/L and/or severe ECG changes, and/or profound weakness or paralysis of skeletal muscle. Thus, severe hypokalemia represents a significant risk factor for the development of paresis or paralysis of respiratory muscles that might lead to respiratory failure.

558 A 44-year-old woman was brought to the hospital with progressive weakness and shortness of breath of 4 weeks' duration. Previous history was significant for dry mucous membranes for which a workup yielded a diagnosis of Sjögren's syndrome. Physical examination disclosed a major decrease in muscle strength of all extremities accompanied by reduced deep tendon reflexes. Other abnormalities were not found. Laboratory data were as follows: hematocrit of 48%, plasma creatinine concentration of 1.3 mg/dL, and blood urea nitrogen (BUN) concentration of 20 mg/dL. Serum electrolyte values were as follows: $[Na^+]_p$ of 136 mEq/L, $[K^+]_p$ of 1.7 mEq/L, $[Cl^-]_p$ of 116 mEq/L, total carbon dioxide (TCO_2) of 10 mmol/L, and anion gap of 10 mEq/L. ABG values were as follows:

pH	6.96 ($[H^+]$ 110 ~ nmol/L)
PCO_2	45 mm Hg
PO_2	70 mm Hg

What is the most likely pathogenesis of the progressive weakness and shortness of breath? What is the specific diagnosis of this patient?

❑ The patient's symptoms and findings on physical examination with respect to the neuromuscular system are best explained by hypokalemia due to potassium depletion. Her previous history was negative for a poor dietary potassium intake, gastrointestinal fluid loss, excessive sweating, and medication that can result in high urinary potassium excretion (eg, diuretics). Since the patient did not have previous episodes of muscle weakness or paralysis and laboratory data revealed additional distinct abnormalities, the diagnosis of familial hypokalemic periodic paralysis is ruled out. Consequently, increased renal potassium excretion is the most likely cause of hypokalemia, and the pathogenesis of the clinical syndrome is best explained by a primary renal disease. The overall renal function (glomerular filtration rate [GFR] assessed by the patient's BUN and plasma creatinine levels) was not significantly depressed; however, severe acidemia due to a mixed metabolic acidosis and respiratory acidosis was present. The greatest alteration in the acid-base composition was a decreased $[HCO_3^-]_p$ that was associated with a normal plasma anion gap (normal plasma unmeasured anions), indicating that the decrease in HCO_3^- stores was not the result of titration by an excessive retention of anions (high anion gap metabolic acidosis due to renal failure, ketoacidosis, etc). The patient's hyperchloremic metabolic acidosis was not accompanied by the expected hypocapnia (secondary respiratory response to a primary metabolic acid-base disturbance) since the PCO_2 was in the upper limit of normal; consequently, the acid-base diagnosis is that of a mixed acid-base disturbance in which hyperchloremic metabolic acidosis is accompanied by respiratory acidosis. The respiratory depression is best explained by dysfunction of respiratory muscles, leading to flaccid paresis or paralysis, caused by hypokalemia and potassium depletion. The specific diagnosis that defines the overall clinical syndrome, including the hypokalemia and the severe acid-base disturbance, is a form of renal tubular acidosis.

PULMONARY-RENAL SYNDROMES

559 What is the so-called uremic lung?

❑ *Uremic lung* is a condition characterized by pulmonary edema caused, at least in part, by increased permeability of the alveolar capillary membrane. This entity is associated with normal or mildly elevated pulmonary wedge pressure and responds promptly to dialysis. Patients with uremia might have an abnormal alveolar-gas exchange caused by the combined effects of low-pressure pulmonary edema (uremic lung) and high-pressure pulmonary edema (secondary to circulatory overload associated with fluid retention and extracellular fluid volume expansion). The perihilar vascular congestion of the uremic lung is responsible for the "butterfly wing" distribution observed on radiologic evaluation of the chest.

560 What diseases must be considered in the differential diagnosis of pulmonary-renal syndromes?

❑ The pulmonary-renal syndromes can be caused by a wide variety of conditions that include Goodpasture's syndrome, Wegener's granulomatosis, systemic vasculitis, polyarteritis nodosa, systemic lupus erythematosus, and uremia associated with pulmonary edema (eg, uremic lung). The differential diagnosis of the pulmonary-renal syndromes requires a comprehensive evaluation of the patient's history, physical examination, and laboratory data, including in many instances the performance of pulmonary and renal biopsy. The presence of a pulmonary-renal syndrome is always indicative of a serious disease that can lead to death or permanent organ damage secondary to respiratory and renal failure.

561 What is Goodpasture's syndrome?

❑ *Goodpasture's syndrome* is a condition characterized by the acute development of a severe disease involving the lung and the kidney (ie, a pulmonary-renal syndrome) that can lead to death or permanent organ damage secondary to respiratory and renal failure. The patients most commonly afflicted are young men who present with hemoptysis, caused by a diffuse hemorrhagic pneumonitis, followed by evidence of acute glomerulonephritis (eg, hematuria, edema, hypertension). Antibodies against the basement membrane of the lung and glomeruli (ie, anti–glomerular basement membrane [GBM] antibodies) can be demonstrated in serum and biopsy samples (lung and kidney). Immunofluorescent staining of biopsy specimens may exhibit IgG deposition in a characteristic linear pattern.

HYPERVENTILATION SYNDROME

562 How common is the hyperventilation syndrome of functional origin? What is the underlying mechanism?

❑ The *hyperventilation syndrome* (of functional origin) is a unique form of dyspnea affecting 6% to 11% of the general population. The basic mechanisms responsible for initiating and sustaining the hyperventilation syndrome are unknown. Although stressful situations disturb the pattern of breathing in normal subjects, it is unclear whether the response of patients with the hyperventilation syndrome is qualitatively or only quantitatively different from that occurring in normal subjects. It has been suggested that the hyperventilation syndrome reflects an overresponsivity of the respiratory system to stress, and indeed, patients with a chronic anxiety state have elevated respiratory drive. The respiratory centers of patients with hyperventilation syndrome also appear to have a hypocapnic "set-point" since they reestablish the previous hypocapnic set-point within 5 minutes of breathing room air following normalization of PCO_2 using carbon dioxide–enriched gas mixtures. Furthermore, patients display an increase in end-tidal carbon dioxide pressure ($P_{ET}CO_2$) of 12 mm Hg during sleep, but hypocapnia recurs within 1 hour of awakening. It must be recognized that it is remarkably easy to maintain hypocapnia once it has been established, only requiring an occasional deep sigh to be superimposed on a normal breathing pattern, since a single deep inspiration and expiration can lower $PaCO_2$ by 7 to 16 mm Hg.

563 What are the causes of the hyperventilation syndrome? Name common organic causes of this syndrome.

❑ Multiple causes of functional and organic origin are responsible for the development of the hyperventilation syndrome. One of them is psychogenic hyperventilation, a functional condition that is almost invariably attributed to anxiety. However, many of such patients do not have a detectable psychiatric disorder. Organic causes of hyperventilation include neurologic disorders, salicylate intoxication, hepatic failure, severe pain, asthma, interstitial lung disease, and pulmonary vascular disease.

564 What signs and symptoms are observed in patients with the hyperventilation syndrome?

❑ Dyspnea is observed in 50% to 90% of patients with the hyperventilation syndrome. Characteristically, these patients explain the dyspnea as "a sense of being unable to take a deep enough breath" (air hunger) or a sense of suffocation or oppression in the chest. Unlike the dyspnea of patients with cardiovascular or pulmonary disease, this form of dyspnea has a less clear-cut relationship to exercise and is less likely to improve with rest. Indeed, it may actually develop shortly after activity has ceased rather than during it. Chest pain is frequently a presenting symptom and it may mimic angina pectoris. Tetany is an uncommon feature, despite statements to the contrary. It has long been recognized that patients with the hyperventilation syndrome have an increased frequency of sighings, up to 100 sighs/hr in patients with a chronic anxiety state, whereas normal subjects only take up to 4 sighs/hr.

565 What are the clinical manifestations of respiratory alkalosis? How important is alkalemia in the severity of the signs and symptoms?

❑ The symptoms and signs of primary hypocapnia frequently occur in the acute phase, but they are seldom evident in chronic respiratory alkalosis. Manifestations such as numbness and paresthesias of the extremities, chest oppression, circumoral numbness, light-headedness, and mental confusion might develop in any situation in which a rapid decrement in $PaCO_2$ occurs to levels half-normal or lower. Less frequently, other manifestations might develop, including muscle cramps, increased deep tendon reflexes, carpopedal spasm, and generalized seizures. Since blood pH levels do not exceed 7.55 in most patients with primary hypocapnia, severe manifestations of decreased systemic acidity are usually absent. Severe alkalemia, however, might be produced, especially with maladjusted ventilators, with some psychiatric conditions, and with lesions involving the CNS.

566 Does the diagnosis of respiratory alkalosis always require that $PaCO_2$ levels be lower than normal?

❑ No. Although the level of $PaCO_2$ is lower than 35 mm Hg in patients with simple respiratory alkalosis who are at rest and at sea level, higher levels might be observed in special circumstances. For example, the presence of an element of respiratory alkalosis might still be recognized at higher levels of $PaCO_2$ in patients with metabolic alkalosis in whom a normal $PaCO_2$ is inappropriately low for this primary metabolic disorder.

Part IV: Management of Respiratory Failure

21. Oxygen Therapy

PRINCIPLES OF OXYGEN THERAPY

567 How should oxygen be administered and what level of PaO_2 is desired in the management of hypoxemic respiratory failure?

❑ Oxygen should be administered by the simplest method and at the lowest inspired fraction (FiO_2) that gives the desired results in patients with hypoxemic respiratory failure. A PaO_2 of 60 mm Hg is a desirable level because it achieves approximately a 90% hemoglobin saturation. Higher PaO_2 adds little to oxygenation and is associated with a risk of oxygen toxicity to the lung if it requires a high FiO_2. Administration of oxygen can be accomplished by soft nasal prongs, simple face masks, and face masks with inspiratory reservoir bags. If the previous measures fail to provide adequate oxygenation, mechanical ventilation should be instituted.

568 What FiO_2 is advisable to prescribe in patients with hypoxemia?

❑ One should always be mindful of the risk of oxygen toxicity, which increases as a function of the level of FiO_2 and the duration of exposure. As a rule, the lowest possible FiO_2 (preferably $<60\%$) that achieves the desired hemoglobin saturation should be used, and supplemental oxygen should be withdrawn when the risk of hypoxemia has passed.

569 Explain further the rationale for the recommendation of maintaining a PaO_2 of about 60 mm Hg during oxygen therapy.

❑ Since a PaO_2 of 58 mm Hg achieves a SaO_2 of 90%, maintaining a PaO_2 of about 60 mm Hg will secure an adequate SaO_2. However, a decrease in PO_2 significantly below 60 mm Hg substantially reduces the oxygen content of blood as the oxyhemoglobin dissociation curve becomes steep below this PO_2 level. Consequently, efforts should be made to maintain PaO_2 at about 60 mm Hg during oxygen therapy.

570 How is the FiO_2 selected for use in mechanical ventilation? Is the response to a high FiO_2 independent of the underlying disease?

❑ Many predictive equations have been created to aid in the selection of a satisfactory FiO_2, but none is sufficiently accurate to substitute for a trial-and-error approach. The FiO_2 is deliberately set at a high value (often 1.0) to ensure adequate oxygenation, and is adjusted depending on the results of arterial blood gas (ABG) analysis performed after 20 minutes. Generally, a PaO_2 of 60 to 90 mm Hg is sought, as this PO_2 achieves near maximum oxygen saturation. The response to a change in FiO_2 depends on the underlying pathophysiology, because shunt responds less well to increased FiO_2 than hypoventilation or $\dot{V}A/\dot{Q}$ mismatch.

571 What are the guidelines with respect to both the level of FiO_2 and the application of positive end-expiratory pressure (PEEP) in patients receiving mechanical ventilation? How does PEEP improve oxygenation?

❑ Using the lowest FiO_2 that achieves a PaO_2 of 60 mm Hg is recommended. If the PaO_2 is higher than 60 mm Hg, the FiO_2 should be decreased accordingly. Addition of PEEP may help to improve oxygenation by opening previously closed alveoli due to the larger lung volume that results from the application of this therapeutic modality. PEEP should be added to patients in whom the FiO_2 cannot be lowered to or below 0.6 (therefore allowing a decrease of the FiO_2 below the toxic range).

572 How is oxygen administered to patients with acute hypercapnic respiratory failure?

❑ Adequate oxygen delivery is critical while a competent airway is being restored in a patient with acute respiratory failure.

In patients with airway obstruction caused by a foreign body, if its removal is not feasible immediately and if the patient's condition is critical, translaryngeal oxygenation, "jet ventilation," or cricothyrotomy should be performed. If the patient is in a coma, severely obtunded, extremely hypercapnic ($PaCO_2$ >80 mm Hg), or severely acidemic (blood pH <7.10) because of respiratory failure, assisted ventilation should be initiated promptly. If none of these conditions is in effect, and if the patient has stable cardiovascular status, oxygen can be delivered by mask, nasal cannula, or nasal prongs. As a general rule, however, mechanical ventilation should be employed if conservative therapy fails to correct hypoxemia and hypercapnia promptly. High inspired oxygen tension should be provided to all patients with acute respiratory acidosis. Indeed, maximal PaO_2 levels must be ensured for those found apneic, in cardiac arrest, or unconscious from carbon monoxide poisoning. An oxygen flow at 6 L/min delivered by mask or nasal cannula is appropriate under such circumstances. For less critically ill patients, nasal prongs offer advantages in comparison with masks, because they can be left in place while the patient coughs up secretions, eats, or drinks. The use of PEEP or continuous positive airway pressure (CPAP) can enhance the effect of a given level of oxygen administration in patients with acute respiratory distress syndrome (ARDS), atelectasis, pulmonary edema, or other diffuse pulmonary diseases.

573 What are the main indications for supplemental oxygen administration in patients with cardiorespiratory failure?

❑ Administration of supplemental oxygen in patients with cardiorespiratory failure is of significant therapeutic value in the following conditions: (1) pulmonary edema due to heart failure as well as that secondary to noncardiac conditions (eg, fluid overload); (2) heart failure precipitated by pulmonary infection or infarction; (3) decompensated cor pulmonale with significant hypoxemia, which worsens pulmonary hypertension; (4) heart failure due to any cause that is accompanied by SaO_2 below

90%; and (5) acute myocardial infarction accompanied by hypoxemia (ie, $PaO_2 \leq 60$ mm Hg), in the initial 24 to 48 hours.

574 Might oxygen supplementation be harmful to patients with heart failure? What is the role of oxygen administration at night in patients with severe heart failure?

❑ Yes. Oxygen supplementation to patients without arterial hypoxemia or in the absence of significant tissue hypoxia due to heart failure might increase systemic vascular resistance and blood pressure (thereby augmenting left ventricular afterload), leading to a slight reduction in cardiac output. Tissue oxygen delivery does not significantly increase by augmenting the fraction of oxygen in the inspired air in the absence of arterial hypoxemia. In addition, FiO_2 of 60% or higher has the potential for inducing oxygen toxicity in any patient, independent of the presence of heart failure. Thus, oxygen supplementation should be prescribed when the potential advantages outweigh disadvantages. Hypoxemia, especially during sleep, is relatively common with severe heart failure. Such blood gas abnormality is generally secondary to the combined effects of pulmonary edema and Cheyne-Stokes respiration.

575 What are the indications of hyperbaric oxygen therapy?

❑ Decompression sickness represents the only condition in which the efficacy of hyperbaric oxygen therapy has been rigorously established. Other indications of hyperbaric oxygen therapy include intravascular air embolism, carbon monoxide poisoning, gas gangrene, osteomyelitis, radiation necrosis, cyanide poisoning, wound healing, burns, selected infections, severe anemia, and cerebral edema.

MODES OF OXYGEN DELIVERY

576 How should supplemental oxygen be administered?

❑ The method for supplemental oxygen delivery depends on whether the patient breathes spontaneously, is apneic, or is already undergoing mechanical ventilation. Supplemental oxygen might be satisfactorily administered to most patients breathing spontaneously by delivering 2 to 4 L of oxygen per minute by facial mask or nasal prongs or catheters. A higher administration rate might be used if the previous regimen fails to correct arterial hypoxemia. Oxygen-rich mixtures might be provided with mechanically controlled ventilation after endotracheal intubation in patients with severe pulmonary edema refractory to more conservative measures or depression of spontaneous respiration (eg, drug overdose, cerebrovascular accident). Application of PEEP might further improve the patient's oxygenation (see pertinent questions).

577 Explain the use of simple masks for oxygen delivery.

❑ Simple masks consist of a cone-shaped piece that fits over the patient's nose and mouth. It has open ports on each side for exhalation; air will be entrained through these ports if the patient's inspiratory flow exceeds the flow of oxygen into the mask. The cone of the mask acts as a reservoir and predisposes to carbon dioxide rebreathing. To minimize this risk, oxygen flow rates of 5 L/min or higher are employed, thus making the simple mask unsuitable to deliver a low FiO_2. The delivered FiO_2 is approximately 35% to 50% with oxygen flow rates of 5 to 10 L/min but varies greatly with the breathing pattern. Unlike nasal cannulae, masks must be removed when patients are eating or receiving airway care.

578 What is a partial-rebreathing mask?

❑ The face piece of a partial-rebreathing mask is similar to that of a simple mask except that it has an attached reservoir bag. When the patient inhales, gas is drawn from the mask, the reservoir bag, and potentially, room air through the exhalation ports. On expiration, the initial third of the exhaled gas (which has a high oxygen but low carbon dioxide concentration) enters the bag. Provided the oxygen flow rate is adjusted to prevent collapse of the reservoir bag during inspiration, an FiO_2 of up to 60% can be delivered.

579 What is a nonrebreathing mask?

❑ The structure of this mask is similar to that of the partial-rebreathing mask, except that it has two valve attachments. One set of valves is at the exhalation ports to prevent entrainment of room air during inspiration but permit the escape of gas during exhalation. Another valve, located between the mask and the reservoir bag, permits gas to enter the mask from the bag but prevents gas flowing from the mask to the bag during exhalation. With a snug fit and adjustment of the oxygen flow rate to prevent the bag from collapsing on inspiration, an FiO_2 of almost 1.0 can be delivered. This may be difficult to achieve in critically ill patients, and the FiO_2 may be considerably lower than 1.0 (commonly no higher than 0.7). The rebreathing mask is used almost exclusively in the delivery of anesthesia.

580 What is an air-entrainment (''Venturi'') mask?

❑ The Venturi mask operates on the Bernoulli principle whereby a jet of gas creates a low, lateral pressure that entrains air. A precise FiO_2 can be obtained by controlling the size of the jet or the air entrainment port, provided that the total flow of gas from the unit exceeds the patient's peak inspiratory flow. A minimum oxygen flow rate of 4 L/min is needed to deliver 24% oxygen and 6 L/min to deliver 28% oxygen. Masks designed to deliver 32% to 35% oxygen do not provide a predictable FiO_2 at the trachea because of an inadequate total flow rate.

581 Explain the use of nasal cannulae for oxygen delivery.

❑ Supplemental oxygen is most commonly delivered by nasal cannulae as they are simple to use, relatively comfortable, and inexpensive. They provide an FiO_2 of 24% to 50% with flow rates up to 6 L/min (the usual rate of delivery is 1 to 4 L/min). At low flow rates, there is no need for routine humidification, but with prolonged use, especially at high flow rates, local irritation and drying of the mucous membranes may develop.

582 What are the effects on arterial oxygen levels of the various modes of delivery of supplemental oxygen?

❑ When oxygen is delivered by nasal cannulae or a face mask, the actual FiO_2 delivered to the trachea is frequently unpredictable because it is dependent on the rate of oxygen administration, the size of the oxygen reservoir, and the patient's inspiratory flow rate. For example, when oxygen is supplied at 1 L/min to a patient who is breathing 10 L/min, the resulting FiO_2 is approximately 0.28, that is, $FiO_2 = [1 + (0.21 \times 10)]/11 = 0.282$. While a number of predictive equations have been created to aid with the selection of an optimal FiO_2, none is sufficiently accurate to replace a trial-and-error approach. The response to an increase in FiO_2 depends on the pathophysiologic mechanism responsible for the hypoxemia. In patients with hypoxemia secondary to a $\dot{V}A/\dot{Q}$ mismatch, small increases in FiO_2 cause significant improvement in PaO_2. With a large shunt (50% of the cardiac output), an increase in FiO_2, even to 1.0, causes virtually no increase in PaO_2. In patients who suddenly deteriorate, the FiO_2 is initially set at a very high value, often 1.0, to ensure adequate oxygenation. An ABG sample is obtained after a 20- to 30-minute period, and the FiO_2 is adjusted according to the patient's PaO_2. Patients with hypoxemia of more gradual onset can be managed in a more controlled manner with lower levels of FiO_2.

RISKS OF OXYGEN THERAPY. OXYGEN TOXICITY

583 Elaborate on the risks of ventilatory depression resulting from oxygen therapy. Is this problem limited to patients with chronic obstructive lung disease (COPD)?

❑ Patients with severe hypercapnia and neurologic stupor (carbon dioxide narcosis) as a consequence of injudicious oxygen therapy continue to be admitted to intensive care units. It has been estimated that in approximately 90% of patients with COPD, severe hypercapnia develops when oxygen is administered in an uncontrolled manner, and about 30% rapidly become unconscious. When oxygen is administered in a controlled manner, the increase in $PaCO_2$ is usually slight, about 1 to 5 mm Hg for a 10 mm Hg increase in PaO_2, but the increase is much larger in some patients. Although oxygen-induced hypercapnia has been associated mostly with COPD, other conditions including neuromuscular diseases are also predisposed to develop ventilatory depression with oxygen therapy.

584 Explain the management of ventilatory depression resulting from oxygen therapy. Is discontinuation of oxygen therapy the best measure to correct oxygen-induced hypercapnia?

❑ Clinicians should focus on the patient's PaO_2 rather than the $PaCO_2$ in the management of oxygen-induced hypercapnia. An increase in $PaCO_2$ of only 3 to 4 mm Hg can produce appreciable respiratory discomfort under conditions of constant mechanical ventilation, whereas similar increases are not distressing during spontaneous ventilation. Indeed, patients can tolerate remarkably high $PaCO_2$ values (eg, 250 mm Hg) without serious sequelae (but could be very uncomfortable), provided they do not have hypoxemia. Clearly, oxygen therapy can precipitate carbon dioxide narcosis, but withdrawing supplemental oxygen completely is a mistake that unfortunately is sometimes made. Instead of total withdrawal of oxygen therapy, every effort should be made to improve the patient's respiratory status. In patients with COPD, such efforts include the use of bronchodilator therapy and assistance with clearance of secretions. Unfortunately, there are no pharmacologic agents that will achieve a satisfactory improvement in neuromuscular performance in patients with neuromuscular disease.

585 What is oxygen toxicity?

❑ *Oxygen toxicity* is an iatrogenic condition caused by prolonged administration of supplemental oxygen at high concentration. This entity is characterized by an initial acute exudative phase and a late chronic proliferative phase. Manifestations of oxygen toxicity include an increased alveolar-arterial oxygen (P_{A}-aO_2) gradient, interstitial and alveolar edema, and depression of several parameters of respiratory function including vital capacity, diffusion capacity, and lung compliance.

586 Explain further the risks of oxygen toxicity and when might these toxic effects develop.

❑ Administration of a high FiO_2 might cause a number of disturbances including tracheobronchitis, decreased ciliary motility, impaired macrophage function, and lung injury resembling that associated with ARDS. Exposure to an FiO_2 of 1.0 (ie, pure oxygen) for up to 24 hours does not pose a significant clinical risk, although prolonged exposure to this concentration is clearly toxic. An FiO_2 of 0.5 is generally considered safe for several weeks if necessary in the management of hypoxemia. For FiO_2 values between 0.5 and 1.0, the duration of safe exposure before the onset of toxicity is unknown, but there is more to fear from severe hypoxemia in critically ill patients than the potential threat of oxygen toxicity.

587 How can oxygen toxicity be prevented?

❑ Oxygen toxicity can be prevented with the use of the lowest possible oxygen concentration in the patient's inspired mixture needed to achieve and maintain a PaO_2 just over 60 mm Hg. Oxygen therapy that increases PaO_2 to higher levels does not significantly augment the oxygen content of the blood and increases the risk of oxygen toxicity.

22. Artificial Airways

TYPES

588 Explain the various measures to establish a patent airway in a patient with acute hypercapnic respiratory failure or at risk of developing this condition. What is the Heimlich maneuver?

❑ In a comatose patient, hypopharyngeal obstruction is commonly observed due to backward positioning of the mandible and tongue, and the possible presence of dentures, foreign bodies, food particles, vomitus, or secretions. Restoration of a patent airway can often be accomplished by positioning the patient on the side, hyperextending the head, displacing the mandible forward, and cleaning the oropharyngeal content manually or by suction. Acute asphyxiation from aspiration of a foreign body should be treated by subdiaphragmatic abdominal thrust (the Heimlich maneuver). At times, laryngoscopy or bronchoscopy might be required, particularly if the obstruction is in the lower portion of the upper airway. In an apneic patient, ventilation must be immediately restored by either mouth-to-mouth breathing or the use of mechanical devices of pharyngeal intubation. Tracheal intubation should be performed at the earliest possible time, for it isolates the airway, minimizes the risk of aspiration, and facilitates oxygenation, ventilation, and removal of secretions. Although a tracheotomy is the most reliable way of securing an adequate airway, it has limited indications and should not be attempted by untrained persons.

589 What artificial airways are interposed between the patient and the mechanical device when ventilatory support is provided? Name the short-term and long-term devices and compare their properties.

❑ Tracheal tubes inserted through the nasal or oral routes are used in most patients at the initiation of mechanical ventilation. Tracheotomy, the other alternative to create an artificial airway, is commonly performed if ventilator support is anticipated to be required for a prolonged period. The latter technique improves patient's comfort and provides a more secure airway allowing chronic ventilation at home or in a long-term care facility. Either type of artificial airway requires the use of cuffs for the application of positive-pressure ventilation. The overall rate of complications of tracheotomy is comparable to that of endotracheal tube placement.

---

590 Compare nasal and oral placement of an endotracheal tube (cannulation).

❑ Endotracheal intubation can be performed through the nose or the mouth. Nasal intubation is usually performed by a blind technique without the use of a laryngoscope. As such there may be less of a tendency to gag or vomit, and it can be performed in patients with cervical injury when manipulation of the neck is prohibited. However, the diameter of a nasal endotracheal tube is usually less than that of an oral tube, which causes increased resistance and work of breathing during spontaneous respiration. The small diameter combined with an increased angle of curvature increases the difficulty of suctioning or performing bedside fiberoptic bronchoscopy in a patient with a nasal endotracheal tube. The larger diameter of an oral endotracheal tube circumvents these problems and also has the advantage of avoiding nasal, sinus, and eustachian tube complications. However, fixation of an oral tube is more difficult, and the position needs to be changed from side to side at least daily to limit local pressure complications.

---

591 Compare the resistance to airflow of normal airways to that of endotracheal tubes of different sizes.

❑ Normal airway resistance is usually less than 2 cm H_2O/L/sec but endotracheal tubes have considerable higher airflow resistance. The resistance of endotracheal tubes is approximately 20,

10, and 6 cm H_2O/L/sec for tube sizes 6, 7, and 8, respectively. As expected, a large tube has less airflow resistance than a small one.

592 What is the effect of intubation on the humidity of inspired air? How is humidity and temperature of inspired gas maintained in this condition?

❑ Once the patient is intubated, the abilities to humidify and warm up the inspired gases and to cough are compromised; thus these functions must be replaced. The inspired gas temperature should be maintained at 34 to 37°C and the relative humidity at 100%. Whereas inspired air usually contains 10 mg of water per liter and its relative humidity is 50%, it contains about 43 mg of water per liter after it has reached the small airways. The water spent to humidify the inspired gas amounts to 300 to 600 mL in 24 hours. Proper humidification of the inspired gas prevents this insensible water loss so that fluid therapy should take into consideration the decreased requirement for water. Furthermore, excessive humidification that results from ultrasonic nebulization of the inspired air, especially in children, might cause significant positive fluid balance.

593 When should tracheotomy be performed in patients receiving mechanical ventilation? What are the advantages of a tracheotomy in comparison to laryngeal intubation?

❑ The optimal timing of a tracheotomy is a subject of controversy. The indication to perform a tracheotomy should be individualized and not undertaken simply because an endotracheal tube has been in place for a certain time. If prolonged ventilator support is anticipated, a tracheotomy should be considered early in the patient's course because this access to the airway is more comfortable than a laryngeal tube and facilitates oral hygiene and nutrition.

594 What are the techniques of surgical airway access?

❑ The techniques of surgical airway access are (1) standard tracheotomy (ie, it provides temporary tracheal access through an incision that enters the trachea between the cartilaginous rings), (2) percutaneous tracheotomy (procedure relatively simple and fast, performed in the intensive care unit), (3) cricothyroidotomy (ie, placement of a tracheal airway through the cricothyroid space), and (4) minitracheotomy (ie, insertion of a 4-mm tube that accommodates a 10F suction catheter). Cricothyroidotomy is the preferred procedure for placement of an emergency airway in patients who cannot undergo translaryngeal intubation.

COMPLICATIONS

595 What are the main diagnostic features of intubation of the right main bronchus, kinking of the endotracheal tube, bronchospasm and mucus plugging, pulmonary embolism, and pulmonary edema in a patient receiving mechanical ventilation?

❑ The corresponding diagnostic features for these conditions are as follows: (1) Intubation of the right main bronchus produces decreased air entry over the left lung, increased plateau pressure caused by diminished thoracic compliance, and hypoxemia; (2) kinking of the endotracheal tube leads to increased peak pressure and a higher gradient between peak and plateau levels of airway pressure; (3) bronchospasm and mucus plugging cause diffuse wheezing over both lung fields, increased peak pressure, and a higher gradient between peak and plateau levels of airway pressure; (4) pulmonary embolism is characterized by hypoxemia without changes in peak and plateau airway pressure; and (5) pulmonary edema produces diffuse rales over both lung fields, increased plateau pressure, and hypoxemia.

596 Is laryngeal injury commonly observed as a complication of airway intubation? How might the risk of laryngeal injury be reduced?

❑ Laryngeal ulceration occurs in almost all patients receiving endotracheal intubation. Damage is most severe in the posterior region, because most pressure is applied on this area as a result of the shapes of the tube, glottis, and spine. The risk of serious damage increases with the diameter of the tube and length of time that the patient is intubated. The laryngeal injury is usually transient, and most ulcers heal spontaneously. Chronic damage of the airway including obstruction (usually caused by granuloma formation) occurs in less than 3% of patients. Because intubation can cause multiple and sometimes serious complications, it should be done under controlled conditions by an experienced physician.

597 How commonly does intubation of a main-stem bronchus occur? What are its causes and consequences?

❑ Intubation of a main-stem bronchus occurs in up to 10% of patients and is the result of improper placement of the tube, inadequate external fixation, and excessive neck movement (ie, neck flexion causes a 2-cm displacement toward the carina). Atelectasis occurs in the contralateral lung (most commonly the left lung because of intubation of main-stem right bronchus) and is typically associated with a decrease in breath sounds. However, auscultation is unreliable in up to 60% of patients and a chest roentgenogram should be always obtained to confirm the position of the tube. The tube tip should be positioned at 3 to 4 cm from both the carina and cords, usually between vertebral bodies T2 and T4.

598 What is the rate of complications involving the endotracheal tube? Explain these complications.

❑ Almost two-thirds of all intubations performed in the intensive care unit are associated with some complication. Placement of an endotracheal tube can cause tooth avulsion (oral tube), nasal bleeding (nasal tube), pharyngeal perforation, vocal cord hematoma, pulmonary aspiration, arrhythmias, or cardiac arrest. While the tube is in place, laryngeal injury with posterior glottic ulceration, laryngeal hematoma, or subglottic stenosis can occur, but most of those lesions heal spontaneously and serious sequelae are uncommon. The cuff can cause tracheal mucosal ulcers, tracheal dilation, or (rarely) tracheoesophageal fistula or tracheal rupture. An additional problem posed by the tube in place is the increase in airway resistance, which is primarily related to tube diameter and the corresponding airflow rates. Although this is of little importance during assist-control (AC) or controlled mechanical ventilation (CMV), it becomes critical during spontaneous breathing or intermittent mandatory ventilation. Problems after extubation include laryngeal incompetence with aspiration, stridor, laryngeal granulomas, and stenosis, tracheal stenosis, and tracheomalacia (usually mild). To minimize the risk of complications, only tubes with high-volume, low-pressure cuffs should be used, and the cuff pressure should be monitored to ensure that the lowest pressure necessary to seal the airway is being used.

---

599 Enumerate the complications associated with endotracheal intubation according to the time of their development.

❑ The complications that can develop as a result of endotracheal intubation are conveniently classified as occurring (1) during placement (ie, tooth avulsion, nasal bleeding, pharyngeal perforation, cord hematoma, and aspiration), (2) while in situ (ie, posterior glottic ulcer, laryngeal hematoma, subglottic stenosis, tracheal dilation, tracheoesophageal fistula, cuff herniation, bronchial intubation, sinusitis/otitis, and increased work of breathing), and (3) following extubation (ie, stridor, laryngeal granuloma, laryngeal stenosis, tracheal stenosis, and tracheomalacia).

600 How common is sinusitis as a complication of airway intubation? Is the risk of sinusitis similar in patients receiving intubation with a nasal tube and those receiving it with an oral tube?

❑ Forty-two percent of patients intubated with a nasal tube and only 6% of those intubated with an oral tube for more than 5 days have been found to have sinusitis. Therefore, nasal intubation represents a significant risk factor for the development of sinusitis of bacterial origin.

601 Explain the importance of cuff pressure with respect to endotracheal tube complications.

❑ When the pressure in the cuff of a tracheal tube exceeds the critical pressure for perfusion of the tracheal mucosa (about 25 mm Hg), serious injury of this structure becomes likely. To minimize the risk of ischemic injury, the lowest possible cuff pressure needed to achieve a seal should be used (preferably <15 mm Hg).

602 What type of cuff can reduce tracheal damage associated with mechanical ventilation? Describe the high-volume ''floppy'' cuff.

❑ The high-volume floppy cuff inflated just enough to prevent any leak (ie, minimal occlusion technique) or allowing a leak of only about 50 mL (ie, minimal leak technique) during inspiration helps to reduce tracheal wall damage at the cuff site.

603 Elaborate on the complications arising from tracheotomy tubes. Should performance of a tracheotomy be delayed after 2 weeks of endotracheal intubation?

❑ Tracheotomy complications can be observed (1) during surgery (eg, hemorrhage, subcutaneous emphysema, pneumothorax), (2) while the tracheotomy cannula is in situ (eg, stomal infection and bleeding, cuff problems, innominate artery rupture and fistula), and (3) following extubation (eg, decannulation difficulty, tracheal stenosis, tracheal granuloma, tracheomalacia). Complications that can develop with a tracheotomy are generally more serious than those with endotracheal intubation; they include stomal infection and bleeding, innominate artery perforation and fistula, cuff complications similar to those with an endotracheal tube, and stomal-site tracheal stenosis following decannulation. A tracheotomy should not be performed simply because an endotracheal tube has been in place a certain number of days. Endotracheal tubes are satisfactorily tolerated for up to 3 weeks or longer, but if mechanical ventilation is likely to be required for a long period of time, tracheotomy should be considered early in the course because it aids in long-term airway management.

604 Explain further the complications of a tracheotomy.

❑ A serious complication of a tracheotomy is innominate artery rupture, which occurs in less than 0.5% of patients and has a mortality of approximately 90%. Other important complications include the development of tracheal stenosis occurring at two different sites. Stenosis can develop at the site of the tracheal tube cuff because pressure within the tracheal tube cuff exceeds the critical pressure for perfusion of the tracheal mucosa (25 mm Hg). This injury, which is also frequently observed with endotracheal intubation, has become less common with the use of high-volume, low-pressure cuffs and frequent monitoring of intracuff pressure. Stenosis can also occur at the site of the tracheotomy stoma because of excessive traction.

23. Mechanical Ventilation

GOALS, INDICATIONS, AND CARE OF PATIENTS

605 What are the main types of ventilator support?

❑ Mechanical ventilation can be performed with either positive-pressure ventilators (ie, lung inflation is caused by positive inspiratory airway pressure) or negative-pressure ventilators (ie, lung inflation is caused by the application of subatmospheric pressure outside the chest cavity, resembling the changes in pleural and alveolar pressures of spontaneous respiration). There are multiple models of positive- and negative-pressure ventilators that are tailored to satisfy the specific needs of patients with respiratory failure. In a modern intensive care unit, negative-pressure ventilators are rarely if ever used.

606 Name the major goals of ventilatory support (ie, mechanical ventilation).

❑ The major goals of mechanical ventilation are to correct severe respiratory failure unresponsive to conservative measures, relieve respiratory distress, decrease the oxygen cost of breathing, improve pulmonary gas exchange, reverse respiratory muscle fatigue, enable the lungs to heal, and avoid complications. In addition, mechanical ventilation is to secure adequate oxygenation and carbon dioxide removal, as safely and comfortably as possible, while the patient's underlying condition resolves spontaneously or responds favorably to treatment.

607 Enumerate the objectives of mechanical ventilation.

❑ The objectives of mechanical ventilation are to (1) improve pulmonary gas exchange (ie, reverse hypoxemia, relieve acute respiratory acidosis), (2) mitigate respiratory distress (ie, decrease oxygen cost of breathing, reverse respiratory muscle fatigue), (3) correct pressure-volume abnormalities (ie, prevent and reverse atelectasis, improve pulmonary compliance, reduce further lung injury), (4) permit lung and airway healing, and (5) avoid complications derived from or associated with respiratory failure.

608 Elaborate further on the objectives and limitations of mechanical ventilation. How important is it to avoid high inflation pressures?

❑ Mechanical ventilation can be lifesaving in patients with acute severe hypoxemia or worsening respiratory acidosis (or both) that is refractory to more conservative measures. In patients with severe cardiopulmonary distress for whom the effort of breathing is intolerable, mechanical ventilation substitutes for the action of the respiratory muscles (in some patients the respiratory muscles account for as much as 5% of total oxygen consumption). In such circumstances, mechanical ventilation allows precious stores of oxygen to be rerouted to other tissue beds that may be vulnerable. In addition, the reversal of respiratory muscle fatigue, which may have a role in the development of acute ventilatory failure, depends on adequate rest of the respiratory muscles. Positive-pressure ventilation can reverse and prevent atelectasis, and by allowing inspiration at a more compliant region of the pulmonary pressure-volume curve, it can decrease the working of breathing. Improvements in pulmonary gas exchange and pressure-volume relations and relief from excessive respiratory work provide an opportunity for the lungs and airways to heal. However, positive-pressure ventilation can also decrease cardiac output and initiate or aggravate alveolar damage. The dangers of ventilator-induced lung injury have led to a reappraisal of the objectives of mechanical ventilation. Rather than strive for normal ABG values, it is probably better to accept a certain degree of respiratory acidosis, and possibly even hypoxemia, to avoid high inflation pressures. Likewise, it may be better to risk oxygen toxicity than to use high pressures to achieve a decrease in the FiO_2.

609 What elements might help decide initiation of mechanical ventilation in the absence of respiratory arrest?

❑ If apnea is present, the need for immediate initiation of mechanical ventilation is obvious. In the absence of respiratory arrest, the indication of mechanical ventilation is based on recognizing the presence of inadequate ventilatory effort, or substantial hypoxemia and hypercapnia unresponsive to conservative measures.

610 Enumerate specific conditions that require immediate application of mechanical ventilation.

❑ Mechanical ventilation must be initiated in all patients presenting with clinical or laboratory evidence of severe respiratory failure, actual or imminent. Consequently, the indications include (1) apnea or respiratory arrest (eg, spontaneous, secondary to administration of paralyzing drugs), (2) progressive worsening of ABG levels with severe hypercapnic encephalopathy (eg, coma), and (3) severe hypoxemia unresponsive to other therapeutic measures.

611 What is the rationale to initiate mechanical ventilation in patients with hypoxemic respiratory failure without hypercapnia?

❑ The rationale supporting the use of mechanical ventilation in patients with hypoxemic respiratory failure without hypercapnia is to improve oxygenation by opening previously closed airways (recruitment of alveoli) as a result of the increase in lung volume obtained with this treatment. Thus, application of mechanical ventilation in this condition is not intended to increase alveolar ventilation but to augment mean lung volume.

612 What are the effects of mechanical ventilation on hypoxemia caused by inefficient gas exchange?

❑ Inefficient gas exchange with resulting hypoxemia is usually secondary to $\dot{V}_A/\dot{Q}$ mismatch or a right-to-left intrapulmonary shunt. In contrast to hypercapnic acidosis caused by ventilatory pump failure, hypoxemia is a less clearly defined indication for mechanical ventilation, because it can frequently be corrected by more conservative measures, such as supplemental oxygen. In the presence of a $\dot{V}_A/\dot{Q}$ inequality (eg, obstructive or infiltrative lung diseases), mechanical ventilation has a variable effect on hypoxemia as it may either improve or worsen the $\dot{V}_A/\dot{Q}$ mismatch. Mechanical ventilation is usually indicated in this setting to maintain adequate $\dot{V}_E$ and prevent hypercapnia, and impaired oxygenation is corrected by increasing the FiO_2. Conversely, in the presence of hypoxemia secondary to a nonanatomic shunt (eg, cardiogenic or noncardiogenic pulmonary edema), mechanical ventilation is beneficial because it recruits previously collapsed or fluid-filled lung units.

613 Provide commonly observed examples of respiratory failure caused by an abnormal central drive requiring mechanical ventilation. Should airway intubation be performed?

❑ Self-administered narcotic and sedative drug overdoses as well as iatrogenic excessive sedative therapy are the most commonly observed examples of respiratory failure caused by central nervous system depression. A less commonly encountered form is a cerebrovascular accident (ie, stroke) involving the brain stem. Because these patients may be unable to protect their upper airway as a result of diminished or absent gag reflex, the trachea may need to be intubated to minimize the risk of aspiration of oral and gastric contents. Subsequently, the presence of a laryngeal tube may help the monitoring of spontaneous tidal volumes and respiratory rate and initiation of pulmonary ventilation if central hypoventilation develops.

614 Enumerate clinically relevant causes of respiratory failure due to "alveolar conditions" (other than COPD in which alveolar destruction is the main problem) that might require mechanical ventilation. What are the specific criteria that mandate initiation of ventilatory support?

❑ Patients with pulmonary edema of cardiac origin, noncardiogenic pulmonary edema (ie, ARDS), extensive pneumonias, or diffuse alveolar hemorrhage who develop hypercapnia ($PaCO_2$ >45 mm Hg) or severe hypoxemia (PaO_2 <50 mm Hg) unresponsive to 100% oxygen delivered by a tight-fitting face mask require immediate application of mechanical ventilation. Alveolar-filling conditions due to any cause generally lead to hypoxemic respiratory failure so that carbon dioxide retention, if present, only occurs in very advanced stages.

615 What disorders of the chest wall and peripheral nervous system commonly lead to respiratory failure requiring mechanical ventilation? When should ventilatory support be initiated?

❑ Myasthenia gravis, Guillain-Barré syndrome, flail chest secondary to trauma, and severe kyphoscoliosis represent the most commonly observed causes of respiratory failure resulting from disorders of the peripheral nervous system and the chest wall. Monitoring the vital capacity in patients with neuromuscular weakness or diseases of the chest wall allows early recognition of impending respiratory failure. Elective tracheal intubation and initiation of mechanical ventilation are indicated when the vital capacity decreases to levels below 1 L and 15 mL/kg of body weight despite the normalcy of ABG levels. If $PaCO_2$ is above 45 mm Hg because of respiratory acidosis (ie, blood pH is decreased) or the vital capacity decreases below 10 mL/kg, the risk of sudden death caused by respiratory failure is substantial; consequently, intubation and mechanical ventilation should be immediately performed.

616 Why does ventilatory function tend to improve over time in patients with severe spinal cord injury?

❑ It is well recognized that pulmonary function improves in the months following spinal cord injury. Patients with lesions below C5 may have a vital capacity of about 30% of predicted in the first week after injury that increases to about 45% by the fifth week and about 60% by the fifth month. This improvement is caused by a change from muscle flaccidity associated with the initial phase of spinal shock to spasticity of the paralyzed intercostal and abdominal muscles that develops thereafter.

617 What is the management for respiratory muscle fatigue? Is resting of respiratory muscles salutary in COPD? What is the role of aminophylline in the therapy of respiratory muscle fatigue?

❑ Muscle rest during mechanical ventilation is the only satisfactory method of managing respiratory fatigue. However, the absence of contraction may also result in muscle atrophy and decreased future respiratory muscle performance. In fact, muscle rest appears to produce no benefits on respiratory muscle function of stable patients with COPD, although this remains controversial. The role of respiratory muscle training in the management of ventilator-dependent patients remains unknown. Although aminophylline increases respiratory muscle strength and may protect against fatigue, the improvement is quite small, and the usefulness of aminophylline for this purpose is questionable in view of the considerable risk of toxicity.

618 What are the effects of the intake of carbohydrates and other nutrients in the ventilatory requirements?

❑ An increase in ventilatory requirements can result from inappropriate nutritional support. If carbohydrate is administered in excess of metabolic demands, it is converted to fat for storage, which markedly affects the respiratory quotient (ie, rate of carbon dioxide production relative to oxygen consumption). Carbohydrates and fats are metabolized with respiratory quotients of 1.0 and 0.7, respectively, whereas the respiratory quotient of lipogenesis is 8.0. If a patient is unable to increase alveolar ventilation due to severe respiratory compromise, hypercapnia will ensue if the patient receives excessive nutritional support (especially of carbohydrates that have the highest respiratory quotient) at the time of being weaned from the ventilator.

---

619 What are the mechanisms responsible for the development of severe dyspnea that mandates the use of ventilator support in patients with acute respiratory failure?

❑ Multiple afferent stimuli arising from receptors located in several body regions may result in severe dyspnea and contribute to acute respiratory failure that mandates the use of ventilatory support. The development of hypercapnia and hypoxemia leads to stimulation of ventilation that is mediated by central and peripheral chemoreceptors. Lung inflammation and abnormalities in respiratory mechanics activate stretch receptors, irritant receptors, J-receptors, and mechanoreceptors. Increased respiratory muscle contractions can activate diaphragmatic afferent receptors. All of these factors cause stimulation of the respiratory centers, which leads to intolerable dyspnea and prompts the physician to use ventilator support.

---

620 Enumerate major aspects of the care of patients receiving ventilator support. What are the major risks of these patients?

❑ Patients receiving mechanical ventilation commonly share risk factors that require appropriate management, including (1) the need to be admitted and to remain in intensive care units or comparable areas because they are critically ill, clinically unstable, and predisposed to sudden death caused by undetected disconnection from the ventilator; (2) medication to prevent stress erosions of the gastric mucosa that may lead to hemorrhage or gastric perforation; (3) adequate intake of nutrients because these patients are unable to spontaneously ingest a well-balanced diet; and (4) careful monitoring of body weight and fluid balance because salt and water retention (commonly observed problem) can further aggravate the hypoxemic respiratory failure.

VENTILATORS

621 What are the main types of ventilators?

❑ Ventilators are best classified according to the method by which pressure is applied to achieve lung inflation. Thus, the two main types are negative-pressure ventilators and positive-pressure ventilators. Negative-pressure ventilators, which reproduce the bellows function of the chest wall, were initially preferred and their development received considerable impetus from the pioneering field of thoracic surgery in the early part of this century. During the poliomyelitis epidemic in the 1950s, the superiority of positive-pressure over negative-pressure machines was recognized, and today ventilator support is provided almost totally with positive-pressure ventilators. The introduction and development of critical care medicine over the past 30 years has been intertwined with improved ventilator design, and the technological advances of mechanical ventilation have been associated with the proliferation of intensive care units.

622 How do positive-pressure ventilators operate?

❑ Almost all modern ventilators operate on the principle of intermittent positive-pressure ventilation (IPPV), which produces lung inflation by generating and applying positive pressure to the airways. These ventilators are classified according to their cycling mechanism: pressure cycled, volume cycled, or time cycled. Another form of positive-pressure ventilation, known as *high-*

frequency ventilation, had brief popularity in the 1980s, but never gained widespread acceptance.

623 What are the main properties of positive-pressure ventilators? Explain the volume-cycled and pressure-cycled models of ventilators.

❑ Positive-pressure ventilators operate as either volume-cycled or pressure-cycled models. Volume-cycled mechanical ventilators deliver preset tidal volumes reliably despite abnormalities in the patient's respiratory mechanics. Pressure-cycled mechanical ventilators have a preset inspiratory pressure that interrupts the inspiration once this value is reached, independently of the tidal volume. Consequently, most adult patients that require mechanical ventilation are supported by volume-cycled models that secure the constancy of tidal volume (however, if the peak airway pressure required to deliver the preset tidal volume is excessively high, a "pop-off" valve will decrease the tidal volume to reduce the risk of lung injury from high pressure). The inability of pressure-cycled ventilators to deliver constant tidal volumes represents a limitation for their use in patient management; this limitation can be overcome by careful monitoring.

624 Explain the principles of operation of a pressure-cycled ventilator.

❑ All of the early positive-pressure ventilators were pressure cycled. In such ventilators, gas is allowed to flow into the lungs until a preset airway pressure limit is reached, at which time a valve opens and allows expiration to occur. A major pitfall of pressure-cycled ventilators is that the volume delivered by the ventilator varies with changes in airway resistance, lung compliance, and integrity of the ventilator circuit. Airway obstruction or decreased lung compliance will result in a low tidal volume and premature cycling of the ventilator. Most ventilators currently used have features of pressure-cycled, volume-cycled, and time-cycled ventilation.

625 Explain the principles of operation of a volume-cycled ventilator.

❑ Volume-cycled ventilators were developed in the 1950s and are currently the most popular type. In such ventilators, gas flows to the patient until a preset volume is delivered to the ventilator circuit, even if this entails the generation of a very high airway pressure. To minimize the risk of barotrauma, a safety or ''pop-off'' pressure limit is set; when exceeded, the excess volume is vented to the atmosphere. Guaranteed delivery of a predetermined volume to the patient with volume-cycled ventilators should not be assumed and exhaled volume should be monitored; the exhaled volume will be lower than the preset value in the presence of a circuit leak from the ventilator.

626 Explain the principles of operation of a time-cycled ventilator.

❑ Time-cycled ventilators allow gas to flow to the patient until a preset inspiratory time is reached. Desired tidal volume is attained by adjustment of inspiratory time and flow rate. Because they can generate high airway pressures, time-cycled ventilators can be used interchangeably with volume-cycled ventilators in the management of seriously ill patients, although the volume delivered varies with changes in lung mechanics.

627 What commonly observed conditions may have increased peak but normal plateau pressures during positive-pressure mechanical ventilation? How effective are pressure-cycled models to ventilate patients with abnormal respiratory compliance?

❑ Patients with severe asthma have high resistance to airflow (reduced dynamic compliance) but normal static compliance. Consequently, peak proximal airway pressures are increased but plateau pressures are normal in severe asthma. On the other hand, patients with pneumonia have normal resistance to airflow (normal dynamic compliance) but decreased static compliance. Therefore, both peak and plateau pressures are abnormally high in pneumonia. Patients with abnormally high airway resistance (eg, severe asthma) as well as patients with a severe reduction in static compliance (eg, pneumonia) generally require high airway pressure during mechanical ventilation so that pressure-cycled models have some limitations (that can be overcome modifying the ventilator setting) to deliver the appropriate tidal volume.

628 How much is the tubing compliance of ventilators?

❑ It is important to recognize that part of the volume generated by the ventilator does not ventilate the patient but instead expands the connecting tubing. The tubing compliance in most ventilator circuits is 2 to 3 mL/cm H_2O of peak pressure and varies with tubing structure, length, and diameter.

629 How do negative-pressure ventilators operate?

❑ Ventilation is achieved with the classic model of negative-pressure ventilators by placing the entire body up to the neck in an iron lung or tank respirator. Intermittent application of subatmospheric pressure creates a pressure gradient that promotes air entry into the lungs in a manner similar to that of spontaneous breathing. Minute ventilation can be altered by a change in the negative pressure or the respiratory rate. Unfortunately, negative-pressure ventilators have many limitations: Only a fixed respiratory rate can be used, satisfactory nursing care is not possible while the patient remains in the tank, and adequate ventilation is unlikely in the presence of increased airway resistance or reduced lung compliance. The performance of negative-pressure ventilators is adequate in patients who have normal lungs, and many patients afflicted by poliomyelitis during the epidemic of the 1950s still use these ventilators.

630 What are the old and current models of negative-pressure ventilators?

❑ The classic ''iron lung'' (tank respirator) was the prototype of negative-pressure ventilators. Models that are currently used include the thoracoabdominal cuirass, poncho wrap, pulmo wrap, and zip-suit. An advantage of these respirators is that the patient can receive ventilatory support without insertion of an airway tube. Since most negative-pressure ventilators operate as pressure-cycled models, they share all the limitations that characterize these respirators (eg, inability to deliver a constant tidal volume when the patient's respiratory mechanics is characterized by high resistance to inflation of thorax and lungs). See more details in the answers to pertinent questions.

631 Explain the use of the cuirass ventilator.

❑ A modified approach to negative-pressure ventilation was attempted with the introduction of the cuirass ventilator. This model of ventilator consists of a rigid shell placed around the rib cage with an attached hose connecting the inner surface to an electric pump that is intermittently activated. The cuirass is most commonly used in patients with kyphoscoliosis and respiratory failure, especially during sleep. However, many such patients prefer the delivery of positive-pressure ventilation through a nose mask or even a permanent tracheostomy and a small domiciliary positive-pressure ventilator. A close fit of the shell to the chest wall may be difficult, especially in patients with musculoskeletal deformity, and a customized cuirass may need to be constructed. Other problems with the cuirass include unreliable generation of negative pressure, difficulty in adjusting inspiratory flow, and skin chafing resulting from an improper seal.

MODES OF VENTILATOR SUPPORT

632 What is the major difference among the various modes of ventilator support? Name the most commonly used modes of mechanical ventilation.

❑ Ventilator modes differ from each other in the nature and amount of spontaneous breathing performed by the patient. The most commonly used modes of ventilatory support include assist-control (AC) ventilation, synchronized intermittent mandatory ventilation (SIMV), and pressure-support ventilation (PSV).

633 What are the main features of commonly used modes of ventilator support?

❑ Commonly used modes of mechanical ventilation are AC ventilation, intermittent mandatory ventilation (IMV), and PSV. In the AC mode, the ventilator delivers a breath either when triggered by the patient's inspiratory effort or independently if such an effort does not occur in a preselected time. In the IMV mode, the patient receives periodic positive-pressure breaths at a preset volume and rate from the ventilator, and, in addition and unlike in AC ventilation, the patient can breathe spontaneously. Spontaneous breathing is achieved with the IMV mode through a demand valve that can produce a considerable increase in the work of breathing. In the PSV mode, a fixed amount of pressure augments each breath. Airway pressure is maintained at a preset level until the patient's inspiratory flow falls to a certain level (eg, 25% of peak flow). Tidal volume is determined by the level of PSV, patient effort, and pulmonary mechanics. Newer ventilator modes such as airway pressure release ventilation and extracorporeal carbon dioxide removal are experimental models that have not been evaluated in a large number of patients to establish their efficacy and safety.

634 Compare the different modes of positive-pressure ventilation (eg, AC ventilation, IMV, PSV, controlled ventilation).

❑ The two major forms of positive-pressure mechanical ventilation are the controlled and the assisted modes. In the controlled mode, spontaneous breathing is inhibited (therefore leading to atrophy of respiratory muscles) whereas in the assisted mode, the patient's inspiratory efforts are preserved and participate in the patient's total ventilation. Consequently, assisted is generally preferred over controlled ventilation. The most commonly used forms of positive-pressure ventilation in patients having spontaneous respiratory efforts include AC ventilation, IMV, and PSV. With AC ventilation, the ventilator delivers a breath either when triggered by a patient's inspiratory effort or independently if such an effort does not occur within a preselected period. With IMV, the patient receives periodic positive-pressure breaths from the ventilator at a preset volume and rate, and spontaneous breathing is also allowed. Spontaneous breathing is achieved by means of a demand valve that can considerably increase the work of breathing. PSV differs from AC ventilation and IMV in that the physician sets a level of pressure (rather than volume) to augment every spontaneous effort. Airway pressure is maintained at a preset level until the patient's inspiratory flow falls below a certain level (eg, 25% of peak flow). Tidal volume is determined by the level of pressure set, the patient's effort, and pulmonary mechanics.

635 What are the main features of controlled mechanical ventilation (CMV)?

❑ During CMV the ventilator delivers a preset number of breaths per minute of a preset volume. Additional breaths cannot be triggered by the patient as in the case of the AC mode. Although one can achieve a spontaneous breath by opening a valve in the system, the necessary negative inspiratory pressure prevents the existence of adequate sustained spontaneous ventilation and leads to air hunger. These disadvantages have relegated CMV to be used in patients who are apneic secondary to brain damage, sedation, or muscle paralysis.

636 What are the main features of AC ventilation?

❑ In the AC mode, the ventilator delivers a breath either when triggered by the patient's inspiratory effort or independently if such an effort does not occur within a preselected period of time, and the patient's triggering effort can exceed the preset rate. If the patient's spontaneous rate falls below the preset backup rate, controlled ventilation is provided until the patient's spontaneous rate exceeds the backup rate. Fine-tuning of the sensitivity of the patient triggering mechanism is imperative, because the ventilator may "autocycle" if it is too sensitive, whereas a very large negative pressure may be required if it is not sensitive enough.

637 What are the main features of IMV and SIMV with a demand circuit?

❑ The patient receiving IMV can breathe spontaneously but in addition receives periodic positive-pressure breaths at a preset volume and rate. Use of IMV might be of value in patients who demonstrate significant hemodynamic deterioration during positive-pressure ventilation, provided they are not adversely affected by the associated increase in the work of breathing. Also, it appears that the reduction in overall peak airway pressure with IMV may decrease the risk of ventilator-induced barotrauma. SIMV is dependent on a demand valve that senses a fall in airway pressure or the generation of airflow and opens to allow spontaneous inspiration. Unfortunately, ventilators incorporating SIMV demand-valve circuits and technologically advanced monitoring systems proliferated before their limitations had been adequately assessed. It has now been repeatedly demonstrated that the excessive reduction in airway pressure necessary to activate the demand valve, combined with the inadequate delivery of instantaneous gas flow, can cause a twofold or greater increase in the work of breathing.

638 What are the main features of PSV? How reliable is PSV in the management of patients with acute respiratory failure?

❑ PSV adds a preset pressure to each spontaneous inspiratory effort. In contrast, AC ventilation and IMV add a preset volume (not pressure) during inspiration. PSV resembles AC ventilation because both methods support a breath initiated by the patient, yet with PSV (which assists every breath) it is not possible to set a backup rate to ensure a minimum level of ventilation (AC permits this selection). Tidal volume decreases with PSV if the patient increases airway resistance or decreases lung compliance because this method adds a preset pressure but not a preset volume. PSV is not a reliable mode to sustain a fixed minute ventilation in patients with unstable respiratory drive (eg, drug overdose, because with PSV the patient must initiate the inspiratory effort) or patients prone to changes in lung mechanics (eg, ARDS, COPD, asthma, because the abnormal lung mechanics decreases delivered tidal volume). Consequently, PSV is often used in combination with IMV, securing that a volume-preset breath is delivered at set intervals and PSV reinforces each intervening spontaneous inspiratory effort. The switch from the inspiratory phase to the expiratory phase of the respiratory cycle during pressure support is dependent on the peak inspiratory flow rate. When the patient's inspiratory flow decreases below a preset level (eg, 5 L/min), pressure augmentation is interrupted and expiration begins.

639 Compare the work of breathing during CPAP ventilation using a demand-valve circuit versus a continuous-flow circuit.

❑ The work of breathing of patients receiving CPAP differs with the use of a demand-valve as compared to a continuous-flow circuit. A considerable drop in inspiratory airway pressure is required to open a demand valve, with consequent increase in the work of breathing of patients using this device.

640 What new methods of mechanical ventilation are currently available?

❑ New methods of ventilatory support are constantly being introduced. These include inverse-ratio ventilation, airway-pressure-release ventilation, proportional-assist ventilation, and extracorporeal carbon dioxide removal. Although these techniques are exciting from a theoretical and physiologic viewpoint, there is no firm evidence that they improve outcome in patients.

641 Explain the rationale for the use of high-frequency ventilation.

❑ High-frequency ventilation is based on the concept that the delivery of a low tidal volume at a rapid respiratory rate might reduce the risk of barotrauma and cardiac complications while achieving adequate alveolar ventilation. Three mechanical systems designed for high-frequency ventilation have been developed: high-frequency positive-pressure ventilation (HFPPV), high-frequency jet ventilation (HFJV), and high-frequency oscillation (HFO). In general, a tidal volume close to that of calculated dead space is delivered 60 to 200 times per minute with HFPPV and HFJV; with HFO there is no bulk flow, but gas is moved in and out of the airways at rates of 60 to 3000 cycles/min. Satisfactory gas exchange is possible with the three methods, but the mechanism of their effects on ABGs is incompletely understood. The use of high-frequency ventilation never attained its original promise and the technique is rarely employed in clinical practice.

642 Explain the use of noninvasive ventilation with face or nasal masks.

❑ There is a resurgence of interest in the use of positive-pressure ventilation with face or nasal masks. This approach is particularly helpful in the long-term treatment of patients with chest wall and neuromuscular disorders. It can also improve pulmonary gas exchange rapidly in patients with acute ventilatory failure. As compared with conventional treatment in patients who have an acute exacerbation of COPD, noninvasive ventilation appears to reduce the need for endotracheal intubation and may decrease mortality. Patients need to be selected carefully for this therapy, since the mask can cause claustrophobia, and it may be dangerous in patients who cannot protect their airways (ie, risk of aspiration pneumonia after vomiting) or who have copious secretions. This approach can be time-consuming for nurses and respiratory therapists, although this is disputed. Albeit noninvasive ventilation is very promising, additional carefully controlled studies are needed to define the appropriate indications and contraindications, the optimal duration of therapy, and the morbidity and mortality associated with this approach as compared with standard mechanical ventilation and endotracheal intubation.

VENTILATOR SETTINGS. PERMISSIVE HYPERCAPNIA

643 Outline the ventilator settings and the rationale supporting their selection.

❑ The most important settings of the ventilator include the FiO_2, tidal volume, rate or frequency, trigger sensitivity, inspiratory flow rate, and use of PEEP. The specific settings of the ventilator are based on the patient's size and condition, and they require repeated reassessment. In addition, the ventilator settings partly depend on the specific mode of ventilator used. Details about each of the ventilator settings are provided in the answers to pertinent questions.

644 How are the ventilator settings selected and changed?

❑ The initial ventilator settings are estimated on the basis of the patient's size and clinical condition and are generally altered after obtaining ABG values and other relevant information. Depending on the stability of the patient's clinical condition, the ventilator settings should be assessed repeatedly and may require further adjustments.

645 What level of FiO_2 should be used during mechanical ventilation? What is the rationale for selecting this level?

❑ The risk of toxic effects of oxygen is minimized by using the lowest FiO_2 with which satisfactory arterial oxygenation can be achieved. The usual goal is a PaO_2 of 60 mm Hg or an oxygen saturation of 90%, as higher values do not substantially enhance tissue oxygenation.

646 What tidal volume should be used with mechanical ventilation? What is permissive hypercapnia or controlled hypoventilation? Is permissive hypercapnia a successful therapeutic modality?

❑ Over the past 20 years, it has been customary to use tidal volumes (ie, 10 to 15 mL/kg of body weight) that are two to three times higher than normal. This approach is being challenged by convincing data indicating that alveolar overdistention can produce endothelial, epithelial, and basement membrane injuries that are associated with increased microvascular permeability and lung rupture. To minimize this risk, one would ideally like to monitor alveolar volume, but this is not feasible. A reasonable substitute is to monitor the peak alveolar pressure as estimated from the plateau pressure, which is measured in a relaxed patient by briefly occluding the ventilatory circuit at end inspiration. The incidence of ventilator-induced lung injury increases markedly when the plateau pressure is high. Although data are incomplete, there is a growing tendency to lower the tidal volume delivered to 5 to 7 mL/kg (or less) in order to achieve a plateau pressure no higher than 35 cm H_2O. Since this may lead to an increase in the $PaCO_2$, the strategy is termed *permissive hypercapnia* or *controlled hypoventilation.* It is important to focus on the pH rather than the $PaCO_2$ when using this approach. If the pH falls below 7.20, some physicians recommend intravenous bicarbonate, but this is of unproved benefit and a subject of controversy. In patients with severe asthma requiring mechanical ventilation, uncontrolled studies suggest that permissive hypercapnia results in lower mortality than conventional ventilation, and the same may be true in patients with the ARDS.

647 What is permissive hypercapnia?

❑ Permissive hypercapnia, also known as *controlled mechanical hypoventilation,* is a treatment modality for patients with acute respiratory failure requiring mechanical ventilation, whereby a priority is given to the prevention of excessive alveolar distention over the maintenance of normal alveolar ventilation (ie, PCO_2 of 40 mm Hg). Tidal volumes of 5 to 8 mL/kg are used in permissive hypercapnia as opposed to 10 to 15 mL/kg of conventional mechanical ventilation. $PaCO_2$ is allowed to rise above 40 mm Hg, and no measures are generally taken to prevent the development of acidemia (decreased blood pH).

648 How severe is the carbon dioxide retention and acidemia observed with permissive hypercapnia?

❑ The severity of carbon dioxide retention and of acidemia reported in patients undergoing permissive hypercapnia varies widely in different reports. In a clinical trial involving 50 patients with ARDS, the mean maximum $PaCO_2$ was 62 mm Hg, and the highest value was 129 mm Hg. With respect to the severity of acidemia, the arterial pH was allowed to decrease to about 7.00 without correction in some clinical trials, whereas others recommend maintaining arterial pH at levels higher than 7.20 with the use of intravenous sodium bicarbonate.

649 Why is neuromuscular blockade generally necessary with the use of permissive hypercapnia?

❑ The increased respiratory drive associated with acute hypercapnia is extremely uncomfortable; sedation with narcotics or benzodiazepines or both is necessary, and these patients also commonly require neuromuscular blockade (eg, vecuronium). This poses a risk of sudden death caused by accidental disconnection from the ventilator, and also once the blocking agent is discontinued, prolonged weakness or paralysis lasting several days or weeks may be observed.

650 What are the main adverse effects and contraindications of permissive hypercapnia?

❑ Adverse effects of permissive hypercapnia include those listed below as contraindications as well as clinical (eg, tachypnea, dyspnea, increased work of breathing, headache, sweating) and biochemical (eg, hyperkalemia, reduced oxygen uptake by hemoglobin, altered drug pharmacokinetics) abnormalities. Contraindications to the use of permissive hypercapnia include the presence of (1) cerebral edema, increased intracranial pressure, or convulsions; (2) depressed cardiac function or arrhythmias; and (3) severe pulmonary hypertension (that may precipitate right ventricular failure).

651 Is permissive hypercapnia a better treatment modality than conventional mechanical ventilation for the management of acute respiratory failure?

❑ Limited experience based on uncontrolled clinical trials suggests that permissive hypercapnia is a better therapeutic modality than conventional mechanical ventilation for the management of ARDS and other forms of acute respiratory failure. Mortality in some studies has been lower than that predicted according to the severity of patients' condition. The role of bicarbonate administration to partially correct the diminished cellular and extracellular pH that accompanies permissive hypercapnia remains undefined.

652 How is the respiratory frequency or rate selected during mechanical ventilation? Does the selected rate differ according to the mode of ventilator support?

❑ Choosing the number of breaths per minute delivered by the ventilator depends on the mode of mechanical ventilation being used. With CMV, the rate is chosen on the basis of the selected tidal volume so that the resulting minute ventilation is likely to achieve a satisfactory $PaCO_2$. If IMV is used, it is probably best to set the ventilator initially at a rate close to that being used by the patient at the preselected tidal volume; later, the rate can be reduced, if desired, depending on clinical and laboratory assessment. With AC ventilation, the backup rate should be set in accordance with the patient's needs as it can be higher than the spontaneous rate if an increase in total ventilation is required. Conversely, if the patient's spontaneous rate is adequate, the backup rate should be set at 2 to 4 breaths/min below this value, to prevent serious hypoventilation in the event that the patient fails to trigger the ventilator.

653 What rate or frequency of ventilation should be used during ventilator support? Explain the ventilator rate with AC ventilation, IMV, and PSV.

❑ The rate of ventilation that should be set depends on the mode of support. With AC ventilation, the backup rate should be about 4 breaths/min less than the patient's spontaneous rate; this ensures that the ventilator will continue to supply an adequate volume should the patient have a sudden decrease in output from the respiratory centers. With IMV, the rate should be high at first and then decreased gradually in accordance with the patient's tolerance. With PSV, the rate is not set.

654 What trigger sensitivity should be used with mechanical ventilation? Does the demand valve respond to changes in pressure or airflow?

❑ Most ventilators are triggered by a change in airway pressure, and their sensitivity is usually set a −1 to −2 cm H_2O. With poorly responsive demand valves, however, the actual pressure generated by the patient may be considerably higher. If the trigger setting is too sensitive, the ventilator will cycle too frequently (''autocycle''), and hyperventilation with severe respiratory alkalosis may result. Flow triggering is available with some ventilators, and it appears to require less work by the patient than pressure triggering does.

655 What inspiration-expiration ratio (I/E) is generally used during mechanical ventilation? How might the I/E ratio be modified?

❑ An I/E ratio of about 1:2 is generally used to minimize gas trapping and the associated increase in mean intrathoracic pressure. The I/E ratio may be adjusted directly on some time-cycled ventilators. On volume-cycled ventilators, it is indirectly determined by regulation of tidal volume, ventilator frequency, and inspiratory flow rate.

656 What level of inspiratory airflow should be used during mechanical ventilation?

❑ An inspiratory flow rate of 60 L/min should be used with most patients during AC ventilation and IMV. In patients with COPD, better gas exchange is achieved at a flow rate of 100 L/min, probably because the resulting increase in expiratory time allows more complete emptying of gas-trapped regions. If the flow rate is insufficient to meet a patient's ventilatory requirements, the patient will strain against his or her own pulmonary impedance and that of the ventilator, with a consequent increase in the work of breathing. It is helpful to examine the contour of the waveform for airway pressure when the flow rate and the sensitivity of the trigger are adjusted. Ideally, the waveform should show a smooth rise and a convex appearance during inspiration. In contrast, a prolonged negative phase with excessive scalloping of the tracing indicates unsatisfactory sensitivity and flow settings.

657 What ventilator settings for FiO_2, tidal volume, ventilator rate, and inspiratory flow rate are commonly used in patient care?

❑ Ventilator settings are selected on the basis of a patient's size and condition and are repeatedly reassessed. FiO_2 is initially set at 0.9 to 1.0, and then adjusted to achieve a PaO_2 of 60 to 90 mm Hg. Tidal volume is commonly set at 10 to 15 mL/kg; recent evidence, however, suggests that large volumes may induce or aggravate lung injury, and a smaller volume (7 to 8 mL/kg) may be more appropriate. Ventilator rate depends on the mode of ventilation: With AC, the backup rate should be 2 to 4 breaths/min below the total rate; with IMV, the rate should initially be high and then gradually decreased in accordance with the patient's tolerance; and with PSV, the rate is not set. An inspiratory flow rate of 60 L/min is optimal for most patients, but a higher value may be preferred in patients with COPD to decrease the work of breathing and improve alveolar gas exchange.

658 Should ventilator mode and settings remain constant in the management of respiratory failure?

❑ No. Selecting the mode and settings of the ventilator is a dynamic process that is based on the patient's physiologic response rather than a fixed set of numbers. The settings require repeated readjustment over the period of dependency on the ventilator, and such iterative interaction requires careful respiratory monitoring.

659 How important is the presence of intermittent deep breaths or sighs on pulmonary function of patients breathing spontaneously or receiving mechanical ventilation?

❑ Spontaneous breathing or mechanical ventilation with constant normal tidal volume (5 mL/kg), without intermittent deep breaths or sighs, causes a reduction in lung compliance with consequent hypoxemia, attributable to progressive alveolar collapse. This source of hypoxemia can be prevented or reversed by intermittent sighs, arbitrarily defined as three times normal tidal volume, and an automatic sighing feature is included on most current ventilators. Constant ventilation with large tidal volume (10 to 15 mL/kg) without intermittent sighs is similarly effective and gained popularity in the 1970s and 1980s. Recent evidence has further documented the importance of volume-induced damage to the lung parenchyma, and have led to the current use of lower tidal volume settings (approximately 7 mL/kg).

AUTO-PEEP

660 What is auto-PEEP? What is the effect of auto-PEEP on the patient's ability to trigger the ventilator?

❑ In some patients, especially those with COPD and a high minute ventilation, gas trapping develops in the alveoli, and the patients have PEEP. This so-called auto-PEEP makes triggering the ventilator more difficult, because the patient needs to generate a negative pressure equal in magnitude to the level of auto-PEEP in addition to the level of sensitivity selected. This is one of the factors that may account for a patient's inability to trigger the ventilator despite obvious respiratory efforts.

661 How can auto-PEEP be recognized in mechanically ventilated patients and in those spontaneously breathing?

❑ At normal end-expiration, the static recoil pressure of the respiratory system is zero, whereas a positive value is observed in patients with dynamic hyperinflation. This positive recoil pressure has been termed *auto-PEEP* or *intrinsic PEEP*. In patients receiving mechanical ventilation, it has been termed *occult PEEP*, because, unlike externally applied PEEP, it is not registered on the ventilator pressure manometer, as the latter is open to atmosphere. If, however, the expiratory port of the ventilator circuit is occluded immediately before the onset of the next breath, the pressure in the lungs and ventilator circuit will equilibrate and the level of auto-PEEP will be displayed on the ventilator manometer. None of these methods help detect auto-PEEP during spontaneous breathing. For this purpose, it is necessary to insert an esophageal balloon catheter, and measure the change in esophageal pressure between the onset of inspiratory muscle effort and the onset of inspiratory flow. Alternatively, dynamic hyperinflation during spontaneous breathing can be detected by monitoring the change in end-expiratory lung volume using devices that record motion of the chest wall, such as inductive plethysmography.

662 Is auto-PEEP usually recognized during mechanical ventilation? How can its value be measured?

❑ Auto-PEEP commonly goes undetected because it is not registered on the pressure manometer of the ventilator, as the latter is open to the atmosphere. Occluding the expiratory port of the circuit at the end of expiration in a relaxed patient causes the pressure in the lungs and circuit to equilibrate, and the level of auto-PEEP will be displayed on the manometer.

663 What therapeutic measures might be used to reduce the increased work of breathing caused by auto-PEEP? Might application of external PEEP be of help?

❑ The increased work of breathing resulting from auto-PEEP can be decreased by therapeutic measures that reduce the level of auto-PEEP, including (1) bronchodilator therapy, (2) employment of a large-bore endotracheal tube, (3) decreasing the minute ventilation demand by controlling fever or pain, (4) reducing the ratio of inspiratory time to expiratory time by increasing the inspiratory flow rate, and (5) using nondistensible tubing in the ventilator circuit. Alternatively, a reduction of the increased work of breathing caused by auto-PEEP can be obtained by the application of external PEEP. The rationale for the treatment of intrinsic

PEEP with the application of external PEEP is as follows: If ambient pressure is elevated by the application of external PEEP, inspiration is more easily accomplished because the alveolar pressure required to initiate inspiration is just below the level of external PEEP (rather than below zero). Thus, we have the paradox whereby external PEEP, which is most commonly employed to induce hyperinflation in patients with diffuse microatelectasis, as in the ARDS, is being used to decrease the work of breathing caused by hyperinflation consequent to auto-PEEP. Although external PEEP may help to decrease the work of breathing associated with auto-PEEP, it is important to note that it does nothing to relieve the accompanying hyperinflation. Thus, it is necessary to add other therapeutic measures to reduce the level of auto-PEEP and therefore the hyperinflation.

PEEP

664 Elaborate on the use of PEEP and on the mechanisms of its salutary effects in patient management. Can the addition of external PEEP help patients with auto-PEEP trigger the ventilator?

❑ Few aspects of ventilator management have been more controversial than PEEP. In patients with the ARDS, PEEP usually produces a substantial increase in PaO_2. This is primarily caused by a reduction in intrapulmonary shunting as a result of a redistribution of lung water from the alveoli to the perivascular interstitial space. Contrary to previous thinking, PEEP does not decrease the total amount of extravascular lung water. Provided the improvement in PaO_2 is not offset by a decline in cardiac output, FiO_2 can be decreased, which is the principal therapeutic effect of PEEP. The addition of PEEP also influences lung mechanics. Patients with acute lung injury commonly have a decreased end-expiratory lung volume, and thus tidal breathing occurs on the low, flat portion of the pressure-volume curve. By shifting tidal breathing to a more compliant portion of the curve, PEEP can reduce the work of breathing. In patients with an airflow limitation and auto-PEEP who have difficulty triggering the ventilator, the addition of external PEEP (to a level not exceeding the level of auto-PEEP) can help to counteract this problem, because to trigger the ventilator the alveolar pressure needs to be decreased only below the level of external PEEP, rather than below zero. In addition to the injury induced by high inflation pressures, mechanical ventilation at a low end-expiratory lung volume aggravates lung injury in laboratory animals, possibly because of shear stresses associated with the repeated closing and opening of alveolar units. Adding about 10 cm H_2O of PEEP to splint the lung open appears to reduce this problem. It is not known whether this type of shear injury occurs in patients.

665 What are the goals of PEEP?

❑ There is no consensus as to the goals of PEEP. Some physicians consider PEEP to have no application other than to ameliorate life-threatening hypoxemia and decrease exposure to a potentially toxic FiO_2; they strive for a satisfactory PaO_2 with the lowest level of PEEP. Other physicians believe that PEEP is a panacea for all respiratory ills and that it modifies the natural course of lung disease; they use it even in patients who can achieve a satisfactory PaO_2 with a relatively low FiO_2. However, the prophylactic application of PEEP fails to influence the development of ARDS in patients at risk for this condition.

666 What is the most common indication for PEEP? How should titration of PEEP be accomplished?

❑ The most common indication for PEEP is to ameliorate life-threatening hypoxemia and decrease exposure to a potentially toxic FiO_2. Titration of PEEP should not be guided solely by PaO_2, because improvement in PaO_2 may be offset by a simultaneous fall in cardiac output. Instead, optimal PEEP is achieved by maximizing oxygen delivery at the lowest FiO_2 setting. In general, this goal can be achieved with a PEEP of 5 to 15 cm H_2O.

667 What is the effect of PEEP on PaO_2? How does PEEP improve patient's oxygenation?

❑ PEEP usually improves PaO_2 in patients with acute diffuse pulmonary infiltrates who have hypoxemia associated with reduced lung volume. PEEP raises end-expiratory lung volume by opening airways and recruiting collapsed alveoli, thus enabling inspiration to occur on the steep portion of the pressure-volume curve. These effects combined with the redistribution of excess fluid within the lungs can reduce intrapulmonary shunt, thereby improving patient's oxygenation.

668 What are the effects of PEEP on functional residual capacity (FRC) and on the extravascular water content of the lung?

❑ PEEP generally improves oxygenation in patients with diffuse infiltrative lung disease who have hypoxemia associated with reduced lung volumes, as demonstrated by the presence of a decreased FRC. The low FRC places the end-expiratory level of the patient's tidal breath on the low flat portion of the pressure-volume curve of the lungs. The increased mean airway pressure induced by the application of PEEP raises the FRC by opening airways and recruiting collapsed alveoli, enabling the next inspiration to occur on the steep portion of the pressure-volume curve. These changes, combined with the possible redistribution of excess fluid within the lungs, result in a reduction in intrapulmonary shunt. Claims that PEEP may actually decrease the extravascular water content of the lungs have not been supported experimentally.

669 How should PEEP be employed and be discontinued when already applied? Explain the ''3-minute rule'' approach to reduce or discontinue PEEP.

❑ Institution of PEEP should be done in a systematic manner to (1) ensure that PEEP is the only variable being changed, (2) use stepwise increments of 3 to 5 cm H_2O, (3) minimize the time interval between changes (eg, 20 minutes) to increase the likelihood that the response reflects the action of PEEP rather than a change in the patient's underlying condition (a beneficial response is usually demonstrable within 10 minutes, although the response is sometimes slower), and (4) evaluate the response to each change in PEEP. Many suggestions have been made to determine the optimum level of PEEP but none has been shown to be clearly superior. The best PEEP is achieved when the FiO_2 can be reduced to an acceptable level without compromising oxygen delivery. A methodical approach is also required when PEEP is being reduced or discontinued. Abrupt cessation of PEEP can produce hypoxemia that takes hours or days to reverse or requires reinstitution of PEEP at a higher level than that used before its suspension. A systematic approach, commonly known as the *3-minute rule,* has been developed to achieve a 90% rate of successful PEEP reduction. Baseline PaO_2 is measured, PEEP is reduced by 5 cm H_2O, the PaO_2 measurement is repeated after 3 minutes, and PEEP is returned to the previous level until the PaO_2 measurement is available. If the PaO_2 falls by less than 20% of the baseline value, there is a 90% likelihood of successful PEEP reduction, while reinstitution of PEEP at 3 minutes in a patient failing the test returns PaO_2 to the baseline level.

---

670 How much higher is the peak proximal airway pressure during inspiration than the pressure level at the completion of inspiration in patients with normal and abnormal respiratory function? How are the peak pressure and plateau pressure affected in ARDS?

❑ The peak pressure (Ppeak) during positive-pressure mechanical ventilation is only 2 to 4 cm H_2O higher than that found at the end of inspiration (Pplateau) in subjects with normal airway resistance. Conversely, peak pressures as high as 20 cm H_2O or more are present in patients with abnormally high airway resistance. Patients with ARDS have high peak pressures as well as high plateau pressures because the main defect is an increase in static compliance (consequently, the two inspiratory pressure levels are increased).

671 What is the rationale for adding PEEP to the ventilator support in patients with respiratory failure caused by alveolar-filling conditions? Explain the "recruitment" of alveolar units.

❑ An abnormally high right-to-left shunt of more than 20% and leading to severe hypoxemia is commonly detected in patients with respiratory failure caused by alveolar-filling conditions (eg, ARDS, extensive pneumonia). The addition of PEEP to the mechanical ventilation increases the end-expiratory lung volume or FRC, producing opening of previously collapsed and unventilated alveoli (ie, recruitment of alveolar units) that were the cause of the abnormally high right-to-left shunt.

672 How might high PEEP levels reduce (as opposed to the expected increase) PaO_2 in patients with acute lung injury? Can PEEP increase venous blood shunting?

❑ The expected effect of a gradual increase in PEEP (up to about 20 cm H_2O) is a progressive rise in arterial oxygenation due to opening of previously closed alveoli. However, high PEEP levels may fail to open closed airways but simply overdistend already open alveolar units, increasing the vascular resistance of these regions. Consequently, the blood flow of regions with closed airways might increase, producing arterial hypoxemia caused by augmented blood shunting. The optimal level of PEEP that is associated with the greatest delivery of oxygen to body tissues is variable because of the composite effects of PEEP on both PaO_2 and cardiac output (ie, oxygen delivery is a function of the product of arterial oxygen content and cardiac output).

673 How is the response to PEEP assessed and what are the determinants of such response? What are the determinants of oxygen delivery to the tissues? Explain the effects of PEEP on cardiac output.

❑ The response to PEEP is assessed by the improvement in the delivery of oxygen to body tissues (ie, product of arterial oxygen content and cardiac output). Such response is dependent on the composite effects of PEEP on the PaO_2 (generally it increases) and on the cardiac output (it may decrease significantly). Several factors are responsible for the decrease in cardiac output during positive-pressure ventilation and PEEP. An increase in intrathoracic pressure compresses the vena cava and thus decreases venous return. Alveolar distention compresses the alveolar vessels, and the resulting increases in pulmonary vascular resistance and right ventricular afterload produce a leftward shift in the interventricular septum. In addition, left ventricular compliance is decreased by both the bulging septum and the increased juxtacardiac pressure resulting from distended lungs.

674 What conditions augment the risk of PEEP-mediated complications?

❑ PEEP has a number of adverse effects, many of which are extensions of those observed with mechanical ventilation. Patients with unilateral lung disease or emphysema are especially vulnerable to complications of PEEP such as barotrauma and decreased cardiac output. The combination of a rapid respiratory rate and shortened expiratory time in patients with obstructive lung disease may lead to the unwitting institution of PEEP because obstructed lung units fail to empty adequately (auto-PEEP). This condition may go undetected because the pressure monitor is open to the atmosphere throughout expiration and registers a negligible or zero pressure.

POSTURE DURING MECHANICAL VENTILATION

675 Does patient's posture during mechanical ventilation have any effect on gas exchange?

❑ Yes. Most lung disorders involve this organ in a nonhomogeneous manner. As a result, the body's position can markedly influence gas exchange. If healthier lung areas are placed in a dependent position to receive higher blood flow, the patient's hypoxemia may improve. Consequently, a trial-and-error approach to body positioning, switching from the supine to the prone position, can produce substantial improvement in oxygenation. Changing a patient's posture from supine to semirecumbent also lowers the risk of aspiration of gastric contents.

676 What effect does body position have on arterial oxygenation in patients with acute lung injury (eg, ARDS)? If patients are placed in a lateral position, should the healthier lung be the more dependent one?

❑ Body position might have significant effects on arterial oxygenation in patients with acute lung injury by mechanisms incompletely understood, but most likely primarily related to changes in regional ventilation (ie, ventilation becomes more homogeneous in the prone posture). Considering that the pulmonary disease is diffuse in ARDS, a lateral position is not likely to have a significant effect on arterial oxygenation in these patients but a switch from supine to prone may be beneficial. Conversely, patients with unilateral disease like pneumonia may derive advantages from a lateral position. When the patient with pneumonia is in a lateral position, it is advantageous that the healthier lung receives the largest blood flow; this is accomplished by placing the best lung in the more dependent position. Consequently, the more diseased lung having less alveolar ventilation will also receive less perfusion because of its nondependent position, thereby reducing its detrimental effect on arterial oxygenation. Prior to the implementation of a more intensive therapeutic intervention in a patient with acute lung injury, the possible contribution of a positional effect on arterial oxygenation should be always considered and implemented.

HEMODYNAMIC EFFECTS OF MECHANICAL VENTILATION

677 What are the factors responsible for the hemodynamic abnormalities caused by mechanical ventilation?

❑ At least three factors are involved in the reduction in cardiac output that occurs with mechanical ventilation: decreased peripheral venous return, increased right ventricular afterload, and decreased left ventricular distensibility. Decreased venous return from peripheral tissues is the major mechanism, although it may go unnoticed because positive-pressure ventilation increases all intrathoracic pressures including central venous pressure and pulmonary capillary wedge pressure (PCWP) and clinical measurement of these indices is usually referenced to atmospheric pressure. Cardiac filling during diastole depends on transmural pressures (intracardiac minus pleural), which are often decreased despite elevations of the same indices relative to atmospheric pressure. Pulmonary vascular resistance is elevated as the increase in lung volume stretches the perialveolar vessels, decreasing their lumina and increasing their resistance to blood flow. This increase in right ventricular afterload may shift the interventricular septum to the left, with consequent reduction in left ventricular compliance. In addition, contact between the distended lung and the heart increases juxtacardiac pressure, which further decreases left ventricular distensibility.

678 Elaborate further on the factors responsible for the decrease in cardiac output during positive-pressure ventilation. Does positive-pressure ventilation always reduce cardiac output?

❑ An increase in intrathoracic pressure decreases venous return. Alveolar distention compresses the alveolar capillary vessels, and the resulting increase in pulmonary vascular resistance and right ventricular afterload produces a leftward shift in the interventricular septum. Left ventricular compliance is decreased by both the bulging septum and the increased juxtacardiac pressure resulting from distended lungs. Positive-pressure ventilation usually lowers cardiac output, primarily as a result of decreased venous return. Conversely, positive-pressure ventilation can increase cardiac output in patients with impaired myocardial contractility because it produces a decrease in left ventricular afterload due to increased intrathoracic pressure.

679 What are the most commonly observed factors responsible for the development of adverse hemodynamic effects (eg, hypotension, decreased cardiac output) with positive-pressure ventilation? Can PEEP and auto-PEEP be responsible for hemodynamic disturbances?

❑ Adverse hemodynamic effects resulting from mechanical ventilation frequently develop in the presence of (1) intravascular volume depletion (eg, gastrointestinal bleeding, low fluid volume status); (2) high tidal volume; (3) a high I/E ratio (eg, $\geq 1:1$); (4) addition of PEEP as a therapeutic maneuver; and (5) severe airway obstruction, which causes a delay in alveolar emptying maintaining an elevated alveolar pressure that never falls to a stable baseline (equal to zero) during passive expiration before the next inspiration starts (known as *auto-PEEP* or *occult PEEP*). Adverse hemodynamic effects with positive-pressure ventilation may be also observed in the absence of any of the previously mentioned predisposing conditions.

680 What are the effects of the hemodynamic abnormalities caused by mechanical ventilation on the function of major organs?

❑ The hemodynamic effects of mechanical ventilation may alter renal, hepatic, and cerebral function. Alterations in renal function including a reduction in urine volume and sodium excretion seem to be primarily caused by a reduction in cardiac output (with a consequent decrease in renal blood flow and alterations of its distribution within the kidney). Hepatic dysfunction in ventilated patients usually reflects the severity of the underlying disease and the effect of positive-pressure ventilation on splanchnic blood flow (ie, decreases). In addition, prolonged or exaggerated downward motion of the diaphragm resulting in an increase in intra-abdominal pressure may lead to an increase in portal vein pressure as well as impaired bile and hepatic vein flow. Patients who have sustained a severe head injury often have a coexisting lung injury that necessitates mechanical ventilation, with or without PEEP.

The ventilator-induced increase in pleural pressure elevates superior vena caval pressure and thus decreases cerebral venous outflow, with a consequent increase in intracranial pressure that may aggravate the neurologic disorder. Consequently, intracranial pressure should be monitored in such patients.

---

681 A 57-year-old woman with crippling rheumatoid arthritis is transferred from a chronic-care facility because of bilateral pneumonia and increasing dyspnea. Body weight is 47 kg. The vital signs are as follows: 39°C, pulse of 116/min, respiration of 37 breaths/min, and blood pressure of 112/68 mm Hg. The ABG values are as follows: PO_2 of 42 mm Hg, PCO_2 of 38 mm Hg, and pH 7.23 while breathing 100% oxygen by a face mask. A decision is made to perform mechanical ventilation with the following settings: tidal volume of 1000 mL; ventilator rate of 15/min, inspiratory flow rate of 60 L/min, and PEEP of 5 cm H_2O. The patient's blood pressure falls to 82/48 mm Hg within minutes after initiation of ventilatory support.

What are the cause and the appropriate management for the hypotension observed in this patient during mechanical ventilation?

❑ A decreased systemic venous return secondary to increased intrathoracic pressure led to a fall in cardiac output, which in turn caused arterial hypotension. The high tidal volume (1000 mL) and PEEP (ie, 5 cm H_2O) caused the hemodynamic compromise and the patient's hypotension. Since the patient had significant hypoxemia secondary to an abnormal pulmonary gas exchange, it is appropriate to use a low level of PEEP (5 cm H_2O) to recruit nonventilated alveoli. However, a reduction in the excessive tidal volume to a value of 600 mL should be implemented for correction of the patient's decreased blood pressure. If hypotension persists after a decrease in delivered tidal volume and evidence of extracellular fluid volume excess is absent, administration of intravenous fluids would be appropriate for the management of the decreased blood pressure.

"FIGHTING THE VENTILATOR"

682 What is the initial response of patients to mechanical ventilation? What is the management of patients "fighting the ventilator"?

❑ Mechanical ventilation can be an uncomfortable and frightening experience, and the patient needs constant reassurance. The development of sudden distress in a previously calm patient ("fighting the ventilator") suggests the occurrence of a new and potentially serious complication. The ventilator should be disconnected and the patient given manual ventilation with an FiO_2 of 1.0 while a systematic search is undertaken for the cause (see pertinent question). If the distress is caused by poor coordination of a patient's respiratory efforts with the rhythm of the ventilator, the problem usually can be resolved by careful adjustment of the ventilator settings plus the administration of analgesic and sedative agents in selected patients. In rare instances, a neuromuscular blocking drug may be needed. The duration of such blockade should be kept to a minimum because of the catastrophic consequences of accidental disconnection from the ventilator (ie, sudden death caused by apnea). In addition, recent reports indicate that as many as 70% of patients with certain characteristics may have prolonged weakness after the discontinuation of neuromuscular blocking agents.

683 What are the causes of sudden respiratory distress in a patient receiving mechanical ventilation (ie, patient "fights the ventilator")?

❑ Patient-related causes and ventilator-related causes may be responsible for the development of sudden respiratory distress in a patient receiving mechanical ventilation. Patient-related causes include artificial airway problem, pneumothorax, bronchospasm, secretions, pulmonary edema, dynamic hyperinflation, abnormal respiratory drive, alteration in body posture, drug-induced problems, abdominal distention, anxiety, and patient-ventilator asynchrony. Ventilator-related causes include system leak, circuit malfunction, inadequate FiO_2, inadequate ventilatory support, improper trigger sensitivity, improper inspiratory flow setting, and patient-ventilator asynchrony.

684 What bedside evaluations might be helpful to establish the cause of acute respiratory distress that develops in a mechanically ventilated patient? Name common causes for this condition.

❑ Peak and plateau airway pressures, exhaled volume (ie, measured expiratory volume), tracheal position (ie, possible deviation from normal midline position), and arterial oxygenation are parameters that might help to establish the cause of acute respiratory distress that suddenly develops in patients receiving mechanical ventilation. Plateau pressure is usually measured using the ''inspiratory hold'' option of the ventilator that results in a pause of about 2 seconds at the end of inspiration. Common causes of acute respiratory distress in this condition include rupture of the endotracheal tube cuff, partial extubation, lung atelectasis, pneumothorax, intubation of the right main bronchus, kinking of the endotracheal tube, bronchospasm and mucus plugging, pulmonary embolism, and pulmonary edema.

685 How does examination of airway-pressure wave curves (in which airway pressure and time are plotted on the vertical and horizontal axes, respectively) help to determine whether the patient is fighting the respirator or is completely relaxed? What is a common cause of this problem?

❑ Examination of the shape of the wave curve of airway pressure after the flow rate and the sensitivity of the trigger have been adjusted allows recognition of the patient's work of breathing. An ideal curve observed in a patient with complete relaxation shows that the airway pressure rises smoothly from a zero level and with a convex shape during inspiration. Conversely, a prolonged negative-pressure phase preceding the ventilator-mediated rise in inspiratory pressure as well as scalloping of the tracing indicates that the patient is exerting strenuous inspiratory efforts (eg, fighting the respirator). These abnormalities on the airway-pressure curves are commonly caused by unsatisfactory sensitivity and flow settings.

686 What should the clinician do when a patient fights the respirator (ie, development of sudden respiratory distress in a ventilator-supported patient who had been stable before this event)?

❑ The following steps should be taken in the management of sudden distress in a ventilator-supported patient: (1) Remove the patient from the ventilator; (2) initiate manual ventilation using a self-inflating bag containing 100% oxygen; (3) perform a rapid physical examination and assess monitored indices; (4) check patency of the airway and pass a suction catheter; (5) if death appears imminent, consider and treat the most likely causes, which might include pneumothorax and an obstructed airway; and (6) once the patient is stabilized, perform more detailed assessment and management.

687 What are the main difficulties encountered with the artificial airway and ventilator's circuit during mechanical ventilation? What is the management of these problems?

❑ Problems in the ventilator circuit, such as a narrow endotracheal tube, a poorly functioning demand valve, certain characteristics and locations of the humidifier, and valves with high expiratory resistance, can markedly increase the work of breathing and predispose patients to barotrauma. To avoid such problems, the plumbing of the circuit needs to be evaluated repeatedly by a knowledgeable person. In addition, adequate humidification and suctioning are needed to prevent bronchial secretions from blocking the tracheal tube or producing atelectasis.

688 What neuromuscular blocking drugs are occasionally used to facilitate mechanical ventilation? What are the possible complications of their use?

❑ Nondepolarizing neuromuscular blocking agents such as pancuronium, vecuronium, and atracurium are occasionally used to facilitate application of mechanical ventilation. The most common serious complication is accidental disconnection of the respirator, which might lead to the patient's death (caused by paralysis of the respiratory muscles). In addition, prolonged paralysis or weakness of the respiratory muscles can occur in patients who had received such agents for several days, and this complication can develop with two distinct patterns. One pattern consists of persistent paralysis or weakness for up to a week and is observed in patients with renal failure; this clinical form is thought to be caused by the persistence of active metabolites of pancuronium or vecuronium that block neuromuscular transmission. The second pattern consists of acute generalized myopathy that persists for weeks or months and is observed in patients concomitantly treated with large doses of corticosteroids.

COMPLICATIONS OF MECHANICAL VENTILATION

689 What are the most important complications of mechanical ventilation?

❑ The most important complications of mechanical ventilation include those related to (1) the endotracheal or tracheotomy tubes (eg, disconnection from the ventilator, displacement of the tube producing atelectasis, and laryngeal/tracheal wall damage), (2) infection (eg, ventilator-associated pneumonia), (3) barotrauma (eg, pneumothorax, pneumomediastinum), (4) decreased cardiac output and reduced oxygen content of mixed venous blood, (5) increased intracranial pressure with augmented risk of brain edema and cerebral injury, (6) renal and hepatic dysfunction caused by hemodynamic abnormalities, and (7) the alveolar damage caused by high FiO_2. Oxygen toxicity is not truly linked to mechanical ventilation as it is also observed in patients breathing spontaneously.

---

690 What is the most common form of bronchial obstruction in patients receiving mechanical ventilation?

❑ Malposition of endotracheal or tracheotomy tubes is the most common cause of bronchial obstruction in patients undergoing ventilator support. Since the origin of the right main bronchus from the trachea is less angulated than its counterpart, the airway tube usually slides into the right bronchus, leading to a left-lung atelectasis. Sliding of poorly anchored or excessively long airway tubes into one main bronchus produces blockade of ventilation of the other main bronchus, causing atelectasis and further impairing respiratory function. While breath sounds are typically reduced over the atelectatic lung, this is a very unreliable sign. If endotracheal intubation is suspected, the endotracheal tube should be pulled back a few centimeters, the chest should be reauscultated, and the position of the tube confirmed by radiography. Endotracheal intubation can be prevented by securing the tip of the tube at least 3 to 4 cm from the carina and vocal cords and obtaining a radiograph at the time of intubation. It is estimated that endotracheal intubation occurs in about 10% of ventilated patients.

---

691 How common is the development of pneumonia during mechanical ventilation? Does the presence of pneumonia increase the patient's risk of death?

❑ Pneumonia occurs in approximately 30% of patients receiving ventilatory support and the risk for its development increases with the duration of mechanical ventilation at a rate of about 1%/day. Ventilator-associated pneumonia has a high mortality; patients receiving mechanical ventilation for more than 72 hours who developed pneumonia had a mortality of 71%, as opposed to 29% of those without pneumonia, according to a report of a large group of patients.

692 What kind of infections are commonly observed in mechanically ventilated patients? What precautions should be taken to reduce the risk of development of such infections? Is the condensate in the tubing circuit a source of infection?

❑ Patients receiving mechanical ventilation are especially prone to develop pneumonia, which is associated with high mortality. The increased risk is partly a result of the adverse effects of ventilator management and also reflects the severity of the underlying illness. Respiratory therapy equipment was a major source of nosocomial pneumonia in the 1960s, attributed principally to mainstream nebulizers that generated microaerosols laden with gram-negative bacilli. Although today's ventilators use humidifying cascades that do not generate aerosols, other aspects of ventilator care may contribute to the development of pneumonia. The condensate in the tubing circuit is rapidly colonized with microorganisms, and care should be taken to avoid inadvertently washing it into the patient's airways. Medication nebulizers are also rapidly colonized and should be cleaned after each treatment.

693 What are the manifestations of barotrauma caused by mechanical ventilation?

❑ Asymptomatic pneumothorax, tension pneumothorax with or without circulatory collapse, pneumomediastinum, pneumoperitoneum (retroperitoneal space), and subcutaneous emphysema (torso, neck, face) are manifestations of barotrauma caused by mechanical ventilation. Clinical examination may fail to reveal the existence of barotrauma, which may be recognized by daily chest x-ray studies (eg, presence of air in the mediastinum known as *pneumomediastinum,* detection of a pneumothorax). A pneumomediastinum is diagnosed by the presence of a thin radiolucent line along the left cardiac border (although frequently undetected on routine anteroposterior radiographs). Radiologic evidence of interstitial pulmonary emphysema includes (1) small lucent gas bubbles of uniform size distributed throughout opacified lungs (''vesicular rarefactions''), (2) radiolucent halos of gas around dense vessels, (3) lucent lines streaking toward the hilum, (4) pneumatoceles, and (5) subpleural air cysts or lucent lines.

694 What is a tension pneumothorax? What is the medical importance of its prompt recognition?

❑ The progressive trapping of air into the pleural space observed in tension pneumothorax increases pressure within this cavity, leading to pulmonary collapse and shift of the mediastinum toward the opposite side. The immediate consequences of a tension pneumothorax include cardiorespiratory failure and risk of sudden death, especially in patients with underlying lung disease (eg, COPD, ARDS) and those receiving mechanical ventilation. Consequently, prompt recognition and treatment of tension pneumothorax is of utmost importance for the preservation of cardiorespiratory function.

695 Elaborate on the diagnosis, cardiovascular effects, and therapy of a tension pneumothorax.

❑ Tension pneumothorax occurs when a lung injury permits air to enter but not leave the pleural space. The diagnosis is made on a clinical basis rather than radiologically. The accumulating gas collapses the ipsilateral lung and shifts the mediastinum and its contents into the contralateral thoracic space, thereby resulting in tracheal deviation, distended neck veins, unilateral absence of breath sounds, and respiratory distress. In the past, it had been commonly believed that a tension pneumothorax had a direct mechanical effect on the cardiovascular system whereby positive thoracic pressure caused compression of thoracic veins and led to a decrease in cardiac output and systemic arterial pressure. However, recent studies showed that experimental tension pneumothorax does not directly decrease cardiac output or arterial pressure. Although stroke volume decreases, cardiac output is maintained by a compensatory increase in heart rate. Marked hypoxemia was observed in these studies and was ascribed to a combination of shunt and ventilation-perfusion mismatch. From these studies, it appears that the cardiovascular collapse associated with a pneumothorax is the result of impaired tissue oxygenation secondary to arterial hypoxemia and the failure to mount a compensatory increase in cardiac output. Management of a tension pneumothorax consists of initially inserting a large-caliber needle into the second intercostal space in the midclavicular line of the affected hemithorax. Definitive therapy consists of inserting a chest tube into the fifth intercostal space anterior to the midaxillary line. Persistence of a pneumothorax and evidence of an air leak despite insertion of a chest tube indicates the presence of a bronchopleural fistula; the possibility of a major tracheobronchial laceration should be also excluded.

---

696 What is the management of the adverse hemodynamic effects observed with positive-pressure ventilation? Explain the role of intravascular volume expansion and adjustments in the ventilator settings to correct the patient's hemodynamic status.

❑ Measures that might help to overcome the adverse hemodynamic effects of mechanical ventilation include (1) decreasing tidal volume (eg, 7 mL/kg of body weight); (2) reducing the I/E ratio by decreasing the inspiratory time or using a higher inspiratory flow rate; (3) changing from the assist control (AC) to the intermittent mandatory ventilation (IMV) mode, which may increase cardiac output because of lowering mean intrathoracic pressure; and (4) intravascular volume expansion, which increases venous blood return to the right atrium and therefore may increase cardiac output. These corrective measures are aimed at increasing ''filling pressure'' of the cardiovascular system or decreasing the mean intrathoracic pressure. Most frequently a combined approach that uses several of the previously mentioned measures is needed to overcome the hypotension and reduced cardiac output observed during positive-pressure ventilation.

697 How can injury to the lung by high distending pressures and volumes (ie, barotrauma) be prevented? How common is the development of complications arising from barotrauma secondary to mechanical ventilation? Is recognition of these complications an easy task?

❑ Because the complications of barotrauma are more likely to develop in patients receiving high tidal volume and airway pressures, their prevention is based on using the lowest possible peak airway pressure and smaller tidal volumes. Barotrauma in the form of pneumothorax, pneumomediastinum, or subcutaneous emphysema occurs in 10% to 20% of patients receiving mechanical ventilation. The term *barotrauma* is probably a misnomer, since alveolar overdistention appears to be the primary mechanism of lung injury rather than high peak airway pressure. The classic apicolateral location of a pneumothorax is less common in patients receiving mechanical ventilation (largely because of their posture), with the result that the diagnosis is often missed.

698 Explain further the most important forms of barotrauma during mechanical ventilation.

❑ Application of high pressure to the airways causes the overdistended alveoli to rupture, forcing gas into the interstitial lung tissue. The gas may dissect centrally along the pulmonary vessels to the mediastinum (ie, pneumomediastinum). It may rupture into the pericardial space in neonates, but the tight apposition of the pericardial layers usually prevents this complication from happening in adults. If the gas in the mediastinum is not able to escape into the fascial planes of the neck and upper torso (subcutaneous emphysema) or into the retroperitoneal space (pneumoperitoneum), pressure may build and the gas may escape through the mediastinal pleura, resulting in a pneumothorax. The development of a tension pneumothorax can have potentially lethal consequences in mechanically ventilated patients because of the risk of profound hypoxemia and circulatory failure. Predisposing risk factors for barotrauma include the presence of underlying lung disease, especially ARDS and COPD, and the magnitude of peak airway pressure. The risk of barotrauma with PEEP is less clearly defined, although many patients receiving PEEP frequently have high peak airway pressures caused by the low lung compliance.

699 What are the consequences of a pulmonary air leak during mechanical ventilation?

❑ A pulmonary air leak during mechanical ventilation may lead to a pneumothorax, pneumomediastinum, and subcutaneous emphysema. These complications are generally caused by barotrauma, although this is a misnomer because alveolar overdistention rather than high peak airway pressure appears to be the primary mechanism. If an air leak persists for longer than 24 hours after a chest tube has been inserted, a bronchopleural fistula probably exists. The consequences of such a fistula include failure of lung expansion, loss of tidal volume and PEEP with worsening gas exchange, unwanted cycling of the ventilator because chest tube suction pressure may be transmitted to the airway and trigger the ventilator, and pleural infection.

700 What are the main diagnostic features of rupture of the cuff of the endotracheal tube, partial extubation, lung atelectasis, and pneumothorax in a patient receiving mechanical ventilation?

❑ The corresponding diagnostic features for these conditions are as follows: (1) Rupture of the endotracheal tube cuff or partial extubation leads to decreased measured exhaled volume, reduction in airway pressure, inability to maintain a set level of PEEP, and presence of saliva or vomitus in the airway; (2) lung atelectasis causes dullness to percussion with decreased air entry on auscultation, ipsilateral deviation of the trachea, increased plateau pressure due to diminished thoracic compliance, and hypoxemia;

and (3) pneumothorax is characterized by hyperresonance, decreased air entry, crunching sound over the precordium, contralateral deviation of the trachea, increased plateau pressure caused by diminished thoracic compliance, and hypoxemia.

DISCONTINUATION OF MECHANICAL VENTILATION

701 Do all patients receiving mechanical ventilation experience difficulties to resume spontaneous breathing?

❑ No. Many patients who require brief periods of mechanical ventilation can resume and sustain spontaneous respiration with little difficulty. Before extubation, patients should be assessed while breathing spontaneously either through a T-tube circuit or through the ventilator circuit. Although breathing through the ventilator circuit may reduce the cost by sparing a T-tube setup, it increases the patient's work of breathing and is not recommended.

702 What is weaning from mechanical ventilation?

❑ The process of discontinuing mechanical ventilation is usually referred to as *weaning* in the daily vernacular of an intensive care unit. In the strict sense, the term *weaning* refers to a slow decrease in the ventilator support with the patient gradually assuming a greater importance in overall ventilation. However, the term is commonly used in a broader sense to refer to all methods of discontinuing mechanical ventilation. In keeping with common practice, *weaning* is used in this book to refer to the overall process of discontinuing ventilatory support rather than a slow gradual assumption of spontaneous ventilation by the patient.

703 Explain the relevance of weaning from mechanical ventilation in the overall management of respiratory failure. What are the major determinants of weaning outcome and the parameters to predict success?

❑ Although the majority of patients can be weaned easily from mechanical ventilation, a substantial minority pose considerable difficulty. The latter group of patients are responsible for a disproportionately high health-care cost, and they pose enormous clinical, economic, and ethical problems. The major determinants of weaning outcome are the adequacy of pulmonary gas exchange, respiratory muscle function, and psychological condition of the patient. The ratio of respiratory rate to tidal volume appears to be the most reliable parameter to predict weaning outcome.

704 Name conditions in which abrupt extubation and cessation of mechanical ventilation are possible.

❑ Abrupt extubation and cessation of mechanical ventilation can be safely done in most postoperative patients. It is most important to secure that the patient is able to protect the airways without a tracheal tube and to sustain spontaneous breathing. Quantifiable physiologic parameters can help predict the likelihood of weaning success, as discussed in the answers to pertinent questions.

705 How difficult is discontinuation of ventilatory support? How important is the selection of adequate timing to initiate weaning from a ventilator?

❑ Discontinuation of ventilatory support is difficult in up to 20% of patients. Main causes of a difficult weaning from the ventilator include respiratory muscle dysfunction resulting from an imbalance between respiratory load and the capacity of the respiratory muscles to meet that load, impaired oxygenation, and psychological disorders. Although discontinuation of mechanical ventilation is easy in patients requiring short-term support, it can be quite difficult in patients recovering from a major episode of acute respiratory failure. Weaning such patients from the ventilator is a major clinical challenge and constitutes a large portion of the workload in an intensive care unit. The initiation of the weaning process requires careful timing. If it is delayed unnecessarily, the patient remains at risk for ventilator-associated complications.

If it is performed prematurely, severe cardiopulmonary decompensation may develop and further delay extubation.

706 Are abdominal paradox and rapid shallow breathing good indicators of respiratory muscle fatigue? Is muscle fatigue responsible for weaning failure?

❑ In the past, abdominal paradox and rapid shallow breathing were considered indicators of respiratory muscle fatigue. Accordingly, it was believed that respiratory muscle fatigue was a common cause of weaning failure. More recent studies indicated that fatigue is neither a necessary nor a sufficient condition for the development of abnormal rib cage–abdominal motion or rapid shallow breathing. However, the lack of a relationship between fatigue and abnormal breathing pattern does not exclude fatigue as a mechanism of weaning failure. Unfortunately, we simply do not know whether muscle fatigue really occurs in these patients, and, if it does, how important it is in determining clinical outcome.

707 What factor must be evaluated before tracheal extubation?

❑ In addition to assessing a patient's capacity to sustain spontaneous breathing without distress, the patient's ability to protect the upper airway and clear secretions (ie, effective cough) must also be evaluated before extubation. Patients who can sustain spontaneous ventilation without distress may have difficulty following extubation due to upper-airway obstruction, inability to protect the upper airway, or inability to clear secretions. In contrast to the many parameters that have been introduced to predict the outcome of a weaning trial, indices that reliably predict the likelihood of complications following extubation have not been developed. Instead, evaluation consists of clinical assessment of factors such as the level of consciousness, the amount of secretions, and the patient's ability to cough.

708 What criteria are used to determine the optimal time for removal of the tracheal tube (ie, extubation) after completion of weaning from ventilator support?

❑ Patients having upper-airway obstruction, excessive airway secretions, and poor or absent gag reflexes (ie, high risk of massive aspiration of food or gastric contents) may require continuation of tracheal intubation after discontinuation of mechanical ventilation. If the previously mentioned conditions are not present, a T-tube trial followed by extubation is advisable. Because the patient's swallowing function may be defective for hours or days following tracheal extubation, it is advisable to be cautious with respect to the oral intake of nutrients in these patients.

709 In an intubated patient who is free of distress while breathing spontaneously, how can extubation success be predicted?

❑ Lack of a gag reflex when a tongue blade is vigorously rubbed against the posterior oropharynx is often considered a contraindication to extubation. However, a gag reflex is absent in about 20% of normal subjects, and aspiration pneumonia may still occur when gag reflex is present. Ability to cough is important because the accompanying expulsive forces can normally clear the airways down to the level of the medium-size bronchi. The cough response can be assessed by stimulation of the patient's airways with a suction catheter. Recently extubated patients should be monitored closely to determine whether there is a need for reintubation.

CONDITIONS FOR A WEANING TRIAL

710 What elements must be considered prior to weaning a patient from the ventilator?

❑ The patient's clinical status should be stable and abnormal laboratory indices of a reversible nature should be corrected before assessment for weaning. Not surprisingly, the same criteria used for institution of mechanical ventilation are considered when weaning is contemplated, including the gas-exchange function of the lung and the reserve of the ventilatory pump in relation to patient's requirements. A number of different criteria have been proposed to predict success and failure of a weaning trial, as discussed elsewhere in this book.

711 Explain how the clinical assessment should be performed prior to weaning from ventilator support.

❑ The clinical assessment consists of establishing that the patient is hemodynamically stable, serious arrhythmias are absent, neurologic condition is stable, and complications arising from any associated major organ system failure are controlled (eg, stimulation of ventilatory drive in hepatic failure, fluid overload or hyperkalemia caused by renal failure). All experts agree that assessment for weaning should not be restricted to pulmonary factors and general evaluation of the patient with particular attention to features reflecting tissue oxygenation (such as urinary output) and cardiac function must also be considered.

712 What information regarding ventilatory pump function may help to predict weaning success?

❑ Information regarding ventilatory pump function that was widely used to help predict weaning success included (1) vital capacity higher than 10 to 15 mL/kg of body weight, (2) maximum negative inspiratory pressure more negative than −30 cm H_2O, (3) minute ventilation lower than 10 L/min, (4) maximum voluntary ventilation more than twice the resting minute ventilation, and (5) respiratory frequency (f) to tidal volume ratio (f/V_T) lower than 100 breaths/min/L. However, none of these measurements except for the f/V_T ratio appear to be truly helpful in predicting weaning success.

713 What measurements might help to determine the correct time to initiate weaning from a ventilator? Explain further the use of the ratio of respiratory frequency to tidal volume as a predictor to initiate weaning.

❑ In general, discontinuation of mechanical ventilation is not contemplated in a patient with cardiopulmonary instability or a PaO_2 less than 60 mm Hg with an FiO_2 of 0.40 or higher. However, satisfactory oxygenation does not reliably predict successful weaning. Instead, the outcome of a weaning trial is more commonly determined by the ability of the respiratory muscles to cope with an increased respiratory workload. Measurements of maximal inspiratory pressure, vital capacity, and minute ventilation have traditionally been used to judge a patient's readiness for weaning, but they have limited predictive accuracy. The f/VT ratio during 1 minute of spontaneous breathing appears to be a more accurate predictor to initiate weaning; a value of less than 100 breaths/min/L indicates that weaning is likely to be successful. Indices such as f/VT serve only as a guide, however, and do not replace the need for careful clinical assessment. Mechanical ventilation saves lives but can result in serious complications, and thus it should be discontinued at the earliest possible time.

714 What parameters are truly helpful in deciding whether a patient is ready to undergo a weaning trial?

❑ We do not recommend the use of either minute ventilation or maximum inspiratory pressure in deciding whether a patient is ready to undergo a weaning trial. However, these measurements are useful in a patient who has already failed a weaning trial, in that they help us to understand the reason why the patient failed the trial. Instead, we evaluate for the absence of rapid shallow breathing in deciding to attempt weaning. Rapid shallow breathing can be quantitated as the f/VT ratio, and a value less than 100 breaths/min/L suggests that rapid shallow breathing is absent and that weaning is likely to be successful. If on bedside assessment we consider that the patient has achieved significant clinical recovery and the f/V_T ratio is less than 100 breaths/min/L, we undertake a weaning trial. If we consider that clinical recovery is incomplete and the f/V_T ratio is greater than 100 breaths/min/L, we defer weaning. As in the case of any diagnostic test, the f/V_T ratio is not a perfect discriminator, and the physician should not feel overly constrained by the threshold value; instead the measurement needs to be interpreted in the context of careful clinical assessment.

715 What is the most accurate predictor of success and failure with respect to a weaning trial from mechanical ventilation? How useful is the f/V_T ratio?

❑ Rapid shallow breathing, as reflected by a high f/V_T ratio, appears as the most accurate predictor of failure, and a low value as the most accurate predictor of success, in weaning patients from mechanical ventilation. The traditional predictors of the outcome of weaning from mechanical ventilation that included minute ventilation ($\dot{V}_E$) and maximal inspiratory pressure (P_{Imax}) are significantly less accurate than the f/V_T ratio. Patients having a f/V_T ratio of 100 or more breaths/min/L have a 95% likelihood that a weaning trial would fail, whereas those having a lower value of this ratio have an 80% likelihood of successful weaning. As a predictor, the f/V_T ratio has several attractive features: It is easy to measure, it is independent of the patient's effort and cooperation, it has high predictive power, and fortuitously, it has a rounded-off threshold value of 100, which is easy to remember.

METHODS OF WEANING

716 Explain the use of intermittent mandatory ventilation (IMV) as a method of weaning.

❑ IMV was the first alternative approach to T-tube trials, and it involves a gradual reduction in the support provided by the ventilator and a progressive increase in the respiratory work performed by the patient. To accomplish weaning, the IMV rate is reduced in steps of 1 to 3 breaths/min, and an ABG sample is obtained after about 30 minutes. As the IMV rate is decreased, inspiratory work increases progressively not only for the spontaneous breaths but also for the assisted breaths. Proponents of IMV believe that application of weaning predictors prolongs this process. They advocate monitoring ABGs while lowering the rate of ventilator-delivered breaths, provided arterial pH remains above 7.35.

717 How can IMV be used as a weaning technique?

❑ Although currently used as a primary mode of mechanical ventilation, IMV was introduced as a method of weaning with claims that it was more efficient, safer, and superior to traditional weaning techniques. When used in a weaning trial, the IMV rate is reduced in steps, usually 1 to 3 breaths/min at each step, and ABGs obtained after 30 minutes or more at that setting. If the arterial blood pH remains above 7.35, the IMV rate is commonly reduced until a rate of zero is reached. This method of weaning is guided by the changes in arterial blood pH in response to stepwise reductions in the number of mechanically delivered breaths, and predictions are not based on physiologic measurements. An advantage of IMV as a weaning technique is that unlike the repeated manipulations required with the T-tube system, IMV is performed without changing the breathing circuit. This is an advantage obtained with the use of a continuous-flow IMV circuit; however, the ubiquitous incorporation of demand valves in current ventilator design may result in a twofold or greater increase in the work of breathing during spontaneous breathing through the ventilator circuit. The originators of IMV recommended that the number of breaths from the ventilator should be titrated in accordance with the results of ABG analysis. This can result in a false sense of security, because 2 to 3 positive-pressure breaths/min can achieve acceptable blood gas values, but these data provide no information regarding the patient's work of breathing, which may be excessive.

---

718 Explain the use of pressure-support ventilation (PSV) as a method of weaning.

❑ PSV augments a spontaneous breath with a fixed level of positive pressure that is set by the physician, and the patient can control the respiratory frequency, inspiratory time, and inspiratory flow rate. Weaning from PSV is accomplished by gradually decreasing in steps of 3 to 6 cm H_2O the level of PSV (according to patient's tolerance), and extubation is commonly performed when the PSV level reaches 5 to 8 cm H_2O.

---

719 Explain the major advantages and disadvantages of the weaning technique using pressure support.

❑ With pressure support, the ventilator augments spontaneous breathing with a fixed amount of positive pressure. When pressure support is used for weaning, the level of pressure is reduced gradually in decrements of 3 to 6 cm H_2O, titrated on the basis of respiratory frequency. Several investigators showed that pressure support can be used to counteract the work of breathing imposed by the endotracheal tube and ventilator circuit. This has led to the notion that if a patient can sustain spontaneous ventilation at this "compensatory level" of pressure support, he or she will tolerate extubation. The problem with this strategy is that a compensatory level of pressure support varies between 3 and 14 cm H_2O, and there is no reliable method for accurately determining the required level in an individual patient.

---

720 Explain the use of spontaneous breathing trials as a method of weaning.

❑ The oldest method of weaning is to undertake spontaneous breathing trials of increasing duration several times a day. Typically, this approach begins with brief trials (lasting about 5 minutes), which are gradually increased in accordance with a patient's performance as assessed by bedside clinical examination. The optimal period of rest between these trials has never been defined, but is commonly as short as 1 to 3 hours. When the patient is able to sustain spontaneous ventilation for some fixed time, such as 1 to 2 hours, extubation is performed. Having the patient breathe through the ventilator circuit minimizes financial cost, but this usually results in a marked increase in the work of breathing. Instead, it is preferable to supply an air-oxygen gas mixture through a T-tube circuit. A recent study showed that undertaking a trial of spontaneous breathing once a day was at least as effective as undertaking multiple trials, several times a day.

---

721 Explain the major advantages and disadvantages of the weaning technique that consists of a trial of spontaneous breathing through a T-tube circuit.

❑ The major advantages of a trial of spontaneous breathing through a T-tube circuit are the rapidity of weaning with this technique (faster than other methods), its simplicity, and the absence of an increased work of breathing caused by opening a ventilator's demand value (such valves are not used in a T-tube circuit). The potential disadvantages of this weaning technique include the lack of exhaled volume monitoring, automatic sighs, and alarm systems. The advantages of a T-tube circuit outweigh the disadvantages, making this method the most useful as a weaning technique.

---

722 What method of weaning from mechanical ventilation might more likely succeed in a short trial?

❑ A large prospective randomized study recently performed demonstrated that a once-daily trial of spontaneous breathing led to extubation about three times more quickly than did IMV and about twice as quickly as PSV. Multiple-daily trials of spontaneous breathing were equally successful as a once-daily trial. Patients were randomly assigned to one of four weaning techniques: (1) IMV; (2) PSV; (3) intermittent trials of spontaneous breathing, conducted two or more times a day; and (4) once-daily trial of spontaneous breathing. Patients assigned to a once-daily trial of spontaneous breathing (ie, method having the best results) were disconnected from the ventilator and allowed to breathe spontaneously through a T-tube circuit for up to 2 hours each day. If signs of intolerance developed, AC ventilation was reinstituted for 24 hours, at which time another trial was attempted. Patients who tolerated a 2-hour trial without signs of distress were extubated.

723 What is the best technique to wean patients from a ventilator?

❑ Our preferred method of weaning is to employ a single daily trial of spontaneous breathing through a T-tube circuit. The trial is conducted while a physician is in the intensive care unit, and if the patient can sustain spontaneous ventilation for 30 to 60 minutes without undue distress, we extubate the patient. If the patient develops signs of distress on physical examination, we stop the trial and reinstitute mechanical ventilation. To allow the respiratory muscles to recover from excessive stress, we rest the patient for approximately 24 hours with a high level of ventilator assistance such as with AC ventilation. We reassess the patient the following morning to see whether he or she is ready for another trial of spontaneous breathing.

724 Is the technique of weaning (ie, process of removing patients from mechanical ventilation) the most important determinant for the successful discontinuation of ventilatory support?

❑ No. The most important determinant of success in weaning is resolution or correction of the precipitating cause of the respiratory failure. Consequently, weaning should be attempted only after reversal of the process responsible for respiratory failure.

WEANING FAILURE

725 Describe the characteristic physical signs observed in patients who fail a trial of weaning from mechanical ventilation.

❑ Patients who fail a trial of weaning from mechanical ventilation display characteristic abnormalities in the pattern of breathing, namely rapid shallow breathing; rib cage–abdominal paradox, which markedly decreases the efficiency of respiratory muscle contraction; diaphoresis and nasal flaring; cyanosis; heightened sternomastoid activity; suprasternal and supraclavicular recession; tachypnea; intercostal recession; and tachycardia.

726 What are the blood gas abnormalities and changes in cardiac output commonly observed in patients who fail a weaning trial?

❑ Patients failing a weaning trial from ventilatory support often develop an increase in $PaCO_2$ with or without a significant fall in PaO_2. The maintenance of a constant PaO_2 (in spite of worsening of ventilation-perfusion mismatching in many patients as a result of discontinuation of mechanical ventilation and resumption of spontaneous breathing) is caused by a simultaneous increase in cardiac output. However, abnormalities in gas exchange can be compounded by changes in cardiac performance during a weaning trial. Increases in the work of breathing with markedly negative swings in intrathoracic pressure predispose to an increase in left ventricular afterload. In fact, it has been demonstrated that discontinuation of mechanical ventilation can result in a decrease in left ventricular ejection fraction.

727 What psychological factors can jeopardize the success of a weaning trial?

❑ The patient's dependence on mechanical ventilation can be associated with feelings of insecurity, anxiety, fear, agony, and panic. Many patients believe that they will remain dependent forever on mechanical ventilation and that discontinuation of ventilator support will result in sudden death. The prevalence and nature of psychological disturbances in ventilator-dependent patients and the degree to which psychological factors contribute to ventilator dependency remain undefined.

728 Is depressed respiratory center output the major determinant of weaning failure?

❑ Patients who fail a trial of weaning from mechanical ventilation commonly develop hypercapnia, which naturally raises the suspicion of respiratory center depression. However, indices of respiratory drive are usually increased above the normal range in such patients. Consequently, a decrease in respiratory center output is not primarily responsible for weaning failure. The increase in $PaCO_2$ in these patients is caused by the rapid shallow breathing, with a consequent increase in physiologic dead space.

729 Name conditions that decrease neuromuscular capacity and conditions that increase respiratory muscle load.

❑ Respiratory pump failure may result from reduced neuromuscular capacity (strength), increased respiratory load, or both. Reduced neuromuscular capacity might be secondary to decreased respiratory center output, phrenic nerve dysfunction, and decreased respiratory muscle strength or endurance (eg, hyperinflation, malnutrition, decreased oxygen supply, respiratory acidosis, metabolic abnormalities, endocrinopathy, drug-induced toxicity, disuse muscle atrophy, respiratory muscle fatigue). Increased respiratory load might be secondary to increased ventilatory requirements (eg, increased carbon dioxide production, augmented dead space ventilation, inappropriately high respiratory drive), and increased work of breathing.

---

730 What are the major causes of respiratory pump failure (eg, weaning failure)? Elaborate on the causes of weaning failure secondary to excessive demands on the respiratory system and respiratory muscle dysfunction.

❑ Failure to wean a patient from ventilatory support most often results from incomplete resolution of the precipitating illness or the development of new problems. Weaning failure caused by hypoxemia in a patient who met the oxygenation criteria before the trial usually indicates the persistence of pulmonary disease, and a slightly longer period of mechanical ventilation is desirable to allow further healing. Excessive demands on the ventilatory pump caused by high ventilatory requirements or excessive work of breathing are important determinants of weaning failure. Carbon dioxide production increases with the hypermetabolism of fever and high intake of carbohydrates. The work of breathing may be increased by unnecessary loads imposed on the respiratory system and optimum plumbing of the ventilatory support device is critical. Demand on the respiratory muscles increases as the ventilatory requirements and work of breathing increase. Inadequate energy supplies may result from malnutrition (especially if associated with hypophosphatemia, hypokalemia, or hypomagnesemia) or decreased oxygen delivery to the respiratory muscles as a result of hypoxemia or reduced cardiac output.

---

731 What are the specific causes of respiratory pump failure after mechanical ventilation?

❑ Respiratory pump failure following the use of ventilator support is most commonly due to respiratory muscle dysfunction. Respiratory muscle dysfunction results from an imbalance between respiratory neuromuscular capacity and the load on the respiratory system. Causes of decreased respiratory neuromuscular capacity that are important in the difficult-to-wean patient include dynamic hyperinflation (which decreases the contractile force), malnutrition, electrolyte abnormalities (hypokalemia, hypocalcemia, and hypophosphatemia decrease muscle contractility), respiratory acidosis, and the aftereffects of neuromuscular blocking agents. An increase in respiratory load may result from excessive ventilatory requirements, increased resistance, decreased compliance, and the presence of auto-PEEP (which poses an inspiratory threshold load).

---

732 Summarize the most important determinants of failure to wean patients from mechanical ventilation.

❑ Weaning patients from mechanical ventilation constitutes a major portion of the workload in an intensive care unit, as more than 40% of total ventilator time is consumed by the weaning process. Several pathophysiologic mechanisms may be responsible for weaning failure, but the precise role of each is incompletely understood. Patients who fail a weaning trial commonly develop hypercapnia, which appears to be caused by a decreased tidal volume rather than secondary to a primary decrease in respiratory drive. Respiratory muscle performance is impaired in these patients as a result of dynamic hyperinflation and paradoxical motion of the rib cage and abdomen. Worsening of pulmonary mechanics during a weaning trial can cause further embarrassment of the respiratory muscles. However, the clinical importance of respiratory muscle fatigue as responsible for weaning failure remains unclear.

---

733 What is the treatment of severe respiratory muscle fatigue? What measures might be used in the management of respiratory muscle dysfunction?

❑ Resting the respiratory muscles with the application of mechanical ventilation is the only satisfactory method for the management of severe respiratory muscle fatigue. Although the optimal duration of rest is unknown, it is probably more than 24 hours. Ironically, however, prolonged rest may result in respiratory muscle atrophy. Numerous measures can be used to manage respiratory muscle dysfunction, a condition that can lead to severe respiratory muscle fatigue. Removal of the underlying cause, if possible, should be considered first. In addition, correction of any electrolyte disturbances as well as of appropriate treatment of respiratory tract infections is mandatory. It is also important to reduce the ventilatory load by reversing any abnormalities of pulmonary mechanics. Nutritional supplementation improves respiratory muscle strength in malnourished patients, such as those with anorexia nervosa. Regardless, it is advisable to ensure adequate nutrition in the management of respiratory muscle dysfunction. Other measures might include administration of aminophylline, training of respiratory muscles, and diaphragmatic pacing.

24. Acute Respiratory Distress Syndrome

GENERAL MANAGEMENT

734 Enumerate the major elements in the management of ARDS.

❑ The main elements of the management of ARDS are (1) oxygen administration to maintain a PaO_2 of about 60 mm Hg (usually requiring mechanical ventilation), (2) measures aimed at reversing any condition that may lead or aggravate ARDS (eg, infections, pancreatitis, drugs), (3) careful management of fluid balance in order to avoid fluid excess, (4) hemodynamic support to optimize tissue perfusion including the cerebral and renal circulation, (5) securing proper nutritional status, and (6) reversing and preventing complications (eg, pneumothorax).

735 What is the specific therapy of ARDS?

❑ No therapy has been found to ameliorate the lung injury of ARDS, and thus, management is largely empirical and supportive. For some time it appeared that early application of PEEP might be useful in preventing the development of ARDS in patients at risk, but a recent study found it to be without value. In the past, corticosteroid therapy was part of standard management, but several large studies showed that they are not useful and may even increase the morbidity and mortality of ARDS.

736 Explain the use of supplemental oxygen and PEEP in the management of ARDS.

❑ Supplemental oxygen is required in all patients with ARDS, and care is required to minimize the risk of oxygen toxicity. Mechanical ventilation and PEEP also need careful application to avoid the hazards associated with their use. Although PEEP has not been proved to decrease the mortality from ARDS, it is almost universally employed. In addition, patients who show significant improvement in oxygenation with PEEP appear to have a lower mortality. PEEP may be beneficial by keeping open the airways and alveoli that would otherwise collapse during expiration and be difficult to reinflate due to the loss of surfactant. In addition, PEEP redistributes edema fluid from the alveoli to the interstitium, which may improve gas exchange by converting units from pure shunt to a more normal $\dot{V}_A/\dot{Q}$ ratio. The application of PEEP usually permits a reduction in inspired oxygen concentration. However, the adverse hemodynamic effects of PEEP can actually lead to an overall impairment in oxygen delivery to the tissues, so careful monitoring is required with its use.

737 What are the potential salutary effects of mechanical ventilation in patients with ARDS?

❑ Patients with ARDS who also have poor respiratory effort are at risk of progressive respiratory failure with hypoxemia and hypercapnia. For such patients, mechanical ventilation is a lifesaving procedure. In addition, mechanical ventilation will decrease the work of breathing by respiratory muscles, correct the blood gas abnormalities, decrease sympathetic activation, diminish whole-body oxygen consumption, and thereby reduce circulatory stress. If hypoxemia is not corrected by the institution of mechanical ventilation, and if inspired oxygen of 60% or more is necessary for prolonged periods, PEEP should be instituted.

738 What are the potential counterproductive effects of mechanical ventilation in patients with ARDS?

❑ The relatively high pulmonary volume and airway pressure that accompany mechanical ventilation might be counterproductive because of hemodynamic and nonhemodynamic mechanisms. The hemodynamic complications might be caused by increased pulmonary vascular resistance due to lung volume expansion as well as high alveolar pressure that augments right ventricular afterload, decreases systemic venous return, and reduces cardiac output. Such reduction in right-sided cardiac output will lead to a secondary decrease in left-sided cardiac output so that oxygen transport to peripheral tissues might be significantly reduced. Moreover, the decreased left ventricular output might also produce a fall in blood pressure accompanied by severe renal underperfusion (and possibly a reduction in cerebral and myocardial blood flow). Additional hemodynamic complications arising from the increased right ventricular pressure include displacement of the interventricular septum, which impedes left ventricular filling during diastole, as well as direct compression of the left ventricle by the inflated lung that also reduces diastolic filling. Nonhemodynamic complications of mechanical ventilation arise from barotrauma, which might produce pneumomediastinum, pneumothorax, and subcutaneous emphysema.

---

739 What does the term *baby lung* mean? What effects might high airway pressure during mechanical ventilation have on the baby lung?

❑ Although diffuse radiographic abnormalities suggest a homogeneous pattern of lung injury in patients with ARDS, studies with computed tomography indicate that the early injury is quite heterogeneous. Rather than having stiff, normal-sized lungs, patients with ARDS can be considered to have two distinct functional compartments: a small compartment with relatively normal compliance (baby lung), and a large stiff compartment that has little functional participation. Consequently, the utilization of high pressure during mechanical ventilation may produce barotrauma by causing considerable overdistention of normal lung regions (baby lung).

---

740 Explain the limitations of physical examination, body weight change, chest radiographs, and ventilator adjustments in the absence of precise hemodynamic monitoring (ie, Swan-Ganz catheter) for the management of critically ill patients with ARDS receiving mechanical ventilation.

❑ Noninvasive techniques (eg, physical examination, chest radiographs) have limited value in the management of critically ill patients with ARDS. Detection of pulmonary rales is of very limited importance because their presence is the rule in these patients. Similarly, portable anteroposterior chest x-ray films fail to distinguish pulmonary edema from infection and cannot determine reliably changes in lung fluid content as well as estimate changes in heart size. In addition, the effects of ventilator adjustments may be difficult to interpret because the progressive lung dysfunction is commonly responsible for the need of higher inflation pressures. Changes in body weight are not good indicators of intravascular volume because "third space" fluid sequestration (eg, peripheral edema, fluid accumulation in body cavities) is commonly present in these patients, but are important prognostic indicators (ie, fluid excess is associated with higher morbidity and mortality). Furthermore, worsening of hypoxemia in association with hypotension and oliguria may lead the health care team to prescribe diuretics to correct fluid excess and promote diuresis or, conversely, to administer fluids to expand intravascular volume. The need for more reliable invasive techniques (ie, measurement of pressures in the pulmonary circulation and cardiac output) to properly assess and manage critically ill patients with ARDS is therefore apparent.

741 How effective are the anti-inflammatory agents including corticosteroids in the treatment of ARDS?

❑ None of several tested anti-inflammatory agents has been proved to be effective in the treatment of ARDS. Various trials have shown that corticosteroid therapy does not prevent the development of ARDS, hasten its reversal, or decrease mortality; in fact, corticosteroids may even increase mortality in patients with an elevated serum creatinine level (>2 mg/dL). Promising preliminary findings on the efficacy of therapy with prostaglandin E_1 were not confirmed in a large multicenter trial. Likewise, multicentered studies showed that ibuprofen, a nonsteroidal anti-inflammatory drug, and exogenous surfactant agents are not beneficial.

---

742 Does inhaled nitric oxide have any beneficial effect in patients with ARDS?

❑ Inhalation of nitric oxide in a concentration of 18 ppm by patients with severe ARDS was found to reduce the pulmonary artery pressure and increase arterial oxygenation by improving the matching of ventilation with perfusion, without producing systemic vasodilation. Whether inhaled nitric oxide improves outcome in ARDS remains unknown.

---

743 Explain the management of drowning and near-drowning. What is the prognosis of these conditions?

❑ The most decisive factor in the management of near-drowning victims is resumption of ventilation by using mouth-to-mouth resuscitation. Even in victims with evident aspiration of fluid, time should not be wasted in attempting to drain liquid from the lungs because large volumes are rarely aspirated. In the absence of an effective pulse, closed-chest cardiac resuscitation is required. Admission to a hospital is imperative for all surviving victims because the patient's clinical status may belie life-threatening hypoxemia; supplemental oxygen should be continued until the measurement of PaO_2 indicates a satisfactory level. Intubation, mechanical ventilation, and hemodynamic monitoring will be required in patients who subsequently develop ARDS. Bronchodilators counteract bronchospasm, and bicarbonate administration might be necessary to correct metabolic acidosis. Electrolyte disturbances, hemolysis, or renal failure should be treated appropriately. Prophylactic steroid or antibiotic therapy is not indicated. The prognosis is good for patients who are alert or who have a blunted level of consciousness on admission to the emergency room, but poor for those in a coma.

744 Elaborate further on the prognosis of ARDS.

❑ The overall mortality of patients with ARDS is approximately 50% to 60%. Yet, a lower mortality is found in patients whose disease is caused by drug overdose and a higher one in those with circulatory collapse (shock) and multiple-organ system failure (eg, hepatic, renal). Factors indicative of poor prognosis are related to the status of the respiratory (eg, need for higher inflation pressures caused by decreased compliance, increase in alveolar-arterial oxygen gradient, requiring application of PEEP and higher inspired PO_2), circulatory (eg, arterial hypotension that fails to respond to intravascular volume replacement), and nutritional (eg, low serum albumin) condition of the patient.

745 Is complete recovery of the anatomy and physiology of the lungs observed after an episode of ARDS?

❑ Although many patients experience complete recovery (ie, absence of symptoms and signs of disease, normal results on pulmonary function tests) following an episode of ARDS, the recovery is incomplete in other patients. The latter group may exhibit interstitial fibrosis and emphysematous changes in lung morphology as long-term sequelae, but the functional effects are usually not severe. Because the development of irreversible changes has been proposed to be dependent on the severity and duration of ARDS, intensive treatment of this condition may reduce the risk of long-term pulmonary damage.

FLUID EXCESS IN ARDS AND PULMONARY EDEMA

746 How large should the fluid intake (ie, total volume of fluid administration) be in patients with ARDS?

❑ Since expansion of body fluid compartments must be prevented in patients with ARDS, fluid restriction is desirable. Yet, patients with ARDS are often hemodynamically unstable and prone to hypotension, making it difficult to establish the optimal fluid prescription. If fluid excess is present, negative fluid balance can be accomplished with the use of diuretics or ultrafiltration aimed at removing fluid as much as possible, while maintaining perfusion to vital organs and circulatory support with pressor drugs if necessary. Fluid restriction appears to improve survival in patients with ARDS, presumably by reducing the fluid excess in the lungs.

747 What are the effects of fluid excess (ie, significant positive fluid balance) in the prognosis of ARDS?

❑ Several retrospective studies showed that a large positive fluid balance is associated with increased mortality. In addition, a randomized prospective study showed that achieving a lower positive fluid balance decreased the number of days of ventilator support and intensive care unit stay. Although the ability to achieve a lower positive fluid balance may be the factor that primarily determines prognosis, rather than the therapeutic strategy itself, these findings suggest that minimizing fluid overload may improve survival in patients with ARDS.

748 What is the importance of a positive fluid balance on the prognosis of ARDS?

❑ The airspaces in patients with ARDS are flooded because of leaky pulmonary capillaries. Consequently, recent efforts have focused on reducing such leakage by lowering pulmonary vascular pressures. Several retrospective studies showed that a large positive fluid balance is associated with increased mortality. Furthermore, a randomized prospective study showed that achieving a lower positive fluid balance decreased the number of days of ventilator support and intensive care unit stay. A lower positive fluid balance may be the factor that primarily determines prognosis, rather than the therapeutic strategy itself, and minimizing fluid overload may improve survival in patients with ARDS.

---

749 What are the causes and the management of fluid overload in ARDS? What is the role of aminophylline, dopamine infusion, glucocorticosteroids, albumin, hemofiltration, dialysis, and combination of diuretics?

❑ Fluid overload refractory to conventional diuretic therapy (eg, lack of response to more than 200 mg of furosemide per day) can be due to (1) high sodium chloride intake, detected by measuring urine Na^+ excretion; (2) decreased drug availability at the lumen of the renal tubules (ie, associated severe circulatory failure, renal failure, or liver disease) and managed with massive doses of loop diuretics, combination of diuretics, hemofiltration, or dialysis; and (3) enhanced renal reabsorption of salt and water with low glomerular filtration rate (GFR). These defects might respond to acetazolamide, thiazides, potassium-sparing diuretics, combination of diuretics, aminophylline, intravenous dopamine infusion, and rarely, glucocorticosteroids (that may increase the GFR).

---

750 Is pulmonary congestion caused by fluid excess or left ventricular failure an uncommon and easily recognized complication of ARDS? How useful might be the insertion of a Swan-Ganz catheter in the evaluation of these patients? How can a low cardiac output be detected?

❑ No. Pulmonary congestion caused by fluid excess or left ventricular failure is a commonly present but easily missed complication observed during the course of acute hypoxemic respiratory failure. Its recognition is made difficult because of the unreliability of physical examination (eg, crackles and rhonchi are present even without fluid excess or left ventricular failure, gallop rhythms are difficult to detect in these patients) and radiographic evaluation (eg, edema caused by fluid excess resembles pulmonary infection, and cardiac silhouette appears enlarged even in the absence of heart failure because the portable chest films are taken in the anteroposterior direction and the lungs are commonly at less volume than at full inspiration). If left ventricular failure is suspected, a Swan-Ganz catheter should be inserted to monitor the hemodynamic condition. This tool allows one to evaluate continuously the pulmonary artery pressure and to intermittently assess PCWP and oxygen content of mixed venous blood. An abnormally high PCWP indicates that end-diastolic left ventricular pressure is increased because of fluid excess or left ventricular failure. In addition, the pulmonary artery catheter may allow one to obtain a thermodilution cardiac output measurement. The presence of abnormally low oxygen content of mixed venous blood in association with adequate arterial oxygen content is indicative of a low cardiac output, although this pattern is not commonly observed.

---

751 When should diuretics be used in volume expansion (eg, risk of pulmonary edema)? Name the major classes or types of diuretics for the treatment of volume expansion and compare their potency in terms of the fractional urinary excretion of sodium (FE_{Na^+}) (% of filtered sodium excreted in the urine).

❑ The physician should consider the use of diuretics when dietary sodium chloride restriction and bed rest fail to correct salt and water retention. Diuretics promote natriuresis (increased urine sodium excretion) and diuresis (increased urine volume) by their actions on the renal tubules. Major indications for the use of diuretics include respiratory dysfunction due to pulmonary congestion or edema, deterioration of cardiac function due to fluid overload, and the mechanical effects of massive ascites. Thiazides, loop diuretics, potassium-sparing diuretics, and acetazolamide are diuretics used in the treatment of volume expansion. Thiazides and loop diuretics, the most commonly prescribed agents, can be used in most diseases accompanied by volume expansion. By contrast, potassium-sparing diuretics and acetazolamide are indicated in specific conditions (see pertinent questions). The potassium-sparing diuretics including spironolactone, triamterene, and amiloride are the least potent diuretics, with a FE_{Na^+} between 2% and 3%. Acetazolamide is also a very mild diuretic, with a FE_{Na^+} between 3% and 5%. The most widely used agents are the thiazides and metolazone, with a FE_{Na^+} between 5% and 8%, and the loop diuretics (furosemide, ethacrynic acid, bumetanide), with a FE_{Na^+} between 20% and 25%.

752 What is the role of high-dosage furosemide or ultrafiltration in the management of ARDS with severe and refractory fluid overload?

❑ High-dosage furosemide (250 to 4000 mg/day) in combination with vasodilators such as low-moderate-dosage dopamine (ie, 1 to 5 µg/kg/min intravenously) or inotropic drugs might be useful in patients with ARDS and fluid overload resistant to conventional treatment. A combination of two to four diuretics acting on different segments of the renal tubule (eg, loop agent, thiazide, acetazolamide, potassium-sparing drug) simultaneously administered might produce a substantial natriuresis in patients who failed to respond to a high-dosage furosemide regimen. Ultrafiltration is an effective therapeutic option for fluid removal in patients who fail to respond to diuretics or those with severe renal insufficiency (the response to diuretic agents is poor or absent in this condition). The ultrafiltration technique (eg, arteriovenous or venovenous access to the circulation) is relatively simple and cost-effective, and might achieve sustained symptomatic improvement in selected patients.

753 Elaborate on the management of fluid overload in patients with respiratory failure. How does the presence of renal insufficiency alter the natriuresis induced by thiazides and loop diuretics?

❑ Renal insufficiency blunts the response to all diuretic agents. Thiazides as single agents are not effective diuretic drugs when the GFR is less than 30 mL/min (about one-third of normal level) whereas loop diuretics used at a high dosage might still produce natriuresis. A combination of loop diuretics and thiazides might have synergistic effects on salt and water excretion in patients with an abnormally low GFR. Diuretic drugs are contraindicated in patients with anuria (lack of urine output).

---

754 Explain further the effects of renal insufficiency on the response to diuretics of patients with fluid overload. Elaborate on the use of thiazides, furosemide, ethacrynic acid, and potassium-sparing diuretics.

❑ Renal insufficiency decreases the response to diuretics and increases their clinical toxicity. Yet, diuretics are valuable therapeutic agents in patients with fluid overload and renal insufficiency except for those with end-stage renal failure (state in which diuretics are contraindicated because of absence of meaningful effects and high risks of toxicity). Thiazides are generally of no value when the GFR is less than 30 mL/min and might further decrease overall renal function. Loop agents (eg, furosemide), on the other hand, have diuretic effects in patients with a low GFR, but a higher dosage (eg, 160 to 200 mg/day) is generally required. Ethacrynic acid is not recommended for the treatment of fluid overload associated with renal insufficiency because of the increased risk of ototoxicity. Potassium-sparing diuretics generally are contraindicated in patients with renal insufficiency because of the risk of hyperkalemia. Renal insufficiency is a common associated condition in patients with circulatory failure. It has multiple causes including a reduced blood flow to the kidney due to heart disease, a concomitant vascular illness (eg, atherosclerosis, hypertensive glomerulosclerosis), and associated metabolic or other diseases (eg, diabetic nephropathy) and as a complication of diuretic therapy.

---

755 What are the most salient properties of loop diuretics (ie, agents most commonly used in the management of pulmonary edema)?

❑ Loop diuretics, the most potent drugs of the group, include furosemide (Lasix), ethacrynic acid (Edecrin), and bumetanide (Bumex). These agents inhibit sodium chloride reabsorption in the thick ascending limb of Henle's loop; this action takes place on the luminal membrane after the diuretic reaches Henle's loop by secretion into the proximal tubule and by glomerular filtration. Loop diuretics can also promote diuresis and natriuresis due to increased renal blood flow, partly mediated by increased secretion of vasodilatory prostaglandins. Administration of nonsteroidal anti-inflammatory agents, drugs known to diminish renal prostaglandin synthesis, can decrease the diuretic action of loop diuretics. The onset of action occurs in minutes, with peak effects observed within 2 hours. The duration of action is up to 8 hours. Daily dosages of these drugs are as follows: (1) furosemide, 20 to 80 mg, maximal dose of 1000 mg/day; (2) ethacrynic acid, 50 to 100 but up to 400 mg/day can be given; and (3) bumetanide, 0.5 to 2.0 mg, maximal dose of 10 mg/day. Titration of daily dosage is based on the response to the initial dose, severity of fluid overload, level of renal function, and need for a rapid and large diuresis. The most salient adverse effects of loop diuretics are potassium depletion with hypokalemia, metabolic alkalosis, hyponatremia, and muscle cramps. Furosemide can also cause glucose intolerance, deafness, and thrombocytopenia. Loop diuretics can have synergistic effects with thiazides so that their combination can be useful in the management of edematous patients who fail to respond to a single agent.

---

756 What are the most salient properties of acetazolamide, a diuretic prescribed to correct metabolic alkalosis complicating respiratory acidosis?

❑ Acetazolamide is a carbonic anhydrase inhibitor that diminishes sodium bicarbonate ($NaHCO_3$) reabsorption in the renal proximal tubules. This diuretic has relatively low potency, comparable to that of potassium-sparing diuretics. Because the increased natriuresis is accompanied by urine bicarbonate excretion, acetazolamide may be useful in posthypercapnic alkalosis, metabolic alkalosis due to loop diuretics, thiazides, and other causes. Acetazolamide is generally prescribed at a dosage of 250 mg three times a day for 2 to 4 days. The onset of action occurs in 1 hour, with the peak effect between 2 and 4 hours and the duration of action between 6 and 8 hours. The most significant adverse effects are the development of metabolic acidosis and renal calculi.

757 Describe the effects of acetazolamide on respiratory function, urinary electrolytes, acid-base balance, and extrarenal tissues. What are the indications of this drug in patients with respiratory diseases?

❑ The transport of carbon dioxide in the blood is dependent on the activity of the carbonic anhydrase of the red cells. Consequently, acetazolamide, a potent inhibitor of carbonic anhydrase, creates a disequilibrium in the transport system of carbon dioxide, increasing PCO_2 in the tissues and decreasing its level in the expired gas. The extrarenal effects of acetazolamide also include stimulation of ventilatory drive (useful in acute mountain sickness, and possible useful in respiratory depression and cor pulmonale with hypercapnia) and depression of intraocular pressure (useful in the treatment of glaucoma). Acetazolamide increases the urinary excretion of Na^+, K^+, and bicarbonate (HCO_3^-). The main effect of this drug on acid-base balance is the induction of metabolic acidosis. This acid-base disorder blunts the pharmacologic action of acetazolamide on the proximal nephron, ameliorating the severity of the acid-base disturbance. The systemic acid-base effect of this drug accounts for its use in the treatment of posthypercapnic alkalosis and metabolic alkalosis caused by other diuretics.

HEMOFILTRATION (CAVH, CVVH) IN ARDS AND CRITICALLY ILL PATIENTS

758 Outline the major features of extracorporeal ultrafiltration (intermittent or continuous) and its use in the management of ARDS with severe and refractory fluid overload. Compare the use of ultrafiltration and dialysis.

❑ Extracorporeal ultrafiltration or hemofiltration is a therapeutic modality that allows fluid removal from the circulation (with the use of a filtering-membrane device interposed between an arterial and a venous access or a venovenous access) in patients with severe fluid overload unresponsive to diuretics. Fluid can be removed at rates of up to 500 mL/hr for a 2- to 6-hour treatment (intermittent modality), or at relatively low rates (eg, 100 mL/hr) for prolonged periods (continuous modality for 24 to 72 hours or longer). Ultrafiltration is an effective temporary method for the control of fluid overload that requires close monitoring because of its potential for inducing serious hemodynamic instability and major fluid and electrolyte losses. Patients with intractable fluid overload with significant renal insufficiency should receive ultrafiltration (intermittent or continuous) plus dialysis. Extracorporeal ultrafiltration (or simply ultrafiltration) promotes fluid loss due to a hydrostatic pressure gradient across the semipermeable membrane that separates the blood compartment from the collecting receptacle. In contrast with ultrafiltration, hemodialysis promotes solute removal from the blood compartment to a dialysate fluid that circulates on the other side of the semipermeable membrane, driven by a concentration (chemical) gradient.

---

759 What humoral mediators of lung injury can be removed with ultrafiltration or hemofiltration techniques? What is the role, if any, of hemofiltration techniques in the management of ARDS?

❑ Continuous hemofiltration can remove several humoral mediators of tissue injury in patients with multiple-organ failure. These substances are complement-activating factor, anaphylatoxin, prostacyclin, thromboxane, interleukin-1, interleukin-6, tumor necrosis factor-alpha, platelet activator factor (PAF), leukotrienes, and oxygen radicals derived from activated neutrophils. Yet, in most clinical studies, employing continuous arteriovenous hemofiltration (CAVH) and continuous venovenous hemofiltration (CVVH) also induced changes in the patient's fluid balance; therefore, it is impossible to ascertain the role of each mechanism (ie, removal of mediators of tissue injury versus changes in volume of body fluids) in the overall response to these treatments in

ARDS. It is currently thought by many critical care specialists that CAVH and CVVH are first-choice therapies for the fluid, electrolyte, and humoral derangements observed in patients with multiple-organ failure, especially if vascular instability and myocardial insufficiency are present.

---

760 Elaborate on the mechanisms responsible for the salutary effects of continuous hemofiltration (or ultrafiltration) in the management of ARDS.

❑ Continuous hemofiltration includes several blood-cleansing procedures based on convection forces that allow removal of large volumes of plasma ultrafiltrate. The possible beneficial effect in ARDS might be due to promoting repair of lung injury and reducing extravascular lung water because of several mechanisms, including (1) reduction of hydrostatic pressure within the pulmonary vasculature; (2) increased intravascular colloid osmotic pressure, which in association with diminished vascular pressure helps to reduce ultrafiltration forces, thereby promoting correction of lung edema; and (3) elimination of low- and middle-molecular-weight substances (eg, thromboxane A_2, interleukins) that may contribute to the pulmonary lesions observed in ARDS. The importance of each of these three mechanisms in the potential salutary effects of continuous hemofiltration remains undefined. While the efficacy of hemofiltration in the management of extravascular lung water accumulation caused by an elevation in hydrostatic microvascular pressure (eg, cardiogenic pulmonary edema) has been well documented, the results in pulmonary edema due to increased capillary permeability (eg, ARDS) are still controversial. It must be recognized that hemofiltration might not work in ARDS because of various factors: (1) Hydrostatic pressure is primarily normal; thus, a hemofiltration-induced reduction in microvascular pressure might not be expected to lower fluid filtration rate. (2) There is an impairment in pulmonary microvascular permeability; thus, the hemofiltration-induced increase in intravascular colloid osmotic pressure may not favor fluid reabsorption because a colloid osmotic pressure gradient cannot develop. In spite of the previous statement, hemofiltration techniques (CAVH and CVVH) were shown to decrease PCWP and extravascular lung water in patients with cardiogenic and non-cardiogenic (eg, ARDS) pulmonary edema, but the effects on the latter are less conclusive.

---

761 Explain the use of extracorporeal ultrafiltration techniques in the management of ARDS and pulmonary edema due to multiple causes.

❑ The fluid overload commonly present in patients with ARDS and pulmonary edema caused by many conditions (eg, excessive fluid administration, renal failure) can be effectively managed with ultrafiltration techniques. As previously indicated, there are two main types of extracorporeal ultrafiltration (or simply ultrafiltration) techniques, known as intermittent and continuous. The latter type includes the continuous arteriovenous hemofiltration with (CAVHD) or without concomitant dialysis (CAVH), and the continuous venovenous hemofiltration with (CVVHD) or without concomitant dialysis (CVVH). When concomitant dialysis is applied as in CAVHD and CVVHD, also referred to as *hemodiafiltration,* a circulating dialysate and a reinfusion solution are added to the ultrafiltration circuit. The use of dialysis is required in patients with renal failure (acute and chronic) superimposed on ARDS or pulmonary edema.

---

762 What are the advantages of the continuous ultrafiltration techniques in the management of patients with ARDS and multiorgan failure? Explain the different continuous ultrafiltration techniques (ie, CAVH, CVVH).

❑ The slow and sustained process of hemofiltration applied in the so-called continuous techniques results in relatively good tolerance with respect to hemodynamic stability in critically ill patients and those having end-stage cardiac disease. Two main forms of continuous hemofiltration techniques are available, as follows: (1) CAVH wherein the patient's arterial blood pressure is the driving force of plasma ultrafiltration (a blood pump is not used) and (2) CVVH where a blood pump is required for ultrafiltration to occur. In both types (CAVH and CVVH) of ultrafiltration techniques the following conditions are generally present: (1) low blood flow; (2) low transmembrane pressure; (3) high filtration fraction (approximately 20%); (4) ''filtration pressure equilibrium,'' which might occur due to rising plasma oncotic pressure and decreasing transmembrane hydrostatic pressure; (5) blood clotting, which is likely to occur when filtration pressure equilibrium develops; and (6) filter failure occurring with clotting of the cartridge. CAVH might also represent an afterload-reducing technique for the left ventricle, which could enhance its performance and thereby help fluid removal from the lungs due to reduced hydrostatic pressure in the pulmonary microcirculation. On the other hand, CVVH does not have this property so that the efficacy of CVVH might differ from that of CAVH.

763 Is dialysis a possible cause of hypoxemia?

❑ Yes. The effect of dialysis on PaO_2 is variable and depends on the type of procedure performed (eg, hemodialysis, peritoneal dialysis), the dialysate composition (eg, acetate dialysate in hemodialysis), the dialysate membrane utilized, and the net fluid balance obtained with this treatment modality. Hemodialysis performed with acetate-containing dialysate (in the absence of simultaneous fluid removal) commonly leads to a transient fall in PaO_2 of 5 to 35 mm Hg that resolves within 2 hours after discontinuation of dialysis. This fall in PaO_2 is caused, at least in part, by depression of pulmonary ventilation that develops as a result of arterial hypocapnia secondary to removal of bicarbonate and carbonic acid by the dialysis procedure. The dialysis cartridge also can play a role in the development of hypoxemia since the cuprophane membrane (cellulosic material) used in some devices may produce leukoagglutination in the pulmonary capillaries because of complement activation, leading to widening of the alveolar-arterial (A-a) oxygen gradient. Peritoneal dialysis may produce hypoxemia because of increased abdominal pressure causing atelectasis of lung bases as well as fluid accumulation in the pleural space. If substantial (eg, 2 to 4 L) fluid removal accompanies any type of dialysis procedure (hemodialysis, peritoneal dialysis), and the patient had pulmonary edema before dialysis, correction of the hypoxemia may be observed at the completion of dialysis.

---

764 What type of dialysis (ie, hemodialysis, peritoneal dialysis) is most appropriate in patients with ARDS who require this treatment?

❑ Hemodialysis is preferred over peritoneal dialysis in patients with ARDS and other forms of respiratory failure. Although hemodialysis may transiently worsen hypoxemia, this effect can be counterbalanced by increasing the fraction of oxygen in the inspired air. In addition, dialysis membranes with low biocompatibility (eg, cuprophane) must be avoided because they can activate the patient's complement, leading to abnormalities in the diffusion of oxygen. The possible complications of peritoneal dialysis in patients having impending or actual respiratory failure occur as described below. The introduction of fluid into the peritoneal cavity increases the abdominal pressure, displacing the diaphragm upward and possibly leading to fluid accumulation in the pleural space. The utilization of a hypertonic dialysate (eg, 4.5% dextrose) pulls fluid from the patient's circulation toward the abdominal space, augmenting further the previously mentioned effects on the diaphragm and pleural space. Consequently, the work of breathing increases, possibly leading to worsening of dyspnea and abnormalities of ABGs. Basal atelectasis caused by the augmented abdominal pressure decreases alveolar-capillary oxygen exchange. The impairment of ventilation caused by peritoneal dialysis can develop in patients breathing spontaneously and in those receiving mechanical ventilation.

765 Elaborate on the development of acute renal failure in ARDS. Does the presence of renal dysfunction have any effect on mortality?

❑ The kidney appears to be the most frequently observed extrapulmonary organ to fail in ARDS. Acute renal failure develops in 33% to 50% of patients with ARDS. Possible etiologic factors include hypotension, the use of nephrotoxic antibiotics, mechanical ventilation that interferes with systemic and renal hemodynamics, and the adverse renal effects of hypoxemia and hypercapnia. In addition, the common clinical practice of trying to keep patients with ARDS "dry" (relatively volume depleted) may induce renal insufficiency. The combination of ARDS and acute renal failure is particularly ominous and associated with a mortality rate of 70% to 80%.

COMPLICATIONS

766 What are the main complications of ARDS?

❑ ARDS commonly leads to complications that further worsen the prognosis of this condition. The most important complications include secondary bacterial infection of the respiratory tract, pneumothorax, pneumomediastinum, pulmonary oxygen toxicity, disseminated intravascular coagulation, left ventricular failure (easily missed condition in patients with ARDS), gastrointestinal hemorrhage, renal failure, electrolyte abnormalities, thrombocytopenia, sepsis, and multisystem organ failure. Other complications of ARDS are related to the specific cause of the acute lung injury and to the treatment of this condition (eg, complications of mechanical ventilation).

767 What factors predispose to the development of pneumothorax or pneumomediastinum in patients with ARDS? How is the diagnosis of these complications made?

❑ The treatment of acute lung injury (eg, ARDS) with mechanical ventilators and high inflation volumes predisposes to the development of both pneumothorax and pneumomediastinum. A sudden deterioration in the patient's respiratory status, associated with an increase in the peak and plateau airway pressures, or sudden hypotension should arouse suspicion of a pneumothorax. Additionally, subcutaneous emphysema may be detected, or typical abnormalities may be evident on the chest x-ray film. Suspicion of a pneumothorax, a life-threatening complication, should lead to immediate steps to confirm and treat this complication (eg, insertion of a chest tube). In addition to this dramatic injury, more subtle forms of lung injury with mechanical ventilation in ARDS may result from overdistention of normal lung areas (baby lung) with relatively normal compliance.

768 How important is the development of sepsis and multiple-organ failure in the mortality from ARDS? Compare the role of pulmonary and intra-abdominal infections in ARDS.

❑ Sepsis is present at the time of death in about 75% of patients with fatal ARDS and more than half of these patients had evidence of multiple-organ failure. The source of sepsis is the airways and lungs in the majority of patients. The increased susceptibility to pulmonary infection may be partly due to the presence of an endotracheal tube, alterations in local and systemic host defenses, or the alveolar edema fluid serving as a rich substrate. In contrast to the predominant pulmonary origin of sepsis occurring after the development of ARDS, intra-abdominal infection appears to be the main source of sepsis preceding ARDS.

769 How common is the development of gastrointestinal bleeding in ARDS?

❑ Varying degrees of severity of upper gastrointestinal hemorrhage occur in up to 85% of patients with ARDS. The incidence of gastrointestinal bleeding appears to be related to the severity of the underlying disease responsible for the ARDS.

770 Elaborate further on the mortality of ARDS.

❑ The mortality of ARDS varies with the underlying cause of the acute lung injury. In addition, for a given cause of ARDS, the mortality varies with the characteristics of the patient. This is evident considering that a trauma patient with ARDS having multiple transfusions or sepsis has a lower mortality than does a patient with a medical condition (ie, other than trauma) having multiple transfusions or sepsis.

CARDIORESPIRATORY FAILURE: PULMONARY EDEMA

771 What general measures are required to control the signs and symptoms of heart failure in patients with cardiorespiratory failure?

❑ Control of the clinical manifestations of heart failure include (1) correction of fluid excess, which is the principal cause of most signs and symptoms (eg, edema, dyspnea) in these patients; (2) reduction of the heart's workload by two mechanisms—a decrease in the blood flow demands of peripheral tissues and a decrease in the perfusion pressure that must be generated by the heart to supply the tissues with blood; and (3) enhancement of pumping action of the heart by means of drugs (eg, digitalis, glycosides) or electrical stimulation (eg, pacemaker). These three groups of measures may be implemented on recognition of symptomatic heart failure.

772 How do vasodilators relieve the signs and symptoms of cardiorespiratory failure?

❑ Vasodilators diminish the metabolic cost of cardiac work during systole (by reducing ventricular preload and afterload), allowing the heart to better meet the metabolic demands of the tissues (by increasing regional blood flows). Consequently, vasodilators (as single agents or combined with digitalis or diuretics) can ameliorate or completely correct signs and symptoms of cardiorespiratory failure. Vasodilators exert their actions on arteries, veins, or both arteries and veins, or have additional properties on the circulatory system due to inhibition of the renin-angiotensin system.

773 Classify and name the commonly used vasodilators for the management of patients in cardiorespiratory failure.

❑ Commonly used vasodilators for the management of heart failure and cardiorespiratory failure are conveniently classified as follows:

1. Venodilators (eg, nitrates including nitroglycerin and isosorbide dinitrate) that relax the smooth muscle of systemic veins, distending these vessels and thereby increasing the capacity of the systemic venous bed (also referred to as the *capacitance bed*). Consequently, venodilators redistribute blood from the pulmonary to the systemic circuit, decreasing pulmonary venous congestion and left ventricular preload.
2. Arteriolar vasodilators (eg, Ca^{++} entry blockers, hydralazine, minoxidil) that relax the smooth muscle of systemic arterioles, reducing the systemic vascular resistance, thereby acting as afterload-reducing agents (diminish left ventricular afterload). Consequently, arteriolar vasodilators reduce wall stress of the left ventricle, increasing cardiac output per beat

(ie, larger stroke volume) due to augmented myocardial fiber shortening.

3. Combined arteriolar and venous dilators (eg, nitroprusside, trimethaphan, and alpha-blockers such as prazosin) that relax the smooth muscle of arterioles and veins of the systemic circulation, thereby reducing left ventricular preload and afterload.
4. Combined arteriolar and venous dilators with additional effects on the circulatory system due to inhibition of the angiotensin-aldosterone system (eg, angiotensin-converting enzyme [ACE] inhibitors including captopril, enalapril, and lisinopril). This group of agents has properties comparable to those of the previous group plus those properties related to ACE inhibition (depression of angiotensin II and aldosterone levels).

---

774 How are nitrates used and what effects does each formulation have on cardiorespiratory failure? What is the action of nitrates on the pulmonary circulation?

❑ Nitrates including nitroglycerin and the long-acting preparations (ie, isosorbide dinitrate, erythrityl tetranitrate, and pentaerythritol tetranitrate) dilate systemic veins as their principal action, and to a lesser degree, the pulmonary arterial bed and the systemic arterioles. A continuous intravenous infusion of nitroglycerin (initial dosage of 10 μg/min, which can be increased every 5 minutes by steps of 10 μg/min to a maximum of 100 μg/min) can be used in acute heart failure and pulmonary edema, when venodilation is the desired effect. Nitroglycerin administered sublingually in a dose of 0.4 to 1.2 mg can help in the management of acute pulmonary edema caused by congestive heart failure associated with normal blood pressure; the effects persist for 15 to 30 minutes and left ventricular filling pressure might decrease from about 20 mm Hg to 10 mm Hg. Effects that last at least 3 hours are obtained with topical nitroglycerin when a 0.5- to 4-inch strip of ointment is applied on the chest skin. Alternatively, nitroglycerin patches or disks can be used, and they allow the patient to shower and provide steady absorption. The long-acting nitrate isosorbide dinitrate (Isordil) can be prescribed as a sublingual (eg, 2.5 to 10.0 mg every 2 hours) or oral (eg, 20 to 60 mg every 4 hours) formulation. The side effects of all nitrates include headache, postural hypotension, and methemoglobinemia (rare).

---

775 Describe the main properties of nitroprusside (drug that releases nitric oxide, a potent vasodilator) and trimethaphan (nondepolarizing ganglionic blocking agent), which are relevant for the treatment of cardiorespiratory failure.

❑ Nitroprusside and trimethaphan are mixed vasodilators for intravenous administration. These drugs are potent dilators of both veins and arterioles. Nitroprusside is used at an initial dosage of 10 to 25 μg/min and maximal dosage of up to 300 μg/min. Because nitroprusside is a light-sensitive compound, the drug container must be covered with foil paper during administration. Medical complications of therapy include thiocyanate toxicity and methemoglobinemia. The trimethaphan dosage is 1 to 15 mg/min and complications of therapy include postural hypotension (blockade of sympathetic ganglia interrupts adrenergic tone on arterioles), bowel and bladder atony, and respiratory depression. Consequently, trimethaphan imposes a risk of worsening respiratory function in patients with cardiorespiratory failure who are breathing spontaneously (ie, without mechanical ventilation).

---

776 What patients might respond better to dobutamine than to dopamine and vice versa in the therapy of cardiorespiratory failure?

❑ When the main goal of therapy is to improve ventricular function by direct inotropic stimulation, dobutamine is preferred to dopamine because this drug is a more cardioselective agent. The increase in cardiac output observed at any level of heart work (assessed as the product of heart rate and systolic pressure) is greater with dobutamine than with dopamine. Thus, in patients with acute or refractory heart failure and cardiorespiratory failure, especially with sinus tachycardia but without hypotension, dobutamine is the preferred drug. On the contrary, dopamine is a better therapeutic choice in patients with heart failure and hypotension because this agent has significant direct vascular effects. The vasoconstrictor effects of a high-dosage regimen of dopamine might help to restore the undesirably low blood pressure of hypotensive patients. Once hypotension is corrected with high-dosage dopamine, decreasing its rate of administration can improve renal and mesenteric perfusion due to selective dopaminergic vasodilation (this property is absent with dobutamine administration).

---

777 What are the specific measures aimed at reversing the syndrome of cardiorespiratory failure in patients with acute cardiogenic pulmonary edema? Is morphine sulfate always indicated in the management of cardiogenic pulmonary edema?

❑ Several measures should be immediately implemented in patients with acute cardiogenic pulmonary edema, including the following:

1. Oxygen-enriched inspired air by nasal cannula or facial mask for patients with adequate respiratory effort. Alternatively, mechanical ventilation after intubation can be used in patients with poor or absent respiratory effort.
2. An upright position of the patient's chest if respiratory effort is adequate. The patient should sit up in the bed or in a chair with the legs hanging down to decrease venous return to the heart.
3. Furosemide at a dosage of 40 to 60 mg intravenously over a 2-minute period.
4. Morphine sulfate at a dosage of 3 to 5 mg intravenously over a 3-minute period while watching for possible respiratory

depression. If respiratory depression develops, the morphine should be discontinued and a morphine antagonist administered immediately. Morphine should not be used in patients with poor respiratory effort or hypercapnia, abnormal mental status, intracranial bleeding, chronic pulmonary disease, or bronchial asthma.

5. Nitroglycerin (eg, 0.3 to 0.6 mg sublingually or 5 μg/min intravenously titrated upward in 5-μg/min increments at 3-minute intervals as needed) or nitroprusside (same intravenous dosage as nitroglycerin), which reduces cardiac preload or afterload, relieving the symptoms of pulmonary edema. Patients with hypertensive heart disease leading to pulmonary edema might be significantly improved with intravenous nitroprusside. Arterial blood pressure should not fall below 100 mm Hg during treatment with vasodilators.
6. Digitalis, which might be useful in patients with atrial fibrillation or flutter or other supraventricular tachycardias and very high ventricular rate; in addition, this drug might improve sinus rhythm in patients who had not been taking this drug and who present with severe aortic valve disease, hypertension, or decreased ejection fraction.
7. Inotropic agents (eg, dobutamine or amrinone) if there is no response to previous measures, presumably due to myocardial failure.
8. Ultrafiltration (intermittent or continuous), an effective modality for rapid fluid removal in patients who fail to respond to diuretics.

The use of aminophylline in the management of acute pulmonary edema is controversial and many experts recommend to avoid this drug.

778 How does morphine provide symptomatic improvement in patients with acute pulmonary edema?

❑ The salutary actions of morphine in acute pulmonary edema are due to (1) diminished cardiac preload mediated by the combined effects of augmented capacitance of systemic veins ("pharmacologic phlebotomy") and depression of respiratory effort that reduces mean negative intrathoracic pressure—the reduced preload causes a diminished venous return to the heart, ameliorating pulmonary edema; (2) afterload-reducing effect on the left ventricle secondary to decreases in arteriolar resistance and blood pressure; and (3) symptomatic improvement by ameliorating dyspnea because of depression of respiratory drive.

779 What criteria might be used to decide whether digitalis should be administered to patients with acute pulmonary edema with sinus rhythm who have been receiving an unknown dosage of digitalis?

❑ Digitalis preparations should not be administered to patients with features consistent with digitalis intoxication, including paroxysmal atrial tachycardia with atrioventricular block, nonparoxysmal atrioventricular junctional tachycardia, frequent ventricular premature contractions, ventricular tachycardia, or a history of previous digitalis intoxication including nausea or vomiting. If these signs and symptoms are absent, digitalis preparations might be administered to patients with acute cardiogenic pulmonary edema. The decision to prescribe digitalis is usually based on clinical and electrocardiographic (ECG) evaluation because measurement of plasma glycoside levels takes too long for results to be useful in the management of acute pulmonary edema.

780 A 70-year-old man with a previous history of hypertension and arteriosclerotic heart disease is brought to a hospital emergency room with severe shortness of breath, central cyanosis, and diaphoresis. He had three "small" myocardial infarctions in the previous 6 years, and he had been in stable congestive heart failure for 18 months preceding the current episode. Over the 48 hours before being brought to the hospital he had remained indoors, sitting up on a sofa, because of dyspnea of increased intensity. Current medication included verapamil, 180 mg, and hydrochlorothiazide, 25 mg, daily. On arrival to the emergency room, he is gasping for air, with extreme cyanosis and severe agitation. His blood pressure is 164/114 mm Hg and his pulse is 110 beats/min and regular. Neck veins are distended, and examination of the heart reveals a diffuse apical impulse in the anterior axillary line, and a protodiastolic as well as a presystolic gallop (combined S_3 and S_4 gallop). Prominent moist rales are present throughout both lung fields. Presacral and pretibial (+++) edema is present. The room-air ABG values and other laboratory data are as follows:

pH	7.36
PCO_2	44 mm Hg
$[HCO_3^-]_p$	24 mEq/L
PO_2	32 mm Hg

Plasma chemistries are as follows:

$[Na^+]$	130 mEq/L
$[K^+]$	3.2 mEq/L
$[Cl^-]$	84 mEq/L
Total CO_2	26 mmol/L
Glucose	152 mg/dL
BUN	59 mg/dL
Creatinine	2.6 mg/dL
Anion gap	20 mEq/L

The ECG reveals an "old," inferior-wall myocardial infarction and diffuse anterolateral ischemia. Cardiac enzymes (creatine phosphatase [CPK]-MB) are within normal limits.

What is the most likely cause of this patient's severe respiratory distress that requires specific therapy?

❑ The severe shortness of breath, central cyanosis, and diaphoresis present on arrival to the emergency room are most likely due to severe left ventricular failure with acute cardiogenic pulmonary edema. The profound impairment in alveolar gas exchange is responsible for the hypoxemia (PO_2 of 32 mm Hg) and central cyanosis (evident on examination of the tongue). The persistent and intense respiratory effort is secondary to postcapillary pulmonary hypertension with alveolar transudate accumulation as well as to the accompanying hypoxemia, and accounts for the shortness of breath. The sympathetic activation that accompanies the patient's hemodynamic crisis explains the diaphoresis.

781 What is the cause of this patient's cardiogenic pulmonary edema?

❑ The cardiogenic pulmonary edema present on arrival at the hospital emergency room is best explained by a combination of hypertensive and ischemic heart disease. The high blood pressure (ie, 164/114 mm Hg) observed in association with symptomatic left ventricular failure and diminished cardiac output indicate a severe increase in systemic vascular resistance. Thus, the augmented left ventricular afterload has played a role in the precipitation of symptomatic heart failure. The previous history of myocardial infarction with a current ECG documenting this earlier injury, in association with acute ischemic changes (likely due to the sum of effects of coronary artery disease, increased oxygen consumption secondary to augmented left ventricular afterload, and decreased PaO_2), support a role of cardiac ischemia in the pathogenesis of acute pulmonary edema. An additional factor that might partly account for the presence of pulmonary edema as well as the state of overall extracellular fluid volume expansion is the associated renal insufficiency (as demonstrated by BUN of 59 mg/dL and creatinine level of 2.6 mg/dL), which further predisposes to salt and water retention in this patient with congestive heart failure.

782 What is the most likely explanation for the room-air ABGs obtained at the emergency room?

❑ The severe hypoxemia (ie, PO_2 of 32 mm Hg) indicates a major impairment of alveolar gas exchange due to extensive alveolar edema. The expected response to this degree of hypoxemia is primary hyperventilation causing hypocapnia (decreased PCO_2), yet this patient exhibits hypercapnia (a PCO_2 of 44 mm Hg is clearly abnormally high in association with a PO_2 of 32 mm Hg). Carbon dioxide retention might be explained by the combined effects of respiratory fatigue following prolonged hyperventilation and a severe abnormality in alveolar gas exchange due to pulmonary edema. Because this patient is known to have had congestive heart failure for 18 months, he should have developed a chronic respiratory alkalosis due to sustained hyperventilation; thus $[HCO_3^-]_p$ should have been substantially lower than 24 mEq/L (level measured on arrival to the emergency room). Although the acute carbon dioxide retention due to pulmonary edema superimposed on chronic respiratory alkalosis increases the $[HCO_3^-]_p$ somewhat, its level should still be below normal. Consequently, it appears that chronic diuretic treatment with hydrochlorothiazide has produced a mild metabolic alkalosis that properly explains the measured $[HCO_3^-]_p$ of 24 mEq/L.

783 How should this patient's pulmonary edema be managed? Should morphine be used in the management of this patient?

❑ The patient's pulmonary edema requires immediate application of multiple measures, including (1) oxygen-rich mixtures such as 2 to 4 L of oxygen per minute by nasal cannula, with close observation for the possibility of respiratory depression requiring laryngeal intubation and mechanical ventilation; (2) intravenous administration of 40 mg of furosemide to reduce left ventricular preload and induce natriuresis and diuresis; (3) intravenous infusion of nitroprusside at initial rate of 5 to 10 μg/kg/min and further adjustments as needed to decrease afterload and reduce systolic blood pressure to under 120 mm Hg—alternatively, nitroglycerin can be administered by either sublingual or intravenous routes. The relatively high PCO_2 (ie, 44 mm Hg) observed in this patient contraindicates the use of morphine since this drug will most likely produce further ventilatory depression.

FAT EMBOLISM. VENOUS AIR EMBOLISM

784 What is the treatment of fat embolism syndrome?

❑ Management of fat embolism syndrome consists of general supportive care. Particular attention should be paid to proper traction and immobilization of fractured extremities; patients whose fractures are not properly immobilized may have further episodes of fat embolization. Early orthopedic consultation should be obtained to determine the need for surgical stabilization of fractures. In a prospective study, prophylactic administration of methylprednisolone (7.5 mg/kg every 6 hours for 12 doses) was found to decrease the incidence of the syndrome; 9 of 41 in the control group and 0 of 21 in the steroid-treated group developed the syndrome. There is no evidence to support the use of corticosteroids once the syndrome has developed. Likewise, there is no evidence to support the use of the other agents in the management of the syndrome, such as heparin, alcohol, low-molecular-weight dextran, or hypertonic glucose and alcohol.

785 What is the treatment of venous air embolism?

❑ If air embolism is suspected, the patient should be placed in the left lateral decubitus position, which facilitates an air bubble to flow toward the apex of the right ventricle. Closed-chest compressions should be initiated, and aspiration of air through a right atrial or pulmonary artery catheter can be effective. The administration of 100% oxygen helps to decrease the size of the emboli by causing resorption of nitrogen in the air.

25. Obstructive Airway Disease

ASTHMA

786 What is the single most important class of drugs for the management of acute asthma? Is frequent administration of the drug (ie, bronchodilator) more important than the total dose? Name commonly used preparations.

❑ Sympathomimetic aerosols (inhaled agents) comprise the therapy of choice for acute asthma. Sequential administration of isoproterenol (1.25 mg) by hand nebulizer every 20 minutes for 3 doses achieves at least as much bronchodilation as subcutaneous epinephrine (eg, 0.3 mg) with the same rapidity of onset but with less potential for toxicity. Contrary to conventional thinking, the inhalational route is at least as effective in patients with severe airway obstruction (FEV_1 <1.0 L) as in those with milder disease. Indeed, when used as single agents, isoproterenol aerosol produces greater bronchodilation than does subcutaneous epinephrine in patients with severe airway obstruction, whereas the response to the two agents is similar in patients with milder disease. In addition, the response to nebulized isoproterenol is similar irrespective of whether the patient has been receiving chronic inhaled sympathomimetic therapy, indicating that sympathomimetic "tolerance" is not an important problem in the acute setting. Failure to achieve a maximal response to inhaled sympathomimetic therapy usually indicates suboptimal dosing rather than the need for an additional agent. Frequency of administration appears to be more important than the total dose delivered; studies have shown greater bronchodilation with sequential aerosol inhalation (every 10 to 20 minutes) than with the same dose given as a bolus. While most studies of the therapy of acute asthma have employed isoproterenol, it is reasonable to expect a similar response with metaproterenol (Alupent, 0.3 ml of 5% solution) or albuterol (Ventolin, 0.5 ml of 0.5% solution). If a metered-dose inhaler (MDI) is employed, the patient requires careful instruction in its use, and many patients will not be able to master the proper technique. However, a MDI used in conjunction with a spacer system (eg, Inspir-Ease) is as equally effective as a handheld nebulizer.

787 Does the use of beta-2-adrenergic agonists increase asthma mortality?

❑ It has been suggested that regular use of beta-2-adrenergic agonists in asthma may be detrimental to overall control and that acute overuse may contribute to asthma mortality. Yet, regular or excessive use of beta-2-adrenergic agonists may just be a marker for more severe disease, but not the cause of higher asthma mortality.

788 What is the recommended therapy of mild and moderate asthma?

❑ The management of mild asthma commonly requires inhalation (1 to 2 puffs) of a beta-2-adrenergic agonist or cromolyn, or both drugs, preceding allergen exposure and exercise. In addition, the development of symptoms indicates the need of an inhaled beta-2-adrenergic agonist, 2 puffs repeated every 3 to 4 hours as needed. The management of moderate asthma requires a more elaborate treatment program than does that of mild asthma. Initial treatment of moderate asthma includes an inhaled beta-2-agonist plus an inhaled corticosteroid or cromolyn, four times a day for each of them. If symptoms persist, one or both of the following drugs can be prescribed: high doses of inhaled corticosteroids or sustained-release theophylline. A short course of oral corticosteroids followed by inhaled corticosteroids is recommended for moderate asthma not responding to the previously outlined treatment plan. Currently, there is significant controversy with respect to the use of inhaled steroids, which are considered first-line therapy of asthma (even of mild degree) by many specialists. Home measurements of peak airflow can help to evaluate the severity of airway obstruction, response to treatment, and the possible need of emergency care.

789 What is the management of stable severe asthma and acute severe asthma?

- ❑ Patients with stable severe asthma in the absence of acute exacerbations require therapy that includes an inhaled beta-2-agonist and inhaled corticosteroids (3 to 6 puffs four times a day, according to the strength of the preparation). In addition, patients might require oral sustained-release theophylline. Intensification of this therapy including a short course of oral corticosteroids is indicated for acute exacerbations (ie, acute severe asthma). Patients with moderate or severe asthma may benefit from peak airflow measurements at home to monitor the degree of airway obstruction and to suggest alterations in therapy or the possible need of emergency care including hospitalization.

790 An 18-year-old woman with asthma has been requiring an inhaled beta-agonist (terbutaline) four times daily to control symptoms (with incomplete resolution) for the past 4 weeks. Previously, she had used the inhaler occasionally, up to twice weekly.

What is the most appropriate therapy for her condition? Is it useful for the patient to monitor her own airflow at home?

- ❑ Since the patient failed to respond to a beta-agonist inhaler as a single agent, the addition of an inhaled corticosteroid (eg, beclomethasone) is indicated. The anti-inflammatory action of corticosteroids acting on the airways should help to control the patient's symptoms. However, the inhaled beta-agonist must be continued on an as-needed basis to supplement the inhaled corticosteroids. Measurement of peak expiratory flow with a handheld meter allows the patient to monitor her condition at home, helping the physician in the management of the patient's symptoms. In addition, a more complete spirometric evaluation can be performed in the physician's office or hospital setting.

791 What is the role of corticosteroid (inhaled and systemic) administration in the treatment of obstructive lung disease?

❑ Therapy with corticosteroids is very effective in many patients with asthma and in a minority of patients with COPD. Inhaled corticosteroids such as beclomethasone, flunisolide, and triamcinolone acetonide (Beclovent, Aerobid, and Azmacort, respectively) are useful in the management of mild to moderate asthma and in some patients with COPD. Systemic corticosteroids represent a major therapeutic tool for acute exacerbations of both asthma and COPD. An initial daily dose of 60 mg of prednisone or equivalent administered every 6 hours is usually effective but high parenteral doses of 125 mg of methylprednisolone (Solu-Medrol) every 6 hours may be required. In addition, systemic corticosteroids may be useful in the chronic management of a small minority patients with obstructive lung disease (eg, COPD).

792 What is the mechanism of action of corticosteroids in patients with airway obstruction?

❑ The mechanism of action of corticosteroids in patients with airway obstruction is unknown. Currently, it is thought that corticosteroids bind to cytoplasmic receptors that transport the steroid into the cell nucleus where an interaction with DNA initiates protein synthesis and, in particular, synthesis of lipomodulin. Lipomodulin is a selective inhibitor of phospholipase A_2, which generates arachidonic acid from membrane phospholipids. This effect inhibits the release of a plethora of mediators from inflammatory cells. Corticosteroid therapy has been shown to provide significant improvement in airflow in patients with acute asthma who are responding poorly to conventional therapy. The delay before demonstrable benefit suggests that the improvement is due to resolution of an inflammatory component rather than augmenting beta-agonist responsiveness (although a small component of the latter cannot be excluded). In patients responding to conventional therapy, steroids appear to have no additive effect. In chronic stable asthmatics, corticosteroids are useful in the management of patients who have a suboptimal response to sympathomimetic agents. This effect appears to be due to augmentation of sympathomimetic action, possibly by decreasing the tachyphylaxis induced by excessive sympathomimetic therapy.

---

793 What is the rationale for the use of corticosteroids in the management of obstructive lung disease? What patients benefit most with this medication?

❑ The anti-inflammatory properties of corticosteroids are largely responsible for their efficacy in the management of obstructive lung disease since airway inflammation is present in most patients with this condition. The efficacy of inhaled corticosteroids is maximal in patients with new-onset asthma and in those with COPD who have airway hyperreactivity. Corticosteroids have been shown to be more effective than beta-agonists in improving airflow and decreasing the frequency of exacerbations in patients with asthma. In addition, systemic corticosteroids are most useful in the management of acute flares of asthma and COPD.

---

794 What is the role of the intravenous administration of corticosteroids in the management of acute asthma? How rapid is the response to corticosteroids? Provide details of preparations commonly used and dosages.

❑ Corticosteroids hasten the resolution of airway obstruction that is refractory to conventional therapy. In addition, these drugs decrease the rate of relapse in patients with recurrent asthma. The precise indications for corticosteroid therapy are controversial but it seems appropriate to initiate this medication in patients whose FEV_1 is less than 40% of predicted after 1 hour of aggressive bronchodilator therapy. The optimal dosage of hydrocortisone is unknown, but a 2-mg/kg bolus followed by 0.5 mg/kg/hr by intravenous infusion achieves an excellent response. Corticosteroids have a slow onset of action. While subjective improvement may be noted after a few hours, significant bronchodilation is not observed before 6 hours, and maximal effect is achieved at 20 hours. Methylprednisolone, 0.8 mg/kg initially followed by 0.1 mg/kg/hr, probably achieves a similar effect to hydrocortisone.

795 What are the local and systemic adverse effects of corticosteroids used in the management of obstructive lung disorders? How can these complications be prevented?

❑ Local effects of inhaled corticosteroids including hoarseness, sore throat, and thrush are generally avoided by rinsing the mouth and throat after inhalation and by using spacer devices for delivery of the medication. Systemic effects observed with long-term corticosteroid therapy include augmented susceptibility to opportunistic infections, bruisability, accelerated bone turnover, and depressed adrenal responsiveness. Considering the importance of the systemic effects of corticosteroids, prolonged administration of these drugs should be limited to patients exhibiting objective benefit.

796 How important is oxygen supplementation in the therapy of acute asthma? Should oxygen therapy be routinely used in acute severe asthma?

❑ Patients with acute asthma rarely develop life-threatening hypoxemia, and correction of hypoxemia does not abolish dyspnea. Nevertheless, it is prudent to administer supplemental oxygen by nasal cannula or face mask, especially considering that sympathomimetic agents have effects on the pulmonary vasculature that may exacerbate hypoxemia by worsening ventilation-perfusion mismatching.

797 How important is it to measure airflow in patients presenting with an acute asthma attack? Is measurement of ABGs a better predictor of the severity of airway obstruction?

❑ It is imperative to obtain an objective measure of airflow obstruction such as FEV_1 or peak expiratory flow rate (PEFR) in patients with an acute asthma attack. These tests are safe, easy to perform, and tolerated by almost all patients. In an emergency room setting, FEV_1 and PEFR have been shown to accurately predict the need for hospital admission; patients with an FEV_1 or PEFR lower than 40% of predicted after 1 hour of intensive therapy require admission. In contrast, PaO_2 correlates poorly with the severity of airway obstruction. Measurement of $PaCO_2$ is more useful than PaO_2 in assessing the severity of an asthma attack. During an episode of acute asthma, $PaCO_2$ is typically decreased but returns to normal or becomes elevated as the attack increases in severity. Virtually all patients with significant hypercapnia ($PaCO_2$ >45 mm Hg) have a FEV_1 or PEFR lower than 25% of predicted.

798 Should antibiotics be routinely administered to patients with acute asthma?

❑ Factors capable of precipitating an acute asthmatic attack should be sought, and if infection is suspected, antibiotics should be administered. However, the routine administration of antibiotics has no beneficial effect on clinical findings, pulmonary function, or outcome in patients with acute asthma.

799 What are the indications for mechanical ventilation in acute asthma? How common is the application of ventilatory support in asthma?

❑ Mechanical ventilation might be required in patients with status asthmaticus with evidence of exhaustion, myocardial ischemia or arrhythmias, severe alteration in mental status, hypercapnia, hypoxemia that fails upon correction with supplemental oxygen, and lack of responsiveness to maximal therapy. Mechanical ventilation is utilized for the management of acute severe asthma on rare occasions (eg, <3% of patients admitted to the hospital with status asthmaticus).

800 Describe the use of alkali therapy in respiratory acidosis (see also permissive hypercapnia).

❑ Since the predominant adverse effect of hypercapnia is related to an alteration in the pH of body fluids, special attention should be directed at restoring pH values to normal rather than achieving a particular $PaCO_2$ level. The presence of a component of metabolic acidosis is the primary indication for alkali therapy in patients with acute respiratory acidosis. Administration of sodium bicarbonate ($NaHCO_3$) to patients with simple respiratory acidosis not only is of questionable effectiveness but also involves considerable risk. A pH-mediated depression of ventilation, enhanced carbon dioxide production due to bicarbonate decomposition resulting in further aggravation of hypercapnia, and volume expansion causing additional impairment in alveolar gas exchange are the major concerns. Yet, alkali therapy might have a special role in patients with severe bronchospasm of any cause, by restoring the responsiveness of the bronchial musculature to beta-adrenergic agonists. Successful management of intractable asthma in patients with a blood pH below 7.00 to values above 7.20 has been reported. It should be recognized that alkali therapy might be used even if the acidemia is either partially or fully of respiratory origin. In spontaneously breathing patients, however, alkali therapy might depress the respiratory drive and weaken the patient's ventilatory status. In the absence of a complicating element of metabolic acidosis and with the possible exception of the severely acidemic patient with intense generalized bronchoconstriction undergoing mechanical ventilation (see above), there is no role for alkali administration in chronic respiratory acidosis.

801 What is the role of aminophylline in the management of acute asthma? Why has the use of this drug for acute severe asthma decreased sharply?

❑ Aminophylline has been a traditional component in the therapy of acute asthma. Yet, this drug used as a single agent is a weak bronchodilator and has a slow onset of action. In the past, aminophylline was considered to have an additive or synergistic effect when combined with a sympathomimetic agent. It is now known that the sympathomimetic agent exerts the predominant bronchodilator effect, and that the main difference between combined therapy and a sole sympathomimetic agent in the treatment of acute asthma is an increased toxicity with the former approach. Consequently, combined therapy should be reserved for the most severely ill patients, and, even then, the benefit is small.

802 What is the role of chest physical therapy in patients with status asthmaticus or pneumonia? How important is the patient's hydration on the quality and quantity of bronchial secretions?

❑ Chest physical therapy has not proved useful in patients with status asthmaticus or patients with pneumonia who are not producing large quantities of sputum. With respect to the state of hydration, patients with COPD are commonly encouraged to drink large quantities of fluid to facilitate expectoration of augmented but less viscous bronchial secretions. However, neither hydration nor dehydration appears to have any effect on the volume of bronchial secretions, the elasticity of sputum, respiratory symptoms, or FEV_1.

803 Explain the use of cromolyn and nedocromil in patients with asthma.

❑ Cromolyn and nedocromil are anti-inflammatory agents without bronchodilator properties that are useful for prophylaxis but not for the acute management of asthma. These drugs decrease histamine release (presumably because of mast-cell-membrane stabilization) and inhibit airway constrictive reflexes by suppressing neurotransmission in afferent nerves.

OVERALL MANAGEMENT OF STABLE COPD

804 What are the major elements in the management of COPD?

❑ The major elements in the management of COPD are the use of bronchodilators, oxygen administration, proper nutrition, pulmonary rehabilitation, preventive therapy that should include a smoking cessation program, and alpha-1-antitrypsin replacement for patients with deficient levels.

805 Outline some basic concepts pertaining to the management of chronic respiratory failure with carbon dioxide retention (hypercapnic respiratory failure).

❑ Unfortunately, only rarely can one remove the underlying cause of respiratory failure in patients with chronic respiratory acidosis. Nonetheless, maximizing alveolar ventilation with relatively simple maneuvers is often rewarding. In contrast to acute respiratory acidosis, administration of oxygen to patients with long-standing carbon dioxide retention should be carried out cautiously; if ventilator support is needed, we prefer to aim for a $PaCO_2$ approximating the patient's chronic stable value rather than aiming for normocapnia. The specific elements of the management of chronic hypercapnic respiratory failure are examined in the answers to subsequent questions.

806 Briefly review the measures aimed at improving pulmonary function that might be used in patients with COPD and hypercapnic respiratory failure. How important is the dietary chloride content in the management of these patients? What is the risk, if any, of the use of sedatives and tranquilizers in these patients?

❑ Pulmonary infections, perhaps the most common causes of respiratory decompensation in patients with COPD, should be treated vigorously with appropriate antibiotics. Bronchodilator therapy is aimed at correcting the increased airway resistance. Avoidance of all possible mechanisms of bronchoconstriction and bronchorrhea including irritant inhalants (eg, tobacco, industrial or urban pollutants, pollens) and medications (eg, beta-adrenergic antagonists, particularly of the nonselective group) should be pursued aggressively. Elimination of retained secretions (by coughing, postural drainage, and chest physiotherapy) can substantially reduce the work of breathing and improve ventilation. Diuretic therapy might reduce the interstitial and alveolar edema associated with pulmonary vascular congestion and thus improve gas exchange. Special care must be taken to prevent or repair diuretic-induced metabolic alkalosis (or that induced by any other cause such as gastric juice losses); even relative alkalemia can dampen ventilatory drive and exacerbate hypercapnia and hypoxemia. Administration of adequate quantities of chloride (usually as the potassium salt) prevents or corrects this complication. Tranquilizers and sedatives should be strictly avoided in patients at risk of carbon dioxide retention. Administration of benzodiazepine antagonists and naloxone may be necessary in the management of some patients. Potassium and phosphate depletion should be corrected, for they might contribute to the development or the maintenance of respiratory failure by impairing the function of skeletal muscles.

807 Does bronchodilator therapy significantly help relief of airway obstruction in patients with COPD?

❑ In the past, patients with COPD (ie, emphysema, chronic bronchitis) were considered to have "irreversible" or "fixed" airway obstruction that fails to respond to any bronchodilatory drug. However, recent studies showed that in many patients with COPD, airflow increases substantially following administration of a bronchodilator agent. This salutary response is also present in patients with relatively pure emphysema. Furthermore, airway obstruction is generally more intense in patients with COPD in acute respiratory failure than when these patients are in remission. Consequently, an attempt to relieve airway obstruction with bronchodilator drugs is indicated in all patients with COPD.

808 What might explain the presence of a substantial response to bronchodilators in some COPD patients?

❑ Patients with COPD who exhibit marked improvement of airflow obstruction with bronchodilators probably have an asthmatic component (ie, concomitant presence of asthma) to their COPD disease and these patients can achieve significant benefit with the use of these drugs. However, COPD patients with irreversible or ''fixed'' airflow obstruction demonstrated by pulmonary function testing may also respond substantially to bronchodilators and these drugs may also effectively reduce the work of breathing.

809 How is relief of airway obstruction accomplished in patients with COPD?

❑ Relief of airway obstruction in patients with COPD is largely achieved with the administration of bronchodilator agents (ie, anticholinergics, sympathomimetics, xanthines) and corticosteroids. Inhalation of bronchodilators is now preferred over the oral route. Details with respect to the use of various bronchodilator agents currently available are presented in the answers to pertinent questions. Bronchodilatory drugs represent the mainstay of therapy for COPD.

810 What are the major classes of bronchodilator drugs used in the management of obstructive airway disease?

❑ The major classes of bronchodilator drugs include the beta-adrenergic agonists (eg, albuterol), anticholinergic agents (eg, ipratropium bromide), and methylxanthines (eg, aminophylline). The mechanism of action, indications, and possible adverse reactions are examined in the answers to subsequent questions. Patients are commonly prescribed a combination of agents belonging to either two or three classes of bronchodilator drugs.

811 Does cessation of smoking favorably alter the natural history of COPD?

❑ Yes. Cessation of smoking generally produces subjective and objective improvement in respiratory function of patients with COPD. Reversal of accelerated decline in lung function is similar in patients with advanced disease as compared to those having less severe pulmonary dysfunction.

812 List the drugs and other therapeutic measures that might be useful in the chronic management of COPD.

❑ Drugs and other therapeutic measures useful in the long-term management of COPD include anticholinergic agents (inhaled), beta-adrenergic agonists (inhaled), methylxanthines, oxygen (in hypoxemic patients), and pulmonary rehabilitation. Systemic corticosteroids and nocturnal ventilatory assistance may be required in some patients.

813 What mucolytic and expectorant agents can be used in patients with COPD?

❑ Excessive airway mucus production is a common feature in patients with chronic bronchitis. The thick sputum present in many patients is often difficult to mobilize and contributes to airway obstruction and frequent coughing. Bronchial secretions can be diminished with the use of sympathomimetics and theophylline that enhance mucociliary clearance and corticosteroids that reduce airway inflammation. Mucolytics and expectorants aid in altering the viscosity of the bronchial mucus, but their overall efficacy remains unproved. Iodinated glycerol has some short-term benefit in COPD patients, but its long-term effects have not been established. The expectorant guaifenesin appears to have no significant effect. *N*-Acetylcysteine (Mucomyst) acts as a mucolytic and can be administered as an aerosol, but it is rarely prescribed because it can produce severe coughing and bronchospasm. If coughing is troubling and nonproductive during a mild exacerbation of COPD, a trial of antitussive therapy (eg, dextromethorphan) may be warranted.

814 What measures can be used to aid removal of secretions in patients with airway obstruction (eg, COPD)? How useful is chest physical therapy in COPD?

❑ Most patients with an exacerbation of COPD report an increase in airway secretions and some of them experience increased difficulty in expectorating secretions. Chest physical therapy is commonly employed to assist the removal of secretions with methods that include percussion, postural drainage, directed coughing, forced expiration technique, and chest vibration. Nevertheless, the efficacy of chest percussion, postural drainage, and other techniques of chest physical therapy in terms of improving pulmonary function in patients with an acute exacerbation of chronic bronchitis is questionable. Furthermore, bronchoconstriction may even develop in some patients as a consequence of physical therapy. Patients with acute respiratory failure who require mechanical ventilation may benefit from postural drainage and chest percussion if they have large amounts of sputum (≥30 mL/day). However, significant hypoxemia may develop after chest percussion in patients having only thin mucoid secretions and a small volume of sputum production. Vigorous chest physical therapy, consisting of postural drainage, chest percussion, deep inspirations, coughing or suctioning, and use of a bronchodilator, has been shown to be at least as effective as fiberoptic bronchoscopy in reversing acute lobar atelectasis. If chest physical therapy is deemed necessary in a critically ill patient receiving mechanical ventilation, use of a short-acting narcotic (such as fentanyl) may attenuate the associated nonsalutary hemodynamic response. In stable patients with substantial sputum production, the forced expiration technique (one or two forced expirations, without glottic closure, starting from mid to low lung volume) appears to be quite useful in assisting the removal of secretions.

815 What is the therapy of dyspnea?

❑ Treatment of the underlying disease is the cardinal principle in the management of any symptom including dyspnea. Bronchodilators may achieve considerable or complete relief of dyspnea in patients with asthma, but relief is usually incomplete in patients with COPD. Oxygen administration can rapidly relieve dyspnea in patients with severe hypoxemia. Diuretic agents (eg, furosemide) may be very effective in the management of dyspnea of patients with pulmonary edema. Consequently, therapeutic measures for the relief of dyspnea differ in accordance with the cause of this disturbance.

816 What are the effects of diazepam and opiates in the treatment of dyspnea? Explain the use of opiates in patients with COPD.

❑ Because an increased respiratory drive can contribute to the development of dyspnea, a drug-induced reduction in respiratory drive might alleviate respiratory distress. Ideally, such drug should blunt the intensity of respiratory sensation without decreasing alveolar ventilation. Unfortunately, diazepam does not have significant effect on dyspnea and can reduce exercise tolerance as well as produce other side effects (even death) in patients with COPD. Opiates can cause respiratory depression through a direct effect on the brain stem respiratory centers and by decreasing carotid body discharge; these drugs also cause a reduction in metabolic rate and oxygen consumption. Some studies showed that oral morphine (0.8 mg/kg) increases exercise capacity in patients with COPD accompanied by a higher $PaCO_2$, decreases ventilatory requirements for a given workload, and decreases dyspnea for a given level of ventilation. Other studies found that most patients with COPD receiving hydrocodone bitartrate (5 mg four times daily) noted subjective relief of dyspnea. Side effects included constipation and drowsiness. Still other investigators found that opiates in the therapy of COPD may worsen the respiratory condition. Further long-term studies are clearly needed as these drugs pose a considerable risk of addiction and side effects.

817 Outline the management options for COPD according to the severity of the disease and presence of complications.

❑ Several treatment options are available for the stable COPD patient. For mild or moderate disease, inhaled anticholinergic or sympathomimetic agents (ie, metered dose inhaler [MDI]) should be prescribed. For more severe disease, an oral sustained-release theophylline preparation can be added. Bronchodilators may be more effective if delivered as an aerosol with a spacer device. In certain COPD patients, symptoms may persist despite optimal treatment with the previously mentioned drugs and a trial of corticosteroids is warranted. Exacerbations of COPD usually require a combined therapy that includes oxygen, more frequent doses of anticholinergics, sympathomimetics, and intravenous corticosteroids. Antibiotics are prescribed if there is evidence of acute bronchitis or pneumonia. Precipitating causes of respiratory failure such as congestive heart failure, pulmonary embolism, and pneumothorax must be excluded. Increased airway secretions must be properly managed, and if the patient has cor pulmonale, oxygen therapy, diuretics, and possibly digoxin need to be prescribed. With severe respiratory failure in patients with end-stage COPD, any prior directive about life support must be respected. Intubation and mechanical ventilation may benefit potentially reversible conditions, especially if there is respiratory muscle fatigue. Nasal continuous positive airway pressure (CPAP) ventilation may benefit some patients and also avoids intubation.

818 Summarize the major elements in the management of chronic stable COPD. Should these measures be applied at once?

❑ The management of chronic stable COPD requires the application of several measures, each of them having a specific purpose, as follows: (1) removal of underlying causative factors (eg, cessation of smoking, discontinuation of occupational exposure); (2) relief of airway narrowing with inhaled bronchodilators (ie, anticholinergic drugs and beta-adrenergic agonists) and possibly oral xanthines if the response to other measures is insufficient; (3) relief of inflammation of the airways with corticosteroids (eg, aerosol, systemic administration), in some patients; (4) provision of supplemental oxygen (eg, nasal prongs, masks) if indicated (see answer to pertinent question); (5) amelioration of pulmonary hypertension with the possible use of vasodilators (eg, calcium antagonists), diuretics (eg, furosemide), and phlebotomy (decreases abnormally high blood viscosity caused by hypoxemia-induced erythrocytosis); and (6) correction of obesity (if present), to reduce ventilatory requirements. These measures should be applied at once because the aim and effects of each of them differ and none acts as a substitute for another measure.

---

819 What are the indications of continuous low-flow oxygen therapy in COPD?

❑ The indications for low-flow oxygen therapy in COPD include patients whose (1) PaO_2 is equal to or less than 55 mm Hg at rest while receiving optimal medical therapy; (2) resting PaO_2 is 56 to 59 mm Hg in the presence of P pulmonale on the ECG or a hematocrit higher than 56%; and (3) PaO_2 is less than 60 mm Hg during sleep and there is simultaneous evidence of significant cardiac arrhythmia, abnormal sleep pattern, or hypoxic organ dysfunction.

---

820 How important is weight reduction in the management of obese patients with chronic respiratory failure? What is the role of pharmacologic stimulants of ventilation in their management?

❑ Efforts should be made to return overweight patients with chronic respiratory failure toward their ideal weight in order to diminish oxygen consumption and carbon dioxide production. In addition, this measure might affect favorably a variety of other adverse factors associated with obesity, if present, such as central hypoventilation, upper-airway obstruction, increased work of respiratory muscles, and $\dot{V}A/\dot{Q}$ mismatching. The use of pharmacologic stimulants of ventilation has been generally disappointing; yet, a measure of benefit has been derived by some patients with central sleep apnea, obesity-hypoventilation syndrome, and COPD (see details in answer to pertinent question).

---

821 What is the role of immunotherapy for influenza and pneumococcal pneumonia in patients with COPD?

❑ Immunotherapy for influenza is recommended for all patients with COPD. Amantadine may help to reduce the symptoms of influenza A but has no effect on infections by influenza B virus. Pneumococcal vaccine is recommended to prevent acute pneumonia in COPD patients, but its overall benefit has not been fully assessed.

---

822 Explain the indications and recommended dosage of alpha-1-antitrypsin (antiprotease inhibitor [API]) in the replacement therapy of the deficient state or disease.

❑ The protease-antiprotease hypothesis of lung injury is based on the association of API deficiency and the development of emphysema as well as on the observation that the rate of decline of pulmonary function in patients with API deficiency is more rapid than in patients with COPD having normal levels of API. However, not all API-deficient patients develop emphysema. Several alleles for the protease inhibitor have been demonstrated on the basis of protein electrophoretic patterns. The homozygous null allele is completely deficient in API, but patients with the homozygous Z allele have approximately 15% of normal API activity. A normal serum API level ranges from 180 to 280 mg/dL. Although expensive, 60 mg/kg of API can be administered intravenously as a weekly dose in selected patients. The long-term effects of replacement therapy in the API-deficient population with emphysema are unknown.

823 What are the main elements of a pulmonary rehabilitation program? Explain the use of nicotine-containing chewing gum and skin patches in a smoking-cessation program?

❑ Rehabilitation should begin with patient education and behavior modification. Smoking cessation is encouraged through counseling, and in some patients nicotine needs to be prescribed as chewing gum (Nicorette) or skin patches (Habitrol, Nicoderm) to limit the symptoms of withdrawal. Pulmonary function may improve in patients with early COPD after they stop smoking. Other modalities of rehabilitation consist of chest physical therapy to assist secretion removal and exercise conditioning that includes inspiratory muscle training. Pulmonary rehabilitation programs have improved the quality of life and exercise capacity of COPD patients. Yet, a standardized approach to rehabilitation has not been established despite the success of these programs.

BETA-ADRENERGIC AGONISTS

824 What is the role of beta-adrenergic agonists in the treatment of obstructive lung disease? Enumerate commonly used preparations.

❑ Beta-adrenergic agonists with relative beta-2-receptor specificity are indicated in the management of asthma (mild, moderate, and severe forms) and the treatment of both acute exacerbations (first-line medication) as well as the chronic management of chronic bronchitis and emphysema. Inhalation of beta-agonists is preferred to oral administration because it provides equivalent bronchodilation with fewer side effects (ie, tachycardia and tremulousness). Commonly used short-acting (3 to 6 hours) preparations include metaproterenol (Alupent, Metaprel), albuterol (Ventolin, Proventil), and terbutaline (Brethaire). A longer-acting preparation (up to 12 hours) of beta-agonists that may help in the prevention of nocturnal symptoms is salmeterol (Serevent).

825 What adrenoreceptors mediate bronchodilation? What are the cardiovascular effects of stimulation of beta-1- (cardiac), beta-2- (peripheral), and alpha- (peripheral) adrenoreceptors?

❑ Stimulation of beta-2-adrenoreceptors causes bronchodilation and vasodilates systemic arterioles. Stimulation of beta-1-adrenoreceptors augments atrial and ventricular contractility (acting on the myocardium), increases heart rate (acting on the sinoatrial node), and enhances atrioventricular conduction (acting on the atrioventricular conduction system). Stimulation of alpha-adrenoceptors vasoconstricts peripheral arterioles.

826 Explain the hypokalemia caused by activation of beta-2-adrenergic receptors observed in untreated patients as well as those receiving medication for the management of asthma and COPD.

❑ Activation of beta-2-adrenergic receptors is responsible for the so-called stress hypokalemia. The endogenous release of catecholamines due to stress (physiologic conditions and disease states), or an exogenous source of beta-2-adrenergic agonists (eg, therapy of obstructive airway disease) stimulates Na^+-K^+-ATPase in skeletal muscle and other tissues, and results in hypokalemia.

827 How effective are beta-adrenergic agonists in the therapy of obstructive airway diseases?

❑ The beta-adrenergic agonists, available for oral, parenteral, or inhalational use, are effective bronchodilators when prescribed alone or in combination with other agents (eg, methylxanthines). These drugs produce bronchodilation by directly stimulating the beta-2-receptors on the bronchial smooth muscle. The beta-adrenergic agonists that are currently prescribed have a longer duration of action than does epinephrine (the first drug made available for this purpose) and their action is more selective since they are devoid of many of the cardiovascular effects of the natural catecholamine (ie, epinephrine).

828 Explain the use and dosage of sympathomimetic agents in the treatment of COPD.

❑ Inhalation of sympathomimetics or beta-agonists is effective and usually provides the first- or second-line approach to therapy of patients with COPD. Beta-adrenergic effects include beta-1 activity, which leads to cardiac stimulation, and beta-2 activity, which produces bronchodilation and increased mucociliary clearance. A disadvantage of beta-2-agonists is their effect on other muscle receptors that produces tremor. When these agonists are administered by inhalation, beta-2 selectivity is further enhanced and the side effects of tachycardia, tremor, and slight hypoxemia are minimized. Commonly used beta-2-agonists include metaproterenol (Alupent, Metaprel), albuterol (Proventil, Ventolin), terbutaline (Brethaire), pirbuterol (Maxair), and bitolterol (Tornalate). The dosages for MDIs and nebulized solutions are as follows: albuterol—2 or 3 puffs every 4 to 6 hours or 0.3 to 0.5 mL of a 0.5% solution in 3 mL of saline every 4 to 6 hours; metaproterenol—2 or 3 puffs every 4 to 6 hours or 0.3 mL of a 5% solution in 3 mL of saline every 4 to 6 hours; bitolterol—2 or 3 puffs every 6 to 8 hours; pirbuterol—2 or 3 puffs every 4 to 6 hours; and terbutaline—2 or 3 puffs every 4 to 6 hours.

829 Is there any advantage to using MDIs as compared with nebulizers containing beta-adrenergic agonists?

❑ Although nebulizers containing beta-adrenergic agonists have been used widely for treating patients with significant airway obstruction, MDIs can provide equivalent benefit with significant savings. Careful instruction and repeated reminders about MDI technique are needed even for experienced patients.

830 What is the most effective route of administration of sympathomimetic agents in stable patients with COPD?

❑ Sympathomimetic agents inhaled from an MDI are more effective than oral sympathomimetics in stable patients with COPD. Proper patient instruction on the use of MDIs is of paramount importance. MDIs are usually prescribed as 2 or 3 puffs three or four times per day, but several additional puffs or increased frequency of administration may be necessary for acute exacerbations of COPD. If a patient with intense dyspnea is unable to use an MDI properly, sympathomimetics can be inhaled from a nebulizer. The use of a spacer device in combination with an MDI helps to achieve bronchodilation that is at least as marked as that obtained with a nebulizer.

831 Explain the use of sympathomimetic agents as inhaled bronchodilators in the management of COPD.

❑ Patients having COPD most frequently show a significant bronchodilator response to inhaled sympathomimetic agents. Commonly prescribed beta-2-selective agents include metaproterenol, albuterol, terbutaline, pirbuterol, and bitolterol. When used in the recommended dosages, these agents have similar efficacy, duration of action, and side effects. In stable patients with COPD, sympathomimetic agents inhaled from an MDI have been shown to be more effective and cause fewer side effects than the oral administration of these drugs; best results require proper use of the MDI. Patients with acute exacerbations of COPD who are unable to use an MDI properly may inhale sympathomimetics from a nebulizer. Metaproterenol may be prescribed in doses of 0.3 mL of a 5% solution every 4 hours, and albuterol may be given in doses of 0.5 mL of a 0.5% solution every 3 to 4 hours. The use of a spacer device with an MDI is beneficial and the bronchodilation obtained is at least as intense as that obtained with a nebulizer. Side effects of inhaled sympathomimetics, including tachycardia, tremor, and slight hypoxemia, are uncommon.

ANTICHOLINERGIC AGENTS

832 What is the role of anticholinergic agents in the treatment of obstructive lung disease? What are the major categories of bronchodilators available for inhalation therapy in COPD? Explain the use of anticholinergic agents for this purpose.

❑ Anticholinergic bronchodilators are at least as effective as beta-2-agonists in patients with stable emphysema or chronic bronchitis but are less effective in patients with asthma. Two major categories of bronchodilators are available for inhalation therapy: anticholinergic and sympathomimetic agents. The most commonly used anticholinergic agents are atropine and ipratropium. Atropine sulfate, 0.02 mg/kg (up to 2.5 mg) as a single dose, can be given by a nebulizer every 4 to 6 hours. However, side effects are very common at this dosage and the use of this agent as a bronchodilator has not been approved by the US Food and Drug Administration. Ipratropium, a synthetic quaternary ammonium compound related to atropine, is approved for use as a bronchodilator in the United States and the recommended dosage is 2 puffs (36 μg) every 4 to 6 hours. A solution of ipratropium for nebulization is also available and the usual dosage of inhalation solution is 500 μg (1 unit-dose vial) administered three to four times a day by oral nebulization. Side effects of ipratropium are very uncommon and are usually limited to a dry mouth.

833 Elaborate on the efficacy of anticholinergic agents in the therapy of obstructive airway diseases.

❑ Anticholinergic agents represent first-line therapy in COPD. Patients with COPD may experience additional bronchodilation with anticholinergic agents, even after optimal bronchodilation with sympathomimetic agents or theophylline. Anticholinergics exert their effects by competitive inhibition of muscarinic cholinergic receptors, relaxing bronchial smooth muscle. Because cholinergic tone tends to be heightened in COPD, anticholinergic agents are usually beneficial in the management of these patients. Anticholinergic agents are highly specific antagonists of the effect of acetylcholine at parasympathetic muscarinic receptor sites. Thus, they inhibit the bronchoconstricting action of the vagus nerve. These agents are classified as tertiary ammonium compounds, atropine and atropine sulfate, and quaternary ammonium compounds, ipratropium bromide (Atrovent), atropine methylnitrate, oxitropium, and glycopyrrolate. The tertiary ammonium compounds are well absorbed from mucosae and rapidly distributed throughout the body, including the central nervous system. Quaternary ammonium compounds are poorly absorbed, and when given parenterally (not recommended for clinical use), they do not cross the blood-brain barrier to any significant degree.

CORTICOSTEROIDS

834 Do corticosteroids have beneficial effects in patients with COPD? Is long-term treatment with these agents advisable?

❑ Corticosteroids are considered beneficial for the COPD patient with significant bronchospasm (ie, an ''asthmatic component'') or during an acute exacerbation. Methylprednisolone (Solu-Medrol) in a dose of 0.5 mg/kg of body weight given every 6 hours for 3 days can rapidly improve airway obstruction during acute exacerbations of COPD. It is prudent to reserve steroid treatment for patients who present with severe bronchospasm or in those in whom this sign persists despite adequate therapy with sympathomimetics, anticholinergics, and xanthines. Because long-term corticosteroid therapy is fraught with adverse effects, their use should be mostly limited to intermittent bolus administration or inhaled steroid preparations. However, in a small minority of patients with COPD, benefits are obtained with chronic oral use of steroids.

835 What is the role of corticosteroids in the relief of airway obstruction in patients with COPD? Compare the therapeutic effects of corticosteroids in asthma and COPD.

❑ Corticosteroids have been shown to benefit patients with an acute exacerbation of COPD. Methylprednisolone, 0.5 mg/kg intravenously every 6 hours, produces a rapid decrease in airway obstruction as demonstrated by the increase FEV_1. The therapeutic effects of corticosteroids are more intense in patients with asthma than in those with chronic bronchitis and emphysema.

836 What patients with chronic stable COPD might respond favorably to corticosteroid therapy? What are the routes of administration?

❑ Patients with chronic stable COPD exhibiting recurrent episodes of wheezing and a relatively large response (ie, FEV_1 increases more than 20%) to inhaled bronchodilators may respond favorably to corticosteroid therapy. These agents are used preferably by inhalation than by systemic administration (eg, oral). In order to reduce the risk of the side effects of systemic administration of corticosteroids in the small fraction of chronic stable COPD patients requiring this medication, it is recommended that the lowest possible daily dosage be prescribed.

837 What oral preparations of corticosteroids can be used in COPD? Describe the available aerosol preparations of corticosteroids.

❑ Prednisone and prednisolone are the agents most commonly used for oral therapy. The initial dose commonly consists of 30 mg (up to about 70 mg) daily. A detectable benefit may be observed within 1 hour, with maximal improvement in ventilatory capacity at 9 to 10 hours. A clinical response usually requires 4 to 10 days of therapy, and it is common to treat a patient for 2 to 3 weeks before corticosteroids are considered ineffective. The development of highly surface-active topical steroids for aerosol administration, for example, beclomethasone dipropionate (Beclovent, Vanceril), have proved to be very effective in the chronic management of airway obstruction but have no role in the management of acutely ill patients.

---

838 Is the administration of systemic corticosteroids of value in the management of acute exacerbations of COPD?

❑ Methylprednisolone has been shown to decrease airway obstruction in patients with acute respiratory failure secondary to an acute exacerbation of COPD. In addition, corticosteroids have a beneficial effect in the management of a minority of chronic stable patients with COPD.

USE OF XANTHINES

---

839 What are the main properties of the methylxanthines? What is the mechanism of action?

❑ The methylxanthines are drugs with multiple actions that include bronchodilation, cardiac stimulation, and increased diuresis. The most prominent of these actions is bronchodilation, and such effect is used in the therapy of obstructive diseases of the airways. Proposed mechanisms for the cellular basis of action of methylxanthines have included (1) inhibition of phosphodiesterases, thereby increasing intracellular cyclic adenosine monophosphate (AMP); (2) direct effects on intracellular calcium concentration; (3) indirect effects on intracellular calcium concentrations via cell membrane hyperpolarization; (4) uncoupling of intracellular calcium increases with muscle contractile elements; and (5) antagonism of adenosine receptors (G-protein–coupled receptors). A large body of evidence suggests that adenosine receptor antagonism is the most important factor responsible for most pharmacologic effects of methylxanthines in doses that are administered therapeutically or consumed in xanthine-containing beverages.

840 What effects other than bronchodilation can be observed with methylxanthines (eg, theophylline)? How are these agents used in the management of COPD?

❑ Theophylline, the most widely used methylxanthine, can improve cardiac and diaphragmatic contractility, diminish pulmonary vascular resistance, stimulate central respiratory activity, and increase diuresis. Because of its narrow therapeutic range and weak bronchodilator effect in stable COPD patients, theophylline use is waning. For patients with acute exacerbations of COPD, the addition of intravenous aminophylline to a standard regimen of a beta-agonist, corticosteroid, and antibiotic does not improve symptoms, spirometric results, or blood oxygenation. Theophylline is usually relegated to third-line therapy as an oral sustained-release preparation prescribed in doses of 300 to 900 mg/day to stable COPD patients and as an intravenous preparation for use in severe acute exacerbations of COPD.

841 Summarize the action of xanthines in obstructive airway disease.

❑ Xanthines (eg, theophylline) have multiple actions that may explain their beneficial effects in patients with obstructive airway disease. These actions include (1) bronchodilation; (2) increased diaphragmatic contractility; (3) improved tolerance to exercise; (4) stimulation of ventilation; (5) improved cardiovascular function; (6) promotion of better ciliary function of airway lining, facilitating the clearance of bronchial secretions; and (7) anti-inflammatory properties exerted on the respiratory tract.

842 What is the role of methylxanthines in the treatment of obstructive lung disease?

❑ Methylxanthines have been widely used in the past for the management of stable asthma, chronic bronchitis, and emphysema. Administration of extended-release preparations (eg, theophylline [Theo-Dur]) once daily in the evening can help to overcome nocturnal bronchospasm in asthma. Theophylline and related compounds can also be effective in patients with stable COPD because these drugs may (1) improve airflow, (2) enhance functional status even without bronchodilation, (3) augment diaphragmatic strength and endurance, and (4) have beneficial effects on right-sided heart function in cor pulmonale. However, the toxicity of methylxanthines (eg, nausea, vomiting, insomnia, agitation, seizures, arrhythmias) limits significantly the use of these drugs. Furthermore, some experts advise to avoid methylxanthines in the management of serious flares of obstructive lung disease because the risks of serious toxic effects might exceed the potential benefits.

843 Explain the use of theophylline (best-known xanthine) in the management of airway obstruction of patients with COPD.

❑ Theophylline has been a widely used drug to achieve bronchodilation. However, this agent has only a weak bronchodilatory effect in stable patients with COPD. Furthermore, the addition of intravenous aminophylline to an otherwise standard treatment regimen (eg, metaproterenol, methylprednisolone, and an antibiotic) in patients with acute exacerbations of COPD does not improve spirometric values, ABG data, or dyspnea. In addition, the acute bronchodilatory effect of the intravenous administration of both aminophylline and albuterol is not additive, and the cardiac toxicity of this combination of drugs is increased. Consequently, the popularity of theophylline for the management of COPD (especially during acute exacerbations) is waning.

844 What is the effect of aminophylline on the respiratory muscles?

❑ Aminophylline increases diaphragmatic contractility. At the usual therapeutic level, however, aminophylline provides only minimal improvement in ventilatory endurance. Because of the limited effect on muscle endurance as well as its potential toxicity, the role of aminophylline in managing respiratory muscle dysfunction remains controversial. The respiratory muscles can be trained to increase strength and endurance. Strength training with high-load, low-repetition tasks has been used for healthy persons and for patients with COPD, cystic fibrosis, or quadriplegia; however, the level of improvement varies widely among reported studies. Endurance training involving low-load, high-repetition tasks has been tried in healthy persons and in patients with COPD or cystic fibrosis and such training usually causes a 20% to 30% improvement in muscle endurance of respiratory muscles.

845 What are the effects of xanthines (eg, aminophylline) on serum $[K^+]$?

❑ Xanthines, drugs widely used in the treatment of reactive airways due to various diseases including bronchial asthma, ''cardiac asthma,'' and COPD, mimic the effects of beta-2-agonists on $[K^+]_p$. Both drugs produce hypokalemia because of stimulation of Na^+-K^+-ATPase as a result of increased cyclic AMP levels. While beta-2-adrenergic agonists enhance production of cyclic AMP, xanthines inhibit degradation of this compound.

846 What levels of theophylline are associated with optimal results in the management of obstructive airway diseases?

❑ The serum levels of theophylline that result in optimal therapeutic effects are approximately 10 to 15 μg/mL. These levels are associated with maximal benefit and minimal toxicity. The daily dosage of theophylline and other xanthines must be adjusted to achieve serum levels that fall within the previously mentioned therapeutic range. Life-threatening toxic effects are generally not observed in most patients unless levels exceed 20 μg/mL.

847 What factors increase the rate of degradation and excretion of xanthines requiring an upward adjustment in the daily dosage?

❑ An increased maintenance dosage of xanthines may be required in children, smokers of tobacco and marijuana, and individuals eating charcoal-broiled and barbecued meats, and with the use of some concomitant medication (eg, ciprofloxacin, rifampin, carbamazepine, phenobarbital, phenytoin).

---

848 What factors decrease the rate of degradation and excretion of xanthines, requiring a downward adjustment in the daily dosage?

❑ A decreased maintenance dosage of xanthines may be required in infants and elderly patients as well as those with a febrile syndrome (eg, viral and bacterial infections), hepatic dysfunction, or congestive heart failure and with the use of some concomitant medication (eg, erythromycin, quinolone antibiotics, propranolol, allopurinol, oral contraceptives, cimetidine). Failure to recognize the need of a downward adjustment in the daily dosage of xanthines in these conditions is responsible for the development of toxic effects of these drugs (occasionally with serious consequences).

---

849 What are the guidelines for the intravenous administration of aminophylline?

❑ The loading doses are 6 mg/kg and 3 mg/kg in patients not already taking theophylline and those taking this drug, respectively. The maintenance dose is as follows: (1) healthy nonsmoking adult, 0.5 mg/kg/hr; (2) adult cigarette or marijuana smoker, 0.8 mg/kg/hr; and (3) patients with congestive heart failure or liver failure, 0.1 to 0.2 mg/kg/hr. However, the serum levels achieved vary considerably among patients and close monitoring of serum levels is advised.

---

850 What are the toxic effects of theophylline and other xanthines?

❑ The most serious toxic effects of xanthines are seizures and cardiac arrhythmias. Commonly observed untoward effects of these drugs are epigastric pain, nausea, vomiting, and diarrhea. Cardiac manifestations are sinus tachycardia, extrasystoles or premature beats, and multifocal atrial tachycardia. Other toxic effects of these compounds are nervousness, insomnia, headaches, tremor, and seizures.

851 What is the management of theophylline toxicity?

❑ Therapy with theophylline preparation should be discontinued in the presence of toxicity, and treatment with syrup of ipecac to induce vomiting should be considered. Charcoal hemoperfusion (eg, the Redy machine commonly used for hemodialysis in intensive care units has a charcoal cartridge that binds theophylline) causes a rapid reduction in serum theophylline levels, and it is recommended when the serum concentration is higher than 60 μg/mL, even in the absence of signs of toxicity. When the concentration is below 40 μg/mL, the hazards of hemoperfusion outweigh the benefits, and for levels of 40 to 60 μg/mL a decision to institute hemoperfusion must be made on an individual basis. If hemoperfusion is not employed, oral administration of activated charcoal is recommended every 4 hours until the serum concentration falls to less than 20 μg/mL. Peritoneal dialysis or hemodialysis (without a charcoal cartridge) is of limited value in lowering serum theophylline levels. Phenobarbital has been recommended as it increases theophylline clearance, although its efficacy has not been demonstrated. Arrhythmias caused by theophylline appear to be responsive to verapamil (calcium antagonist).

ACUTE EXACERBATIONS OF COPD

852 How serious is the development of acute respiratory failure in patients with COPD? What are the essentials of treatment for this condition?

❑ Acute respiratory failure is a leading cause of death in patients with COPD; however, aggressive management may reverse the precipitating event and reduce short-term mortality. The essentials of treatment for this condition include administration of supplementary oxygen to ameliorate hypoxemia, relief of respiratory acidosis with measures aimed at the precipitating causes as well as the underlying disease, and the use of inhaled anticholinergic and sympathomimetic bronchodilators, and the oral or intravenous administration of corticosteroids to relieve airway obstruction. In addition, broad-spectrum antibiotic therapy should be prescribed if infection is suspected (especially in a severely ill patient), and low-dose heparin may be administered to prevent pulmonary thromboembolism. In selected patients, noninvasive positive-pressure ventilation using a nasal or face mask can increase survival.

---

853 List the major elements in the management of an acute exacerbation of COPD.

❑ The management of an acute exacerbation of COPD includes (1) relief of airway narrowing and inflammation with inhaled bronchodilators (ie, anticholinergic drugs, beta-adrenergic agents) and systemic administration of corticosteroids; (2) eradication of infectious processes responsible for exacerbation, if applicable (eg, broad-spectrum antibacterial agents); (3) provision of supplemental oxygen; (4) reversal of respiratory acidosis with the possible use of mechanical ventilation, if indicated; and (5) correction of other factors that led to the COPD exacerbation (eg, sedatives).

---

854 Is the management of respiratory acidosis similar in all patients with COPD?

❑ The management of respiratory acidosis in patients with COPD differs depending on the cause, severity, and rate of progression of carbon dioxide retention. If respiratory acidosis is detected at the patient's initial presentation, administration of bronchodilators and removal of secretions might help to relieve the acid-base disorder. If respiratory acidosis is caused by the use of narcotic agents, intravenous naloxone (2 mg) might be useful. Respiratory acidosis may also develop because of uncontrolled oxygen therapy; the management of this condition consists of gradual reduction of the concentration of supplemental oxygen aiming at a PaO_2 of about 60 mm Hg. An additional measure to be considered but rarely used in the management of respiratory acidosis in patients with COPD is the administration of analeptic agents (see details on pertinent questions). In a small proportion of patients, mechanical ventilation is required to manage the respiratory acidosis in patients with COPD.

855 Explain the application of specific measures for the management of hypercapnic respiratory failure.

❑ Treatment of hypercapnic respiratory failure must be directed at prompt removal of the underlying cause whenever possible. Immediate therapeutic efforts should focus on establishing and securing a patent airway, restoring adequate oxygenation by delivering an oxygen-rich inspired mixture, and providing adequate ventilation in order to repair the abnormal blood gas composition. As noted, acute respiratory acidosis poses its major threat to survival not because of hypercapnia or acidemia, but because of the associated hypoxemia. At times, prompt removal of the initiating cause might be possible (eg, foreign body in the airway, maladjusted ventilator, tension pneumothorax), thus enabling swift restoration of oxygenation and ventilation. On other occasions, cause-specific measures might also be available (eg, cardiogenic pulmonary edema, pleural effusion, atelectasis, paralytic crisis in myasthenia gravis, hypokalemic myopathy, phosphate-depletion myopathy), but in addition to pursuing them aggressively, nonspecific supportive measures should be taken until the underlying disease can be reversed.

856 Summarize the overall management of acute hypercapnic respiratory failure. What is the role of digitalis in the treatment of cardiorespiratory failure?

❑ Swift restoration of $PaCO_2$ to normal levels is advisable in patients with acute hypercapnia (ie, minutes to hours in duration). Measures against all possible reversible factors responsible for the acute respiratory acidosis should be taken. Thus, bronchodilator therapy (eg, beta-adrenergic agonists, corticosteroids) should be used in patients with bronchospasm. In patients with excessive secretions, bronchodilator therapy, chest physical therapy, and postural drainage are helpful. Pulmonary infections should be treated aggressively. Reversal of the hypercapnia, acidemia, and hypoxemia will usually improve cardiac dysfunction and pulmonary hypertension. Excluding the case of cor pulmonale in association with low cardiac output, administration of digitalis appears to be of no value in the treatment of the depressed cardiac contractility accompanying severe respiratory acidosis. Close monitoring of the patient's fluid status is crucial, for volume overload increases pulmonary capillary blood pressure and predisposes to the development of pulmonary edema. Diuretics should be used, as needed. Nutritional support is important to minimize reduction in the strength and endurance of the respiratory muscles and depression in the body's immunity.

857 How important are inhaled anticholinergic agents, beta-adrenergic agonists, systemic corticosteroids, antibiotics, and methylxanthines in the management of acute COPD exacerbations?

❑ Inhaled anticholinergic agents, inhaled beta-adrenergic agonists, and systemic corticosteroids represent first-line drugs in the therapy of COPD exacerbations. Antibiotics (10-day course) may be useful in patients with purulent bronchial secretions. Methylxanthines are not indicated in the management of acute COPD exacerbations because of the high risk-benefit ratio in this medical condition. As explained elsewhere in this book, methylxanthines are useful in the chronic management of some patients with chronic bronchitis and emphysema.

858 What microorganisms are likely to play a role in the COPD exacerbations? What antibiotics might be recommended for the treatment of this condition?

❑ The airways of the patient with chronic bronchitis provide a rich medium for bacterial colonization. Although viruses do play a major role in the flare-ups of bronchitis in COPD patients, colonizing organisms such as *Streptococcus pneumoniae, Haemophilus influenzae,* and *Moraxella catarrhalis* also have a pathogenic role in exacerbations of airway inflammation. Thus, antibiotics are good adjuncts to therapy during acute exacerbations of COPD and should be administered for 7 to 10 days. Recommended agents include ampicillin (500 mg every 6 hours), amoxicillin (500 mg every 8 hours), tetracycline (500 mg every 6 hours), trimethoprim (160 mg/day) combined with sulfamethoxazole (800 mg/day), and ciprofloxacin (500 mg every 12 hours). For repeated flare-ups, it is sometimes useful to modify the antibiotic regimen. Long-term prophylaxis with antibacterial drugs is generally not advised.

859 What elements favor initiation of a course of antibiotics in patients with a COPD exacerbation? What antibiotics should be chosen?

❑ A course of antibiotics is generally advisable in patients developing an exacerbation of COPD that has one or more of the following signs and symptoms: purulent bronchial secretions, increased volume of bronchial secretions, and development or intensification of dyspnea. Broad-spectrum antibiotics are generally used and the specific selection is based on cost of medication and previous good tolerance to the drug by the patient.

860 What is the role of antibacterial agents in the management of patients with COPD in acute respiratory failure?

❑ Since exacerbations of COPD are commonly accompanied by symptoms of respiratory tract infection, the latter is considered a major precipitating cause of respiratory failure in these patients. However, the role of bacterial infection in these exacerbations has not been well documented and, until recently, there had been no evidence that antibiotic therapy was beneficial. A recent, carefully conducted study found that broad-spectrum antimicrobial agents including trimethoprim-sulfamethoxazole (160/180 mg, respectively, twice daily), amoxicillin (250 mg four times a day), or doxycycline (200 mg initially followed by 100 mg/d) produced a more rapid recovery in PEFR and a faster resolution of symptoms. Although this study dealt with relatively stable patients, it is reasonable to expect that these and other antimicrobial agents will also benefit more severely ill patients with COPD who appear to have an airway infection. In summary, the use of broad-spectrum antimicrobial agents is currently recommended when respiratory tract infection is suspected as the precipitating cause of respiratory failure in COPD patients.

---

861 How useful is the evaluation of sputum stains and cultures in the management of exacerbations of COPD associated with purulent bronchial secretions? What is the treatment of bronchial infection?

❑ Evaluation of sputum stains and cultures is not generally helpful in managing acute exacerbations of COPD because of the high rate of airway colonization. Oral administration of trimethoprim-sulfamethoxazole, amoxicillin, or doxycycline in a 10-day course (one of them) promotes recovery of most patients with acute exacerbations of COPD with increased sputum volume and purulence independent of the specific cause of the bronchial infection.

---

862 How important is nutritional support in the management of patients with COPD in acute respiratory failure?

❑ The precise role of nutritional support in the management of patients with COPD is controversial. Nutritional deprivation has been shown to decrease ventilatory drive, as well as both muscle bulk and strength. However, diets consisting of a high proportion of carbohydrate lead to increased carbon dioxide production and may precipitate ventilatory failure. Although proof of efficacy of nutritional support in the management of patients with acute COPD exacerbations does not exist, it seems prudent to encourage patients to eat as soon as possible. If the patient cannot eat and is likely to require mechanical ventilation for more than 1 day, a small-bore feeding tube should be inserted so that enteral feeding can be instituted (assuming that contraindications to enteral feeding such as gastrointestinal bleeding or ileus are not present).

863 What is the role of analeptic agents in the management of patients with COPD in acute respiratory failure? What drugs have been used for this purpose?

❑ A variety of analeptic agents have been employed with the intention of increasing alveolar ventilation in COPD patients. These drugs exert their actions at all levels of the brain and spinal cord, increasing arousal and sensory responsiveness. The analeptics stimulate breathing but their safety margin is small and unpredictable. Nikethamide and doxapram are the two best-known drugs from this group of compounds. Nikethamide has a short duration of action and its effects seldom last more than 5 to 10 minutes. This agent can be given orally, intravenously, or intramuscularly in doses of 5 to 10 mg. Side effects of nikethamide include hypertension, tachycardia, sweating, vomiting, tremors, rigidity, and convulsions (especially when the drug is repeatedly administered). Doxapram is a more potent and selective analeptic agent, and there is less risk of convulsion with this drug than with nikethamide. The stimulatory effect of doxapram on respiration is mediated through activation of both peripheral and central chemoreceptors. The usual dosage is 1 to 3 mg/min, given by intravenous infusion, and can be titrated to achieve a desired ABG value but not exceeding a total dosage of 4 mg/kg. Side effects of doxapram are similar to those of nikethamide. In controlled studies, doxapram did not decrease the need for intubation and mechanical ventilation in patients with acute respiratory failure. Consequently, the limited therapeutic effects and the substantial potential toxicity have led the majority of physicians to stop prescribing analeptic agents to COPD patients with respiratory failure.

864 What measures might help to prevent the development of complications in patients with COPD in acute respiratory failure?

❑ Optimal management of the acute exacerbations of COPD helps to minimize the risk of complications. In addition, the following specific measures might help to prevent common complications. ECG monitoring, for example, permits detection of cardiac arrhythmias that either might respond to modifications of the primary therapy or require antiarrhythmic measures (eg, drugs, cardioversion, pacemaker). Because of the high risk of pulmonary thromboembolism originated in the systemic venous circulation, low-dose subcutaneous heparin (eg, 5000 units every 8 to 12 hours) should be considered. Similarly, antacids, sucralfate, and H_2-blockers might help to decrease the risk of gastrointestinal hemorrhage.

---

865 A 61-year-old white-collar worker is admitted to the hospital with severe dyspnea, night sweats, and purulent sputum production. Physical examination demonstrates fever (39.0°C), a pulse rate of 108 beats/min, respiration rate of 32 breaths/min, and blood pressure of 120/82 mm Hg. He has intense respiratory efforts including the use of sternomastoid muscles, supraclavicular fossa recession, and diffuse bilateral wheezing. Chest hyperinflation with low flat diaphragms appears on the x-ray film. ABG values are as follows: SaO_2 of 80%, PaO_2 of 46 mm Hg, $PaCO_2$ of 56 mm Hg, pH 7.30, and HCO_3^- of 25 mEq/L.

What therapeutic measures should be implemented immediately?

❑ Controlled oxygen therapy, inhaled anticholinergic agents, and antibiotics represent the main therapeutic measures in the management of this patient. Because hypoxemia is the most life-threatening abnormality, the use of controlled oxygen therapy to relieve hypoxemia without aggravating carbon dioxide retention is of utmost importance in the management of patients with an acute COPD exacerbation. Supplemental low-flow oxygen should be administered by a 24% or 28% Venturi face mask or by nasal cannula at 1 to 2 L/min. The usual therapeutic goal is an SaO_2 of 90%, because higher values do not significantly increase systemic oxygenation and predispose to carbon dioxide retention. The use of antibiotics (eg, amoxicillin) is appropriate in this patient, considering the presence of fever and purulent sputum.

OXYGEN THERAPY IN COPD

866 How can tissue oxygenation be improved in patients with COPD in acute respiratory failure?

❑ Hypoxemia (ie, decreased blood oxygen tension) is most often the immediate life-threatening abnormality of patients in respiratory failure because it causes tissue hypoxia (brain, myocardium, etc); thus, the first priority is to improve blood oxygen levels. The use of controlled oxygen therapy in an attempt to relieve life-threatening hypoxemia without aggravating carbon dioxide retention has been the major mode of therapy for about 30 years. Supplemental low-flow oxygen should be administered with this purpose, either by nasal cannula at 1 to 2 L/min or via a Venturi-type mask set at 24% or 28% oxygen. If the PaO_2 exceeds 60 mm Hg while the patient breathes room air, supplemental oxygen most likely will not cause significant carbon dioxide retention. The usual goal is to attain a PaO_2 of about 60 mm Hg since this PO_2 level results in satisfactory hemoglobin oxygen saturation. In most patients, controlled oxygen therapy does not cause significant carbon dioxide retention. Attention must also be paid to the adequacy of cardiac output and the hemoglobin concentration in all patients with acute respiratory failure since these factors are also major determinants of oxygen delivery to the tissues.

867 What are the indications and importance of supplemental oxygen administration in patients with COPD?

❑ The indications of oxygen therapy in COPD include (1) patients with acute exacerbations of the disease; (2) patients with a PaO_2 lower than 55 mm Hg during steady-state conditions while receiving intensive bronchodilator therapy; and (3) patients with a

PaO_2 lower than 59 mm Hg during stable condition with intensive treatment who concomitantly have polycythemia (hematocrit >55%), edema caused by heart failure, or cor pulmonale (eg, right ventricular hypertrophy diagnosed by ECG). Supplemental oxygen is the only therapy shown to prolong survival in patients with COPD and chronic hypoxemia. Consequently, oxygen administration is of great importance in the management of patients with COPD.

868 How should oxygen be administered to patients with chronic respiratory failure and carbon dioxide retention?

❑ Reduction in ventilatory drive during oxygen administration is a major hazard in patients with chronic respiratory acidosis. Indeed, injudicious use of oxygen therapy can produce further reduction in alveolar ventilation and aggravate hypercapnia dramatically. This risk notwithstanding, careful and controlled oxygen administration by venti-masks (ie, Venturi masks) or nasal prongs can improve oxygenation and symptomatology considerably without substantial aggravation of the hypercapnia. In general, the hypoxic drive to ventilation remains adequate if the PaO_2 does not exceed 60 mm Hg. Nasal catheters or prongs at a flow rate of 2 L of oxygen per minute generally deliver an inspired oxygen concentration of approximately 23% to 28%, which improves PaO_2 values to levels of 50 to 60 mm Hg in many patients with chronic respiratory failure. A higher flow rate of 4 L of oxygen per minute, which can increase the inspired oxygen to approximately 31% to 38%, might be required in patients with more severe hypoxemia. The inspired oxygen concentration obtained with different oxygen flow rates (eg, 2 or 4 L/min) is very variable and, therefore, it is difficult to predict the level of oxygen that reaches the alveoli because the latter is largely dependent on the patient's own inspiratory flow rate. Commonly available venti-masks reliably deliver an inspired oxygen concentration of 28% or 35% and they can be used in the place of nasal catheters. Yet, as noted previously, the considerable advantage of nasal prongs is that they do not interfere with coughing, drinking, and eating. The use of venti-masks is most useful when starting treatment; thereafter, a switch to nasal catheters is appropriate.

---

869 Explain the effects of supplemental oxygen on the $PaCO_2$ of patients with COPD. How severe is the carbon dioxide retention? What are the mechanisms responsible for these effects?

❑ When supplemental oxygen is given to patients with acute respiratory failure secondary to COPD, the $PaCO_2$ usually increases. In most cases, this increase is slight, about 1 to 5 mm Hg for a 10 mm Hg increase in PaO_2. However, a greater increase in $PaCO_2$ occurs in some patients, and uncontrolled oxygen therapy may cause severe retention of carbon dioxide. The degree of increase in $PaCO_2$ is correlated with the baseline PaO_2 and with the increase in PaO_2 during supplemental oxygen therapy. However, the severity of carbon dioxide retention does not correlate with the baseline $PaCO_2$. Patients who have acidemia or abnormal rib cage–abdominal motion (asynchronous or paradoxical breathing) may be at an increased risk for carbon dioxide retention. The mechanism responsible for the increase in $PaCO_2$ is controversial. It was once thought that patients with COPD depend primarily on their hypoxic drive because of an impaired ventilatory response to carbon dioxide. If this was responsible, one would expect a proportional inverse relationship between minute ventilation and $PaCO_2$ on administration of oxygen. However, studies of patients with acute respiratory failure (eg, PaO_2 of 38 mm Hg, $PaCO_2$ of 65 mm Hg, and pH 7.34) demonstrated that administration of 100% oxygen causes substantial increases in the PaO_2 (eg, 225 mm Hg) and $PaCO_2$ (to 88 mm Hg), but the decrease in minute ventilation is quite small (7%) and insufficient to account for the 35% increase in $PaCO_2$. Consequently, other factors appear to play a role in the development of oxygen-induced hypercapnia, as follows: (1) The administration of oxygen may cause the release of hypoxic vasoconstriction in poorly ventilated regions of the lung, resulting in a worsening of the alveolar ventilation-perfusion relationship, and (2) for any given amount of carbon dioxide bound to hemoglobin, the $PaCO_2$ is considerably higher in the presence of a high oxygen saturation than in the presence of a low oxygen saturation (Haldane effect).

870 Does oxygen supplementation consistently help to relieve the dyspnea in COPD? What are the effects of cold airflow on dyspnea?

❑ Supplemental oxygen may result in a decrease in dyspnea and improved exercise performance in patients with COPD. Unfortunately, it is not possible to identify with certainty the patients who are likely to derive relief from supplemental oxygen without clinical testing because even the degree of exercise-induced hypoxemia is a poor predictor. The decrease in dyspnea with supplemental oxygen is proportional to the reduction in ventilation. It has been suggested that relief of dyspnea in patients with COPD at rest with oxygen supplementation is at least in part a placebo effect resulting from wearing nasal cannulae. In fact, patients commonly report a decrease in dyspnea when seated near a fan or open window. In support of the salutary effect of a flow of cold air directed against the cheek is the observation that in healthy volunteers this measure causes a decrease in dyspnea induced by both resistive load and inhaled carbon dioxide in the absence of a significant reduction in total ventilation.

871 Is long-term oxygen therapy advantageous in the management of COPD? What are the indications of home oxygen administration?

❑ Long-term oxygen administration is the only therapeutic measure known to improve survival in hypoxemic patients with COPD. Continuous oxygen therapy for more than 19 hours each day is associated with the best overall survival rate. Supplemental oxygen improves the quality of life, pulmonary hemodynamics, and polycythemia. A patient with COPD who has received maximal medical management and who persistently has a PaO_2 less than 55 mm Hg is a candidate for continuous home oxygen therapy. A patient with a PaO_2 between 55 and 60 mm Hg may benefit from oxygen therapy if there is associated cor pulmonale, polycythemia, or changes in mental status. Patients with COPD may develop a more severe arterial oxygen desaturation during sleep, especially during rapid eye movement (REM) sleep. Nocturnal oxygen supplementation in patients prone to desaturation may improve the quality of sleep and minimize pulmonary arterial hypertension during periods of REM-induced hypoxemia. The administration of oxygen during exercise-induced hypoxemia may also be warranted. During acute exacerbations of COPD, oxygen is most commonly provided by nasal prongs or face mask. With respect to home oxygen administration, regional costs and preferences determine the source of oxygen (ie, liquid, compressed gas, concentrator) and the method of delivery (ie, reservoir cannulae, demand-delivery systems, transtracheal delivery).

MECHANICAL VENTILATION IN COPD

872 What are the indications of ventilator support in COPD?

❑ Mechanical ventilation is required in a small proportion of patients with COPD to manage the respiratory acidosis. If possible, this therapeutic modality should be avoided because these patients are particularly susceptible to the complications of mechanical ventilation. No particular set of ABG values serves as absolute criteria for the institution of mechanical ventilation, and the decision is primarily clinical in nature and based on the patient's mental status (confusion, restlessness), ineffective cough, or apnea. When mechanical ventilation is instituted, care is required to avoid the development of metabolic alkalosis; the goal is to correct pH rather than $PaCO_2$. Although COPD patients may have well-tolerated chronic hypercapnia, they do not exhibit serious acidemia; therefore, a major drop in arterial pH indicates impending severe respiratory failure, necessitating initiation of ventilator assistance.

873 Explain further the indications for the use of mechanical ventilation in patients with COPD in acute respiratory failure. Does mechanical ventilation decrease mortality in these patients?

❑ The management of respiratory failure in patients with COPD may require ventilatory support, although conservative measures represent the standard treatment for this condition. Indications for the use of mechanical ventilation include the presence of severe respiratory distress, apnea, or a progressive increase in $PaCO_2$. Ventilator support should be avoided if possible because COPD patients are particularly susceptible to complications derived from mechanical ventilation. There is not a particular ABG value that serves as absolute criterion for the institution of mechanical ventilation. The decision for initiation of ventilator support is based primarily on the patient's mental status (confusion, restlessness, and stupor caused by hypercapnic encephalopathy) and the presence of apnea or ineffective cough. When mechanical ventilation is deemed necessary, the goal is to correct the arterial blood pH rather than $PaCO_2$. Although patients with COPD requiring ventilator support have a high mortality, mechanical ventilation during the acute episode does not in itself appear to be associated with increased mortality. It is believed that the severity of the disease but not the mechanical ventilation is the reason for the high mortality observed in patients with COPD requiring ventilator support.

874 Elaborate on the rationale for a conservative therapeutic approach (ie, without intubation and mechanical ventilation) in patients with an exacerbation of COPD.

❑ Whereas an aggressive approach that favors the early utilization of ventilator assistance is most appropriate for acute respiratory acidosis, a more conservative approach is advisable in patients with chronic lung diseases because of the great difficulty often encountered in weaning such patients from ventilators. Thus, if adequate oxygenation is attained by conservative therapy (PaO_2 on the order of 50 to 60 mm Hg), persistent hypercapnia is not in itself an indication for mechanical ventilation. As a general rule, if the patient is alert, is able to cough, and can cooperate with the treatment program, mechanical ventilation is usually not necessary. On the other hand, if the patient is obtunded and unable to cough and the carbon dioxide is elevated or increasing rapidly, endotracheal intubation and mechanical ventilation should be instituted. Noninvasive mechanical ventilation with the use of a nasal or facial mask is being used more frequently in an effort to avoid the possible complications of tracheal intubation.

---

875 What is the desired $PaCO_2$ during mechanical ventilation in patients with chronic hypercapnic respiratory failure? What are the risks of rapid correction of hypercapnia in these patients? What is the management of "posthypercapnic metabolic alkalosis"?

❑ In patients with chronic hypercapnia, the minute ventilation delivered by the ventilator should be adjusted to maintain the patient's usual $PaCO_2$. If a patient's hypercapnia is lowered to the normal range, the kidneys compensate by excreting bicarbonate and blood pH is normalized. Consequently, when patients resume their usual level of spontaneous ventilation, acute respiratory acidosis occurs because the level of bicarbonate is inadequate for buffering. If difficulty is expected during weaning, the $PaCO_2$ should be allowed to increase gradually into the hypercapnic range during the period of ventilator support. Overly rapid reduction in $PaCO_2$ in patients with chronic carbon dioxide retention risks the development of sudden, substantial alkalemia with the attendant hazards of a major reduction in cardiac output and cerebral blood flow, cardiac arrhythmias (including predisposition to digitalis intoxication), and generalized seizures. When assisted ventilation is used, blood gases should initially be measured frequently to prevent or correct both overventilation and underventilation. Should "posthypercapnic metabolic alkalosis" develop, it can be managed effectively by the provision of adequate quantities of chloride by the oral or parenteral route.

---

876 What is the role of noninvasive ventilation in the management of acute exacerbations of COPD?

❑ Noninvasive positive-pressure ventilation (NIPPV) is an alternative approach to the standard method of endotracheal intubation followed by mechanical ventilation. The use of artificial airways with the standard approach commonly leads to infectious complications and injury to the trachea. NIPPV uses a nasal or face mask instead of a tracheal tube. Limited experience with pressure-support ventilation delivered with the use of a face mask demonstrated that this method improves physiologic measurements and reduces the need for intubation, the frequency of complications, the length of the hospital stay, and the mortality rate in patients with acute exacerbations of COPD. Unfortunately, we still do not know which patients are best suited for this therapy.

---

877 A 55-year-old man with a previous history of severe COPD reports to the hospital emergency room with severe respiratory distress. The ABG values are as follows: PaO_2 of 48 mm Hg, $PaCO_2$ of 70 mm Hg, and pH 7.21. A follow-up visit for COPD that took place 1 month earlier revealed the following blood gas levels: PaO_2 of 56 mm Hg, $PaCO_2$ of 50 mm Hg, and pH 7.38. Because of a progressive downhill course of his condition despite maximal therapy, mechanical ventilation is performed using the assist-control mode.

What would be a desirable set of ABG values at about 1 hour after institution of mechanical ventilation?

❑ A desirable set of ABGs would be one having $PaCO_2$ and pH values close to 50 mm Hg and 7.38, respectively, which represent the levels that the patient had 1 month before his current hospital admission. Alkalemia (elevated blood pH) must be avoided because it depresses spontaneous ventilation and increases myocardial and neuromuscular excitability. Eucapnia and hypocapnia must be avoided because the patient had chronic hypercapnia, and therefore he will not be able to resume spontaneous breathing, maintaining $PaCO_2$ levels lower than those present before his current hospital admission. A desirable PaO_2 is about 60 mm Hg as this level achieves adequate hemoglobin saturation; such PO_2 must be obtained with the lowest possible FiO_2 (eg, 40%).

878 A 67-year-old man with an acute exacerbation of COPD continues a downhill course despite treatment with supplemental oxygen, bronchodilators, corticosteroids, and antibiotics. Blood gases values are as follows: PaO_2 of 48 mm Hg, $PaCO_2$ of 71 mm Hg, and pH 7.25. The assist-control mode of mechanical ventilation is instituted with FiO_2 of 0.5, tidal volume of 1000 mL, inspiratory flow rate of 80 L/min, backup rate of 15 breaths/min, and PEEP of 5 cm H_2O. Thirty minutes after initiation of mechanical ventilation, the patient develops recurrent episodes of supraventricular tachycardia unresponsive to vagal stimulatory maneuvers and generalized muscle twitching. A new set of blood gas measurements reveals a PaO_2 of 74 mm Hg, $PaCO_2$ of 36 mm Hg, and pH 7.52; auto-PEEP of 2 cm H_2O is detected.

What is the cause of the patient's symptoms?

❑ The recurrent episodes of supraventricular tachycardia unresponsive to vagal maneuvers and generalized muscle twitching are manifestations of acute respiratory alkalosis caused by mechanical hyperventilation.

879 What ventilator setting should be changed to correct the iatrogenic acute respiratory alkalosis observed in the just-described patient?

❑ The ventilator-induced hypocapnia, responsible for the cardiac and neuromuscular symptoms, is best corrected by decreasing the set tidal volume of assist-control ventilation (eg, from 1000 mL to 600 mL). Since every inspiratory effort of the patient is boosted or assisted by the ventilator with this ventilation modality, decreasing the set tidal volume will diminish total pulmonary ventilation and therefore will correct the iatrogenic hypocapnia. Other measures to correct the respiratory alkalosis such as switching from assist-control ventilation to intermittent mandatory ventilation with a lower backup rate, or a decrease in the inspiratory flow rate are less desirable options because these measures can markedly increase the work of breathing. The set tidal volume should use a target arterial blood pH (eg, 7.40) rather than a target $PaCO_2$ since alkalemia is responsible for the increased myocardial and neuromuscular excitability that accompanies acute hypocapnia.

COPD: COMPLICATIONS

880 What are the most important complications observed in patients with COPD who develop acute respiratory failure?

❑ The most important complications observed in patients with COPD who develop acute respiratory failure are cardiac arrhythmias, pulmonary embolism, pneumothorax, gastrointestinal hemorrhage, and renal insufficiency.

881 Is gastrointestinal bleeding a common complication in patients with COPD presenting with acute respiratory failure?

❑ Yes. Upper gastrointestinal hemorrhage (eg, stomach, duodenum) occurs in about 20% of patients with COPD in acute respiratory failure. This complication may have serious consequences because of the reduction of oxygen-carrying capacity of the blood and decreased cardiac output caused by reduced venous return (ie, reduced intravascular volume).

882 How serious is the development of acute renal failure in patients with COPD and acute respiratory failure? What are the consequences and management of this complication?

❑ In the setting of COPD and acute respiratory failure, the development of acute renal failure significantly worsens the patient's prognosis. Predisposing factors of renal failure include hypoxemia and hypercapnia, gastrointestinal hemorrhage, hemodynamic compromise, and antibiotic therapy (eg, nephrotoxicity of aminoglycosides, allergic interstitial nephritis). Fluid overload and hyperkalemia caused by the reduced renal function are commonly observed. The management of these patients may require hemodialysis.

883 What is the most common cause of pneumothorax in COPD? How important is the development of pneumothorax in the symptoms of patients with COPD?

❑ The progressive alveolar destruction that occurs in COPD may lead to the development of thin-walled subpleural blebs. Rupture of a bleb results in a pneumothorax, which produces marked worsening of the patient's symptoms because of limited pulmonary reserve. The use of mechanical ventilation increases the risk for the development of pneumothorax in patients with COPD.

884 What are the factors responsible for the short-term mortality of patients with COPD in acute respiratory failure?

❑ Several factors are important in determining the short-term mortality of patients with an acute COPD exacerbation, including (1) the severity of the COPD; (2) the precipitating illness (eg, acute respiratory failure that is brought on by a massive pulmonary embolus is likely to be associated with a higher mortality than is respiratory failure caused by an exacerbation of chronic bronchitis); and (3) the seriousness of the acute respiratory failure, as determined by arterial blood pH (eg, a pH <7.26 entails worse prognosis). The initial PaO_2 may also be an important determinant of mortality but the $PaCO_2$ appears to be less important. Although mechanical ventilation during the acute episode does not in itself appear to be associated with increased mortality, patients who require ventilator support have an increased mortality due to a more severe disease.

885 What is the short-term mortality of COPD patients in acute respiratory failure? What is the long-term mortality of these patients?

❑ The short-term mortality of patients with COPD in acute respiratory failure according to data reported between 1968 and 1976 was approximately 28%. However, more recent studies reported a mortality of only 7% following an acute COPD exacerbation. The lower mortality in the more recent studies is probably due to the selection of patients who were less severely ill than those reported in prior studies and to improvements in patient care. The long-term mortality for patients with COPD surviving an episode of acute respiratory failure varies widely from 60% or higher at 1 year to less than 30% at 2 years. The major factor that determines prognosis is the severity of the patient's underlying COPD. In fact, acute respiratory failure precipitated by an exacerbation of chronic bronchitis does not appear to modify the patient's long-term prognosis.

COR PULMONALE

886 A 56-year-old-woman with a long-standing history of COPD is admitted to the hospital because of worsening congestive heart failure. She has a 30-year history of smoking one to two packs of cigarettes daily, sputum production for at least 6 months per year in the past 5 years, home oxygen use for 3 years, and congestive heart failure over the last 2 years. Two days before admission she noticed chills and subjective fever (body temperature not measured), yellowish bronchial secretions, a major decrease in urine production, persistent epigastric discomfort, marked swelling of the lower extremities, and progressive somnolence. Physical examination on admission to the hospital reveals an obtunded patient with mild cyanosis. Rectal temperature and respiratory rate are 38.2°C and 22 breaths/min, respectively. Her blood pressure is 142/82 mm Hg and the pulse is 162 beats/min and regular. Neck examination reveals jugular vein distention, and cardiac evaluation discloses a prominent retrosternal and epigastric impulse indicative of right ventricular hypertrophy. Diminished airflow and diffuse wheezing are present in both lung fields. Examination of the abdomen reveals the liver edge at 15 cm below the costal margin, accompanied by hepatojugular reflux and moderate diffuse epigastric pain elicited with palpation of the right upper abdominal quadrant. The liver span in the midclavicular line is 18 cm. Neurologic examination reveals flapping tremor and funduscopic evaluation discloses bilateral papilledema. Room-air ABG and other laboratory data are as follows:

pH	7.28
PCO_2	66 mm Hg
$[HCO_3^-]_p$	30 mEq/L
PO_2	38 mm Hg
$[Na^+]$	137 mEq/L
$[K^+]$	4.1 mEq/L
$[Cl^-]$	93 mEq/L
Total CO_2	32 mmol/L
Glucose	118 mg/dL
Creatinine	1.1 mg/dL
BUN	18 mg/dL
Hematocrit	57%
White cell count	12,800 cells/μL
Neutrophils	78%
Lymphocytes	16%
Monocytes	2%
Eosinophils	0%

The ECG reveals multifocal atrial tachycardia and low voltage in peripheral and precordial leads. Microscopic examination of the sputum reveals an abundant mixed flora that is positive and negative with Gram's stain.

What is the most likely cause of this patient's cardiorespiratory failure?

❑ A respiratory tract infection is the most likely explanation for the cardiorespiratory failure in this patient with long-standing chronic lung disease. This diagnosis is supported by the recent history of chills and fever (although body temperature elevation was not confirmed), fever on admission, yellow bronchial secretions (indicative of an inflammatory reaction with accumulation of white cells), abundance of both gram-positive and gram-negative bacteria on microscopic examination of bronchial secretions, leukocytosis, and neutrophilia. This infectious process increases airway resistance and augments the work of breathing, producing more intense dyspnea. The increased tissue oxygen demands as well as increased carbon dioxide production that accompany a febrile state further increase the shortness of breath. Consequently, hypoxemia and hypercapnia either develop or, if previously present, are aggravated, producing further elevation in pulmonary artery pressure, which promotes the right-sided heart failure observed in this patient.

887 How important is this patient's blood gas abnormalities in the decompensated state of cor pulmonale?

❑ The blood gas abnormalities documented on admission (ie, PO_2 of 38 mm Hg, PCO_2 of 66 mm Hg, pH 7.28) most likely play a prominent role in this patient's decompensated cor pulmonale. Hypoxemia, hypercapnia, and acidemia increase pulmonary vascular resistance, thereby augmenting right ventricular afterload that might precipitate decompensation of cardiac function. The abnormally high airway resistance in a patient with COPD also augments right ventricular afterload. In addition, the increased cardiac output secondary to hypoxemia worsens pulmonary hypertension, and therefore might precipitate right ventricular failure. The critical importance of abnormal blood gas values and respiratory dysfunction on the decompensated state of cor pulmonale becomes apparent by the immediate salutary effects of correction of hypoxemia and hypercapnia on cardiac function.

---

888 What might account for the somnolence, flapping tremor of upper extremities, and bilateral papilledema in this patient with cardiorespiratory failure?

❑ Hypercapnic encephalopathy might properly explain the somnolence, flapping tremor (also known as *asterixis,* a neurologic sign that might be observed in patients with hepatic encephalopathy or uremia), and bilateral papilledema. These manifestations are not present in patients with congestive heart failure without hypercapnia. Effective treatment of cardiorespiratory failure is accompanied by the disappearance of these signs and symptoms.

---

889 Is this patient's cardiac arrhythmia, a multifocal atrial tachycardia, most likely responsible for the state of decompensated hemodynamic condition? Should measures directly aimed at the treatment of the arrhythmia be prescribed?

❑ No. Supraventricular tachyarrhythmias are exceedingly common in patients with chronic pulmonary diseases (eg, COPD), do not generally produce significant hemodynamic compromise, do not require specific treatment, and are most likely due to the blood gas abnormalities and other factors (eg, drugs) present in these patients. Successful management of the cardiorespiratory failure without any maneuvers aimed at correcting the arrhythmia (eg, digitalis, antiarrhythmic drugs) reverses the disturbance of cardiac rhythm in most instances. Furthermore, the application of measures primarily aimed at correcting the cardiac arrhythmia are generally counterproductive because they fail to correct the rhythm disturbance and might increase the patient's morbidity or mortality.

890 What type of arrhythmias are observed in patients with COPD? What are the causes and significance of these arrhythmias?

❑ Patients with COPD may display a wide variety of arrhythmias, including sinus tachycardia (which is the most common type), premature atrial complexes, atrial fibrillation, multifocal atrial tachycardia, premature ventricular complexes, and ventricular tachycardia. The incidence of arrhythmias varies considerably in different studies, depending on the definition of arrhythmia and the mode of detection. Continuous Holter monitoring usually reveals a threefold or higher rate of abnormalities than does routine ECG. About 50% of patients with COPD who have acute respiratory failure display arrhythmias that are probably clinically significant. Ventricular arrhythmias appear to be as common as supraventricular arrhythmias. Several factors may play a role in causing arrhythmias, including the presence of cor pulmonale, hypoxemia (probably a weak determinant of arrhythmias), electrolyte abnormalities, increased levels of catecholamines related to stress, associated ischemic heart disease, medications, procedures such as endotracheal intubation and bronchoscopy, as well as pulmonary artery catheterization. The development of arrhythmias is associated with high mortality during the subsequent 2 years. Death may be a direct effect of the arrhythmia, or more likely reflects the severity of the underlying disease.

891 What is the most appropriate management for this patient having a decompensated state of cor pulmonale with cardiorespiratory failure?

❑ The most important therapeutic measures aimed at ameliorating the state of cardiorespiratory failure include the following:

1. Controlled administration of 24% or 28% oxygen with a Venturi mask (or by nasal cannula at 2 L/min) to improve

PO_2 with periodic evaluation of ABGs. Because this patient has hypercapnic encephalopathy, the possibility of further respiratory depression in response to oxygen administration is high; thus, the likelihood of the need for laryngeal intubation and mechanical ventilation is substantial.

2. Administration of bronchodilator agents including anticholinergic drugs, beta-adrenergic agonists, and corticosteroids, which might play a critical role to improve the patient's signs and symptoms.
3. Administration of loop diuretics to promote a negative salt and water balance, ameliorating the congestive hepatomegaly, peripheral edema, as well as the abnormal alveolar-capillary gas exchange.
4. Administration of antibiotics to eradicate the pulmonary infection (and the febrile syndrome) that appears as the main cause of deterioration of the patient's condition, leading to the syndrome of cardiorespiratory failure.

892 What is the management of pulmonary hypertension?

❑ Several measures should be considered for simultaneous use in the management of pulmonary hypertension including (1) supplemental oxygen if hypoxemia is present; (2) chronic anticoagulation because thrombosis or embolism are commonly present, unless a contraindication exists for this treatment; and (3) vasodilators such as calcium channel blockers, nitrates, hydralazine, adenosine, and prostaglandins. A 12-week prospective study recently demonstrated that continuous intravenous infusion of epoprostenol (prostacyclin) produced symptomatic and hemodynamic improvement as well as better survival than did standard treatment in patients with severe primary pulmonary hypertension.

893 Explain the management of pulmonary hypertension in patients with COPD in acute respiratory failure.

❑ Pulmonary hypertension usually develops as a result of chronic hypoxemia (major pathogenetic factor) in patients with

COPD. Consequently, oxygen administration represents the most important therapeutic tool for the pulmonary hypertension in these patients. Vasodilators, such as hydralazine, nitrates, calcium channel blockers, prostaglandins, and prostacyclin, can decrease pulmonary artery pressure, but they also cause systemic hypotension and have yielded inconsistent results in patients with COPD. Consequently, none of these drugs are routinely indicated in the management of pulmonary hypertension of COPD patients.

894 What are the indications of diuretics and phlebotomy in the management of COPD?

❑ The use of diuretics in COPD patients is reserved for those having left ventricular backward failure (ie, venocapillary pulmonary hypertension, pulmonary edema) or systemic venous congestion and peripheral edema associated with cor pulmonale. The clinician should be very cautious with the use of these drugs because they can cause important side effects. Phlebotomy in the polycythemic patient with cor pulmonale is recommended for patients who maintain a severely elevated hematocrit (>55%) despite long-term oxygen therapy.

895 What medication might benefit patients with predominantly right ventricular failure and significant precapillary and postcapillary pulmonary hypertension? Outline the treatment of cor pulmonale and the role of oxygen supplementation.

❑ Postcapillary (also known as *venocapillary*) pulmonary hypertension might respond to venodilators (eg, nitroglycerin, isosorbide dinitrate) as well as to left ventricular afterload-reducing drugs such as the combined vasodilators (eg, ACE inhibitors, prazosin). Precapillary pulmonary hypertension might be treated with Ca^{++} antagonists, hydralazine, and prostacyclin. In addition, all forms of pulmonary hypertension might be ameliorated by diuretics due to a shift of blood from the thorax to the systemic venous circulation (eg, venodilator effect of furosemide) and reduction of intravascular volume secondary to the negative salt and water balance. Furthermore, correction of the increased airway resistance that frequently accompanies congestive heart failure with bronchodilators (eg, using ipratropium bromide) might help to ameliorate all forms of pulmonary hypertension. Management of hypoxemia, if present, with oxygen-rich inspired mixtures can decrease pulmonary vascular resistance, thereby reducing pulmonary artery pressure. The salutary effects of oxygen administration on hemodynamic parameters of patients with cor pulmonale (eg, patients with right ventricular failure secondary to COPD) might be dramatic, producing brisk diuresis and prompt resolution of anasarca.

896 What are the indications for digitalis (eg, digoxin) in the treatment of COPD?

❑ The use of digitalis preparations is generally reserved for COPD patients with symptomatic left ventricular failure caused by systolic dysfunction or atrial tachyarrhythmias.

897 What are the side effects of aminophylline therapy in patients with respiratory and cardiac diseases?

❑ The side effects of aminophylline include nausea and vomiting, headache, flushing, hypotension, palpitations, and precordial pain. Increased perfusion of poorly ventilated lung alveoli might produce hypoxemia. The most serious toxic effects of aminophylline include convulsions, hypotension (due to systemic vasodilation), and sudden death (complication of ventricular arrhythmias).

898 How common is the development of pulmonary embolism in patients with COPD?

❑ Significant pulmonary embolism occurs in approximately 25% of patients with COPD in acute respiratory failure. Diagnosis is particularly difficult because of the underlying lung disease, and pulmonary angiography may be needed for confirmation of embolism in these patients.

899 What is the management of deep vein thrombosis (DVT) and pulmonary embolism?

❑ Systemic anticoagulation with heparin (eg, 1500 IU/hr) should be prescribed (unless a contraindication exists) in all patients with pulmonary embolism or DVT at or above the popliteal fossa. The activated partial thromboplastin time (aPTT) should be maintained with heparin at 1.5 to 2.5 times the control level. Warfarin may be started simultaneously with heparin and continued for at least 3 months; the dose of warfarin should be adjusted to achieve a prothrombin time of two to three times the control level. The use of a vena cava filter in patients with DVT or pulmonary embolism should be considered if (1) anticoagulation is contraindicated, (2) thrombosis or embolism recur despite adequate anticoagulation, and (3) pulmonary hypertension develops because of embolism.

900 Elaborate on the diagnosis and management of chronic thromboembolism of the pulmonary circulation.

❑ Some patients with recurrent pulmonary embolism develop pulmonary hypertension and cor pulmonale because a substantial portion of the pulmonary vascular bed remains occluded by unresolved clots. Yet, clots dissolve in most patients who survive after pulmonary embolism. Patients with chronic thromboembolic disease of the lungs commonly consult for dyspnea and syncope (caused by pulmonary hypertension), symptoms that are nonspecific and may be confused with COPD, especially when previous episodes of acute pulmonary embolism or DVT had remained unrecognized. Perfusion lung scans of patients with this disease appear distinctly abnormal, making radioisotopic lung scans a helpful diagnostic tool of chronic pulmonary embolism. However, patients with preexisting parenchymal disease, such as COPD, also have abnormal-appearing lung scans, and differentiation of these disorders—even with the addition of a ventilation scan—can be very difficult. Accordingly, pulmonary angiography may be necessary. The treatment for patients with major symptoms includes systemic anticoagulation, vasodilators, and supplemental oxygen if hypoxemia is present. Thrombolytic drugs do not play a significant role in the treatment of chronic pulmonary thromboembolic disease.

26. Infections

PNEUMONIAS

901 How reliable are the clinical signs of infection (eg, fever, purulent secretions) in the diagnosis of hospital-acquired pneumonia? How important is the bacteriologic evaluation of a specimen obtained from the lower respiratory tract in this condition?

❑ The traditionally used clinical signs of pneumonia including fever, purulent secretions, leukocytosis, and new or changing radiographic infiltrates are neither sensitive nor specific for the diagnosis of the nosocomial form of respiratory infections. Consequently, patients suspected of community-acquired pneumonia are commonly treated with an empirical choice of antibiotics. In patients with hospital-acquired pneumonia, depending on its severity, evaluation of specimens obtained from the lower airways is commonly required for the selection of antibiotics.

902 What is the most dependable procedure to isolate the microorganism(s) responsible for nosocomial pneumonia in ventilator-supported patients?

❑ Fiberoptic bronchoscopy with quantitative cultures of specimens obtained from the lower airways using a protected brush provides the most reliable information (although it has some limitations) with respect to the etiology of nosocomial pneumonia in ventilator-supported patients. Bacteriologic evaluation of the sputum is misleading because of the high rate (approximately 100%) of upper-airway colonization in these patients. The clinician should correlate the bacteriologic information with other patient data (eg, fever, purulent bronchial secretions) to establish with confidence the role of any microorganism(s) isolated from the patient's airway on the clinical manifestations.

903 What types of antibiotics are commonly prescribed for the management of respiratory infections in ventilator-supported patients?

❑ Antibiotic therapy used in the management of pulmonary infections in patients receiving mechanical ventilation usually consists of two bactericidal agents, for example, a beta-lactam plus an aminoglycoside, to cover gram-negative bacilli and gram-positive cocci.

904 What is the treatment of community-acquired pneumonia?

❑ Empirical therapy with erythromycin or azithromycin is often used successfully in the management of community-acquired pneumonia. Therapy with only one of the following—trimethoprim-sulfamethoxazole, tetracyclines, or quinolones—is not recommended because many pneumococci are resistant to these drugs. For patients of advanced age or having COPD or other underlying disease, trimethoprim-sulfamethoxazole or a beta-lactam (with a beta-lactamase inhibitor) should be added to erythromycin. For more seriously ill patients, empirical therapy might include erythromycin plus a second-generation (eg, cefuroxime) or third-generation (eg, ceftriaxone) cephalosporin.

905 What is the treatment of nosocomial pneumonia?

❑ A standard empirical treatment is commonly used in the initial management of nosocomial pneumonia. The high prevalence of methicillin-resistant *Staphylococcus aureus* has led to the addition of vancomycin to a combination of beta-lactam and aminoglycoside agents in the therapy of this disease. The clinical response to the initial treatment and the bacteriologic information derived from bronchial secretions will determine whether changes in the initial prescription are necessary.

906 A previously healthy, 71-year-old woman consults for the development over the past 2 days of persistent cough with slight nonpurulent sputum production, fever (39.6°C), and shortness of breath. She has smoked one pack of cigarettes per day for 20 years and drinks alcohol with moderation. Physical examination shows tachycardia (112/min), tachypnea (30/min), and signs of consolidation on the right posterior hemithorax (confirmed by chest x-ray films). Laboratory data reveal leukocytosis with a left shift deviation (white blood cell and neutrophil counts of 20,000/μL and 87%, respectively), and mixed flora is observed on Gram's stain evaluation of sputum.

What is the most appropriate initial treatment of this patient's condition?

❑ A combination of erythromycin and a second-generation cephalosporin is the most appropriate initial treatment for the reasons discussed below. This empirical combination is directed at the microorganisms most likely responsible for the community-acquired pneumonia observed in this elderly patient with a significant smoking history. The mixed flora found in the sputum may not represent the microorganisms responsible for the pneumonia. Consequently, the empirical regimen chosen should cover the most likely bacteria involved in her disease including *S. pneumoniae, H. influenzae, Legionella* organisms, and *Moraxella* species. Erythromycin is effective against *S. pneumoniae* and *Legionella* species, and a second-generation cephalosporin should cover *H. influenzae* and *Moraxella* organisms. Monotherapy with erythromycin, cephalosporin, penicillin (absence of coverage for *Legionella* and gram-negative bacteria), or trimethoprim-sulfamethoxazole (lack of coverage for *Legionella*) is not recommended for the management of this patient.

907 What is the treatment of aspiration pneumonia?

❑ Vigorous suctioning is often recommended after an episode of aspiration, but the rapid distribution of the acid material to the lung periphery together with the instantaneous nature of the injury limits its potential value. As with other causes of ARDS, corticosteroids have been extensively employed in the management of aspiration pneumonia. However, recent prospective controlled trials showed them to be without benefit, and they may even increase mortality; therefore, their use is no longer recommended. Infection commonly complicates the aspiration of gastric contents. There is no evidence that antibiotics given at the time of the acute event decrease lung infection or improve clinical outcome. In practice, patients are frequently treated empirically on the basis of expected bacteriologic patterns, which include gram-positive and gram-negative organisms. If mixed aerobic and anaeorbic infection is considered likely, clindamycin and an aminoglycoside have been recommended to provide broad-spectrum coverage. In addition, patients require general supportive measures common to all causes of ARDS. Various surgical procedures have been employed in some patients with intractable aspiration, including an epiglottic-arytenoid flap operation, glottic closure with suture of the vocal cords, cricopharyngeal myotomy, injection of Teflon into a paralyzed vocal cord, diversion procedures, and even total laryngectomy.

908 What is the treatment of pneumonia secondary to aspiration of oropharyngeal bacteria?

❑ Most community-acquired aspiration pneumonias are responsive to penicillin, and so empirical therapy is usually employed in this setting. Varying the dosages to range from 2 to 20 million units/day has been suggested. Although *Bacteroides fragilis* is usually not sensitive to penicillin G on in vitro testing, most pulmonary infections respond satisfactorily. Chloramphenicol, clindamycin, and metronidazole can be used in the presence of allergy to penicillin, and in a recent study of patients with lung abscesses, clindamycin proved superior to penicillin. In the hospital setting, pneumonia secondary to aspiration of oropharyngeal contents is more likely to be due to mixed aerobic and anaerobic organisms. Rather than choosing empirical antibiotic therapy, obtaining precise baceteriologic diagnosis by using invasive procedures may be preferable in deciding the optimal therapy. Delayed resolution with persistence of a cavity on chest x-ray studies after 4 to 6 weeks is no longer considered an indication for surgery because most resolve with continued antibiotic therapy. Chest physiotherapy is sometimes employed to enhance drainage, although its value has not been scientifically evaluated. There is no evidence that bronchoscopy is of value in assisting drainage, but it should be performed to exclude the presence of tumor if resolution is delayed. It should be also considered if a lung abscess is found in an edentulous patient because many of these patients have an underlying bronchial carcinoma.

909 Briefly explain the main features that accompany the aspiration of foreign bodies. What is the treatment of this condition?

❑ Solid-foreign-body aspiration is much more common in infants and children than in adults. Peanuts, coins, and toys are frequent offenders in children, while meat and bones are the usual culprits in adults. The consequences depend on the nature of the foreign body and the site of occlusion. A large foreign body lodged at the laryngeal aperture causes immediate aphonia, laryngospasm, and stridor followed by asphyxia. More commonly, objects enter the bronchial tree with almost exclusive involvement of the lower lobes, the right being more frequently affected than the left side. Patients may recall the aspiratory event or complain of cough, dyspnea, chest pain, or localized wheezing without knowledge of the precipitative factor. Rigid bronchoscopy is the usual technique of extracting foreign bodies from pediatric patients. In a large number of adults, the fiberoptic bronchoscope has been successfully employed in the removal of foreign bodies. Solid objects may be extracted with a forceps or a wire basket. This approach is less successful with vegetable substances because of the surrounding mucosal reaction. In this situation, it is preferable to direct a Fogarty balloon catheter beyond the object, inflate the balloon, and then draw the foreign body into a larger airway for subsequent extraction using a wire basket.

27. Miscellaneous Conditions

CHEST TRAUMA

910 Explain the development and management of respiratory failure in patients with a flail chest. What is the management of this condition?

❑ Abnormalities of the chest wall (eg, flail chest caused by trauma) are uncommon causes of ventilatory failure. It was formerly considered that the ventilatory failure observed in patients with a flail chest was caused by the paradoxical motion of the rib cage (pendelluft); consequently, mechanical ventilation was used as a pneumatic splint to stabilize the chest wall. It is now believed that the pulmonary dysfunction in patients with a flail chest is secondary to the underlying parenchymal injury resulting from pulmonary contusion. Thus, mechanical ventilation has the same indications in patients with a flail chest as with any other cause of respiratory failure.

911 What are the main features of a ''sucking'' pneumothorax?

❑ An open (''sucking'') pneumothorax can occur with a large penetrating chest injury. If the opening in the chest wall exceeds the laryngeal cross-sectional area, air passes preferentially through the defect with each respiratory effort. This results in complete lung collapse and marked paradoxical motion of the mediastinum with each breath. Management consists of covering the defect with a sterile occlusive dressing. The dressing should be taped on only three sides so that it functions like a flutter valve. Thus, air can leave the thorax during expiration, but it is unable to enter the thorax on inspiration. Securely taping all sides of the dressing can produce a tension pneumothorax if air continues to leak from a pulmonary parenchymal laceration. Definitive surgical closure is usually required at a later time.

SLEEP APNEA

912 What is the treatment of obstructive sleep apnea?

❑ Treatment of obstructive sleep apnea should be directed toward the underlying mechanisms. Obese subjects should be placed on a weight reduction program that includes a reduced caloric intake; however, this approach commonly fails, so surgical techniques such as gastric stapling can be considered in patients with marked obesity (those exceeding 50% of ideal weight). Yet, in patients achieving a substantial weight loss (eg, up to 100 kg) the obstructive sleep apnea syndrome may not improve. Progesterone administration can reduce the number of obstructive sleep apnea episodes in some patients, probably because of the respiratory stimulant properties of this drug. However, progesterone may increase the number of obstructive apneas in other patients because of preferential stimulation of diaphragmatic activity as compared to other respiratory muscles. Administration of drugs including protriptyline hydrochloride, clomipramine hydrochloride, aminophylline, and acetazolamide has limited success in the treatment of obstructive sleep apnea. In selected patients, supplemental oxygen therapy can decrease the severity of the obstructive apneas, presumably from its beneficial effect on the neural pathway that controls the upper airway. In other patients, supplemental oxygen can prolong apnea and worsen cardiac arrhythmias. The use of CPAP and surgical techniques is discussed in the answers to subsequent questions.

913 What is the treatment of central sleep apnea (and hypopnea)?

❑ The treatment of central sleep apnea and hypopnea can include respiratory stimulants such as aminophylline, progesterone, and acetazolamide, and mechanical ventilation. Nasal CPAP, which reverses obstructive apneas by acting as a pneumatic splint, can also be beneficial in patients with central apneas; its mode of action is not known.

---

914 How can positive-pressure ventilation or an airway tube be used in the management of obstructive sleep apnea?

❑ CPAP with a nasal mask is the first-line therapy in patients with obstructive sleep apnea. Positive pressure acts as a pneumatic splint that prevents collapse of the upper airway, reducing the number of obstructive apneas, raising resting lung volume, and improving SaO_2. However, some patients may not comply with nightly use of the appropriate nose mask.

---

915 What is the role of uvulopalatopharyngoplasty in the treatment of obstructive sleep apnea?

❑ Uvulopalatopharyngoplasty is a surgical procedure analogous to an extensive tonsillectomy and adenoidectomy in terms of operative morbidity. It is designed to enlarge the upper airway by removing redundant oropharyngeal tissue from the lateral aspect of the posterior pharyngeal wall and pharyngopalatal arch while preserving the regional muscles. Amputation of the uvula is carried out as another component of the operation. The establishment of a larger upper airspace with uvulopalatopharyngoplasty produces improvement in some patients, but it is not possible to identify which patients are likely to respond. Most studies finding a beneficial response to this therapy were uncontrolled in nature.

---

916 A 62-year-old male truck driver consults because of progressive daytime sleepiness over the past year that was responsible for two collisions with other motor vehicles in the highway within the past 2 months. His medical history is negative for smoking and other significant diseases. Physical examination reveals a thin patient whose oropharynx, chest, and circulatory system are normal. Chest x-ray and ECG results are also normal. Overnight polysomnography demonstrates more than 100 episodes of apnea (ie, cessation of airflow for more than 10 seconds) with arousals on the electroencephalogram (EEG), and arterial oxygen desaturation below 85% and preservation of rib cage and abdominal motions during the apneic periods.

What is the cause of the daytime sleepiness? What is the most appropriate therapy for this patient's condition?

❑ The severe daytime sleepiness of this patient is a manifestation of a sleep apnea syndrome caused by obstruction of the upper airway. The most appropriate therapy consists of nasal CPAP, which overcomes the obstruction by splinting open the upper airway. Nasal CPAP is currently considered the standard initial treatment for patients with moderate to severe obstructive sleep apnea syndrome. Nocturnal supplemental oxygen might help correct the oxygen desaturation but does not decrease the frequency of apneic episodes. Other treatments including the use of progesterone (respiratory stimulant) or protriptyline (antidepressant that suppresses REM sleep during which apneas are most frequent) are not substitutes for nasal CPAP.

CHEYNE-STOKES RESPIRATION

917 Is periodic breathing including Cheyne-Stokes respiration invariably associated with serious cardiac or neurologic disease? What is the treatment of this condition?

❑ Mild degrees of periodic breathing, which can be easily missed on physical examination, are often found in otherwise normal subjects, particularly during sleep. In addition, approximately 30% to 75% of premature infants breathe periodically during their first month of life and sojourners at high altitude often display Cheyne-Stokes respiration during sleep. Consequently, the crescendo-decrescendo pattern of breathing known as *Cheyne-Stokes respiration* is not always a forewarning of the presence of a serious underlying disease. With respect to the management of Cheyne-Stokes respiration, specific therapy is generally not required, although administration of aminophylline, oxygen, and carbon dioxide has been shown to suppress periodic breathing.

918 What is the management of Cheyne-Stokes respiration? What are the advantages of a successful treatment for this condition?

❑ Proper treatment of congestive heart failure can improve Cheyne-Stokes respiration if this is the basis for the abnormal breathing pattern. Administration of supplemental oxygen or 5% to 10% carbon dioxide in oxygen at 2 to 4 L/min (eg, nasal catheter) may eliminate the periodic breathing and frequent arousals in patients with heart failure that failed to respond to other measures as well as in those without a cardiac basis for the abnormal breathing pattern. Amelioration of Cheyne-Stokes respiration helps to achieve better nocturnal sleep, reducing daytime hypersomnolence.

CARBON MONOXIDE INTOXICATION. SMOKE INHALATION INJURY

919 How does carbon monoxide produce its toxic effects? What level of carbon monoxide can lead to serious intoxication?

❑ The toxic effects of carbon monoxide are caused by its combination with hemoglobin at the same place on the hemoglobin molecule as does oxygen, but with an affinity 250 times higher (therefore displacing oxygen from the hemoglobin molecule). In addition, carbon monoxide inhibits the transfer of electrons between the respiratory chain and molecular oxygen, thereby further impairing the synthesis of ATP. A concentration of carbon monoxide of about 0.1% in the inspired air may be lethal because its corresponding pressure is 0.7 mm Hg, a level that can displace all oxygen from hemoglobin because of its 250-fold higher affinity. The carbon monoxide–hemoglobin dissociation curve is of identical shape to that of oxygen but the level plotted on the horizontal axis (abscissa) is 1/250th of that in the oxygen-hemoglobin dissociation curve (eg, 0.4 mm Hg of carbon monoxide pressure saturates 98% of the hemoglobin, a level comparable to that of a PaO_2 of 100 mm Hg).

---

920 Does oxygen administration have any value in carbon monoxide poisoning, a condition associated with normal PaO_2?

❑ Yes. Administration of pure oxygen is of critical importance in the management of carbon monoxide poisoning because oxygen at high alveolar (and thereby arterial) pressure displaces the toxic gas from hemoglobin and facilitates its pulmonary elimination. The half-life for the disappearance of carboxyhemoglobin is 4 hours while breathing room air. This is decreased to 40 to 60 minutes while breathing 100% oxygen and to 20 to 25 minutes while breathing oxygen at 2 to 3 atm.

---

921 How are the PaO_2 and the oxygen content levels of arterial blood affected in a patient with severe carbon monoxide poisoning?

❑ The PaO_2 of a patient presenting with carbon monoxide poisoning is normal in spite of the life-threatening tissue hypoxia detected. However, the oxygen content of arterial blood is seriously reduced because of the displacement of oxygen by carbon monoxide within the hemoglobin molecule. Consequently, measurement of PaO_2 does not provide a reliable indication of the oxygenation defect observed with carbon monoxide poisoning. Determination of the carboxyhemoglobin level allows the practitioner to identify the syndrome and initiate therapy.

---

922 What is the management of smoke inhalation injury?

❑ Management of smoke inhalation injury includes removing the victim from exposure, checking vital signs, and ensuring a patent airway. All fire victims with mental status abnormalities or a high likelihood of smoke inhalation injury should be hospitalized for at least 24 hours. The administration of supplemental oxygen relieves hypoxemia and enhances the dissociation of carbon monoxide from hemoglobin by decreasing the half-time for elimination from 4 hours while breathing room air to 40 to 60 minutes with an FiO_2 of 1.0. To achieve an adequate FiO_2, intubation and mechanical ventilation may be required. Hyperbaric oxygen causes a further reduction in the half-life of carboxyhemoglobin; an FiO_2 of 1.0 at 2 atm decreases the half-life to 20 to 25 minutes. Bronchospasm usually responds to bronchodilators. Corticosteroids are no longer recommended in the management of smoke inhalation injury. Antibiotics should be prescribed only if there is evidence of infection. In the rare cases where ARDS supervenes, the management is identical to that described for other causes. Patients surviving the acute clinical course usually recover completely. Long-term complications including tracheal stenosis, bronchiolitis obliterans, and bronchiectasis are rare.

ACID-BASE AND POTASSIUM DISTURBANCES IN RESPIRATORY FAILURE

923 What is the treatment of respiratory alkalosis (primary hypocapnia)?

❑ Management of primary hypocapnia must be directed toward correcting the underlying cause, whenever possible. Because respiratory alkalosis, especially that of a chronic nature, poses little risk to health and produces few or no symptoms, measures to treat the deranged acid-base composition are not required. The anxiety-hyperventilation syndrome represents an exception in which an active therapeutic approach is rewarding. Providing reassurance, sedation, and ultimately, psychotherapy to the patient is most helpful. Rebreathing in a paper bag or any other closed system provides immediate symptomatic relief that, unfortunately, is short-lasting. When severe and persistent alkalemia due to primary hypocapnia is present, sedation may be needed. Alternatively, correction of the alkalemia might be attained by maneuvers aimed at reducing the $[HCO_3^-]_p$ whenever the direct treatment of hypocapnia is unsuccessful or risky.

924 How important is detection and treatment of metabolic alkalosis in patients with abnormal respiratory function?

❑ Failure to recognize and correct superimposed metabolic alkalosis in patients with underlying pulmonary dysfunction can have important clinical consequences, because relative or absolute alkalemia can lessen an important stimulus to ventilation in such patients. A measurement of urine chloride concentration might help to exclude the presence of the most common forms of metabolic alkalosis, if plasma acid-base values are diagnostically inconclusive. In the absence of recent diuretic administration, the finding of abundant urinary chloride provides a reasonable assurance that a superimposed, chloride-responsive alkalosis is not present.

925 Describe the various therapeutic measures for the management of metabolic alkalosis superimposed on respiratory acidosis.

❑ Besides the administration of chloride salts, under special circumstances other therapeutic measures might be necessary for the speedy correction of metabolic alkalosis in patients with chronic respiratory acidosis. The administration of acetazolamide, an agent that inhibits renal bicarbonate reabsorption, can result in substantial bicarbonate losses in the form of the Na^+ and K^+ salts. The pharmacologic effect of acetazolamide substantially diminishes once the elevated $[HCO_3^-]_p$ is returned to normal; if potassium depletion was initially present, serum potassium should be closely monitored and replacement of this ion must be secured. On occasion, the administration of an acidifying agent such as NH_4Cl or HCl might be required. An alternative therapeutic approach in the treatment of metabolic alkalosis in patients with respiratory acidosis and renal failure is the use of hemodialysis with a low bicarbonate concentration in the dialysate or hemofiltration along with saline solution. Effective treatment of a superimposed element of metabolic alkalosis can result in a significant decline in the $PaCO_2$ level.

926 What is the treatment of lactic acidosis?

❑ Correction of the underlying cause of lactic acidosis is the cornerstone of treatment. The high mortality associated with lactic acidosis can be reduced by securing adequate support of vital functions. The hemodynamic status and tissue perfusion might improve with correction of volume deficit, enhancing cardiac output, and avoiding vasoconstricting drugs (ie, phenylephrine HCl, norepinephrine). Tissue oxygenation must be optimized by correcting anemia or by providing a higher inspired oxygen mixture with or without mechanical ventilation, or by using both methods. Energy stores must be replenished to prevent the development of hypoglycemia. If drugs or toxins are responsible for the lactic acidosis, it is mandatory to remove these agents promptly from the patient's tissues, by whatever means available (ie, hemodialysis or hemoperfusion, if necessary). Sepsis must be treated aggressively. Other measures in the management of lactic acidosis might include alkali therapy as well as the use of dichloroacetate, which enhances the oxidation of pyruvate.

927 Describe the use of $NaHCO_3$ infusions in the treatment of lactic acidosis caused by tissue hypoxia.

❑ The utilization of alkali therapy in the treatment of lactic acidosis is controversial as the rising pH associated with this treatment tends to further increase hyperlactatemia. It has been known for years that acidosis inhibits glycolysis, whereas alkalosis stimulates it and consequently results in elevated plasma lactate levels; this effect, however, is generally mild and usually results in an increase in plasma lactate of only 1 to 3 mEq/L. This pH feedback control is not unique to lactic acid but also occurs with other organic acids, including ketoacids, whose production is inhibited by acidosis, whereas alkalosis stimulates it. Additionally, bicarbonate therapy neither alters the natural course of the deranged metabolism leading to lactic acidosis nor diminishes the mortality of this condition. Yet, most experts advise bicarbonate therapy for lactic acidosis in the presence of extreme acidemia (blood pH <7.20 or $[HCO_3^-]_p$ <10 to 12 mEq/L). Bicarbonate administration, however, has several potential adverse effects that are described elsewhere in this book.

928 A consistent observation during acute HCO_3^- administration is a transient elevation in PCO_2. What is the cause of this phenomenon?

❑ Acute alkalemia is known to depress pulmonary ventilation. Yet, the rise in PCO_2 observed shortly after the intravenous infusion of HCO_3^- is not the result of depressed ventilation but of increased carbon dioxide production. This phenomenon is demonstrated by the associated increase in the level of carbon dioxide in the expired air that occurs during acute alkali administration, which indicates increased carbon dioxide excretion. The increased carbon dioxide production observed immediately after bicarbonate administration is caused by decomposition of bicarbonate in carbon dioxide and water (with an intermediate step in which carbonic acid is generated). This process is initiated by the increase in pH secondary to bicarbonate infusion. Thereafter, the increased pH of body fluids triggers the release of hydrogen ions from proteins and phosphate which interact with the bicarbonate that decomposes in carbon dioxide and water. In addition, tissue metabolism is stimulated in response to alkalemia, leading to an increased cellular production of carbon dioxide. This process is especially relevant to the use of bicarbonate therapy in patients being managed with permissive hypercapnia.

929 What is the role of Carbicarb (0.33 mol/L sodium carbonate and 0.33 mol/L sodium bicarbonate) in the treatment of lactic acidosis caused by tissue hypoxia?

❑ The alkalinizing capacity of Carbicarb is identical to that of $NaHCO_3$, but Carbicarb produces less carbon dioxide. Thus, the potential risk of tissue acidosis due to the H_2CO_3 accumulation associated with alkali therapy appears to be lower, by comparison, when Carbicarb is used instead of pure $NaHCO_3$. However, the use of Carbicarb in clinical practice (eg, treatment of lactic acidosis caused by tissue hypoxia) is not universally accepted.

930 What is the role of dichloroacetate in the treatment of lactic acidosis caused by tissue hypoxia?

❑ Dichloroacetate limits lactate production by stimulating pyruvate dehydrogenase activity resulting in oxidation of pyruvate to acetyl coenzyme A. The usual dose in adults with lactic acidosis is 50 mg/kg of body weight, diluted in 50 ml of normal saline solution for intravenous infusion over a 30-minute period. This dose might be repeated if plasma lactate levels remain substantially elevated. Limited experience with dichloroacetate indicates that this therapy can be beneficial in some instances of lactic acidosis.

931 Should patients at risk of respiratory failure presenting with mild hypokalemia receive potassium supplementation?

❑ Patients with mild asymptomatic hypokalemia ($[K^+]_p$ of 3.0 to 3.5 mEq/L) due to potassium redistribution (ie, stress hypokalemia) who are not receiving digitalis therapy and are free of heart disease or severe liver disease should not receive any form of K^+ replacement therapy. Thus, potassium supplementation, potassium-sparing diuretics, or ACE inhibitors should not be prescribed. However, patients with mild hypokalemia, independent of the pathogenic mechanisms, should receive potassium supplementation if potassium loss (renal or extrarenal) is excessive. This approach is simply aimed at preventing a progressive negative potassium balance in a patient who already has a mild decrement in $[K^+]_p$. Representative examples include patients recovering from surgery who have substantial gastrointestinal fluid and potassium loss and those receiving total parenteral nutrition aimed at promoting tissue anabolism and repair.

932 Compare the risks of K^+ administration by oral and parenteral routes with respect to a safe rate of K^+ repletion and total amount of this ion given.

❑ While 50 mEq of potassium can be safely given as a single bolus dose by oral route, a similar dose administered intravenously requires a constant infusion of 5 hours' duration. The oral route forces administered K^+ to go through the splanchnic circulation in which uptake by the hepatocytes and other cells prevents a large rapid entry of potassium to the systemic circulation. Furthermore, the oral route of K^+ administration triggers insulin release and activates the sympathetic nervous system, thereby increasing internal disposal of the potassium load. Potassium administration by the oral route promotes a smoother repletion of K^+ stores. The protective mechanisms against iatrogenic hyperkalemia during K^+ supplementation described above for the oral route are not available with intravenous administration of K^+, the rate of which should generally not exceed 10 mEq/hr. If the rate of intravenous K^+ administration exceeds 10 mEq/hr because of a life-threatening hypokalemic crisis, continuous ECG monitoring is mandatory. An exception to this rule is the potassium replacement therapy in the recovery from diabetic ketoacidosis.

933 Name a commonly used pharmacologic agent that contains significant amounts of potassium.

❑ The parenteral administration of large doses of penicillin in the form of K^+ salt (K^+ penicillin) represents a source of substantial potassium intake. The potassium content of 1 million units of K^+ penicillin is 1.7 mEq; therefore, a patient receiving 30 million units of penicillin per day will be receiving a supplementary 51 mEq of potassium daily, as a result of this therapy.

934 Should treatment be initiated for mild (less severe degree) hyperkalemia? What therapeutic measures should be initiated for all forms (mild, moderate, or severe) of hyperkalemia?

❑ Hyperkalemia of any severity requires prompt therapeutic intervention because of the potential risk of a life-threatening state caused by cardiac arrest (asystole or ventricular fibrillation) or respiratory arrest (skeletal muscle paralysis). The following measures should be started immediately on recognition of hyperkalemia: (1) discontinuation of all sources of potassium intake, oral and parenteral; (2) interruption of the administration of drugs that can impair K^+ homeostasis leading to hyperkalemia, including beta-adrenergic blockers, prostaglandin inhibitors, and potassium-sparing diuretics; (3) removal of the toxic substances that played a role in the development of hyperkalemia (eg, digitalis drugs); and (4) promotion of a negative K^+ balance by increasing potassium excretion through renal and extrarenal routes.

935 Describe general strategies for the treatment of severe hyperkalemia.

❑ The three following strategies must be considered whenever severe hyperkalemia is present:

1. Counterbalance the effect of hyperkalemia on the excitability of myocardial and skeletal muscle with the administration of drugs. This modality is not aimed at reducing the increased $[K^+]_p$.
2. Modify internal K^+ balance, promoting the translocation of potassium from extracellular fluid to the intracellular fluid. This modality will not alter the total body K^+ stores.
3. Modify external K^+ balance, inducing a net potassium loss from the body.

936 Describe the treatment of hyperkalemia with agents that ameliorate the effects of hyperkalemia on skeletal and cardiac muscle.

❑ Administration of calcium (Ca^{++}) salts (chloride or gluconate) will diminish tissue excitability by widening the difference between resting and threshold potential. When Ca^{++} salts are provided, the resting membrane potential will remain depolarized by the hyperkalemia while the threshold membrane potential will be depolarized by the calcium infusion, enlarging the difference between resting and threshold membrane potential, so its value returns toward normal. Calcium gluconate (20 mL of a 10% solution) can be infused intravenously over a 10-minute period. The intravenous administration of Ca^{++} salts is definitely indicated when $[K^+]_p$ reaches 7.0 mEq/L or when significant ECG abnormalities (absence of P wave, prolongation of QRS complexes, etc) are present. The effects of Ca^{++} infusion are short-lasting, with peak effect noted about 5 minutes after infusion.

---

937 Describe the therapy of hyperkalemia aimed at inducing the translocation of potassium from extracellular fluid to intracellular fluid. Describe in detail the use of insulin and of glucose in the treatment of severe hyperkalemia.

❑ The most important pharmacologic agent that promotes cellular potassium entry is insulin. Because insulin promotes tissue uptake of potassium and glucose, the latter must be infused to prevent hypoglycemia. Considering that hyperglycemia of endogenous and exogenous origin can result in hyperkalemia (especially in diabetics), caution should be exercised as to the rate of glucose infusion. Consequently, a situation that mimics a euglycemic insulin clamp (providing exogenous glucose in adequate amounts to maintain a normal plasma glucose level) must be instituted. A less important strategy that can translocate potassium to the intracellular fluid is $NaHCO_3$ infusion. Insulin can be effectively administered by means of an intravenous bolus of 5 units of regular insulin followed by a continuous intravenous insulin infusion; the latter might consist of 10 units of regular insulin dissolved in 500 mL of a solution of 20% glucose in water, infused at a rate of 100 mL/hr. Plasma glucose and $[K^+]_p$ should be closely monitored with measurements taken every 30 minutes to evaluate the results of therapy and to prevent major changes in plasma glucose. The stated rate of administration of the insulin/glucose mixture can be modified to reach therapeutic goals.

938 What is the effect of $NaHCO_3$ infusion on $[K^+]_p$? What is the role of $NaHCO_3$ infusion in the treatment of hyperkalemia?

❑ The administration of $NaHCO_3$ (alkali) is expected to move potassium into cells inducing hypokalemia by raising extracellular pH. However, the effect of HCO_3^- infusion on $[K^+]_p$ is inconsistent. Furthermore, the mild hypokalemia observed with this alkali infusion has been shown to occur not from the transfer of potassium to the intracellular fluid but rather from the dilution of extracellular potassium due to expansion of the extracellular fluid volume (the currently used ampules of $NaHCO_3$ are 1 N solutions having 1 Eq/L); thus, their osmolality is about six times that of body fluids, therefore promoting fluid transfer from intracellular fluid to extracellular fluid. Hyperkalemia associated with severe acidemia due to metabolic acidosis (primary reduction in $[HCO_3^-]_p$) should be treated with $NaHCO_3$ infusion unless the patient has significant extracellular fluid volume expansion and a high risk of pulmonary edema. However, $NaHCO_3$ infusion is generally an unreliable tool for the control of severe hyperkalemia, especially in patients with renal failure in whom bicarbonaturia and the associated kaliuresis will not develop. Thus, bicarbonate administration should not be considered the primary modality but only a supplementary one in the therapy of severe hyperkalemia. A combined protocol that includes insulin plus glucose administration (primary treatment modality) and alkali infusion (supplemental treatment modality) can be as follows: 1 to 2 ampules (44 mEq/ampule) of $NaHCO_3$, and 10 units of regular insulin added to a solution of 20% glucose in water for infusion at 100 mL/hr.

939 Describe another pharmacologic agent for the treatment of severe hyperkalemia that promotes the transfer of potassium from the extracellular fluid to the intracellular fluid. Explain the time frame of the therapeutic response to insulin and glucose, sodium bicarbonate, and albuterol in the management of severe hyperkalemia.

❑ Cellular potassium uptake is increased with the administration of selective beta-2-adrenergic agonists. Albuterol, a member of this family of drugs, can be administered (20-mg dosage) as an aerosol for inhalation. This treatment modality, although effective, must be considered only as supplementary. The therapeutic response to insulin and glucose infusion and to albuterol is prompt, with a significant hypokalemic effect observed within 60 minutes. By contrast, the effect of $NaHCO_3$ infusion on $[K^+]_p$, if any, requires a few hours.

940 Describe procedures for potassium removal (negative external K^+ balance) in the therapy of hyperkalemia including the use of sodium polystyrene sulfonate (Kayexalate) and dialysis.

❑ The administration of polystyrene sulfonate resins and the performance of dialysis (hemodialysis and peritoneal dialysis) are effective measures for potassium removal in patients with hyperkalemia. Sodium polystyrene sulfonate can be administered orally or in a retention enema (the latter is a more effective route). Optimal action of this resin requires that sorbitol be given concomitantly. A satisfactory formulation for its use in both routes is that of 25 gm of resin, 25 gm of sorbitol, and 100 mL of water. Oral and rectal routes can be used concomitantly, and similar doses can be administered multiple times, even hourly. Sodium polystyrene sulfonate exchanges sodium (Na^+) initially bound to the resin for potassium (K^+) initially present in gastrointestinal fluids. Each gram of resin can induce a net potassium loss of approximately 1 mEq. Severe hyperkalemia accompanied by a preserved renal function can usually be corrected without dialysis. Potassium removal can be achieved when renal function is preserved by inducing an enhanced kaliuresis with the administration of fluids containing sodium chloride or $NaHCO_3$, or both, and with the use of diuretics (acting on the proximal tubule, loop of Henle, and distal tubule, such as acetazolamide, furosemide, and thiazides, respectively). The majority of patients who develop severe hyperkalemia, however, have renal failure, and dialysis is the treatment indicated for this electrolyte abnormality.

28. Respiratory Monitoring

INTRODUCTION

941 What are the goals of respiratory monitoring?

❑ The major goal of monitoring is to implement a system that alerts the attendants of a significant change in the patient's condition, providing an opportunity for the timely institution of lifesaving measures, to aid with diagnosis and therapy, and to create trends that assist in assessing therapeutic response and predicting prognosis. Significant improvements in respiratory monitoring have occurred in recent years based on both technological advances and a better understanding of the pathophysiologic characteristics of respiratory failure.

942 How common is the need of cardiopulmonary monitoring the principal or exclusive reason for admission to an intensive care unit? What is the main purpose of patient monitoring?

❑ As many as 40% of patients are admitted to an intensive care unit solely for monitoring purposes and do not receive active intervention. The major purpose of monitoring is to alert the medical personnel of a significant change in a patient's condition so that lifesaving measures can be instituted and to aid diagnosis and therapy.

943 What are the main variables that require monitoring in patients receiving mechanical ventilation?

❑ Variables that require monitoring in patients receiving mechanical ventilation include (1) gas exchange (ie, PaO_2 or hemoglobin saturation, $PaCO_2$, and pH), (2) airway pressure (ie, peak inspiratory pressure, plateau [end-inspiratory occlusion] pressure, PEEP [external and auto-PEEP, waveform of pressure curve]), (3) breathing pattern (ie, minute ventilation, tidal volume, respiratory frequency, pattern of rib cage–abdominal motion), (4) hemodynamic function (ie, blood pressure, urinary output, cardiac output, pulmonary-artery occlusion pressure), and (5) chest film (ie, endotracheal tube position, signs of barotrauma, signs of pneumonia). In complex situations, such as patients with the ARDS who require high levels of PEEP, a pulmonary artery catheter may be required to help titrate fluid and vasopressor therapy. Monitoring also helps to determine when ventilator support can be discontinued.

944 Enumerate the features of an ideal monitoring system.

❑ An ideal monitoring system must be pertinent to patient treatment, provide data in a way that is easy to interpret, be high in technical accuracy, be specific for the index being measured, be sensitive enough to detect small changes, have good reproducibility, be easy to use, impose low risk to the patient, and be cost-effective.

945 What are the main phenomena examined during respiratory monitoring?

❑ Two major categories of phenomena are examined during respiratory monitoring: (1) oxygenation indices and (2) ventilation indices. The oxygenation indices include ABGs (ie, intermittent blood sampling), SaO_2, transcutaneous oxygen tension, and mixed venous oxygen saturation. The ventilation indices include capnography, transcutaneous carbon dioxide tension, breathing pattern, and evaluation of respiratory center function, respiratory muscle function, and respiratory mechanics.

946 How can monitoring of respiratory muscle strength be performed?

❑ Respiratory muscle strength is assessed by measuring maximum respiratory (inspiratory and expiratory) pressures. The maximum inspiratory pressure (PImax) is highest following complete expiration, whereas the maximum expiratory pressure (PEmax) is highest at total lung capacity (maximal inspiration). The dependence of PImax on patient cooperation can result in poorly reproducible measurements. A two-step modification of the measurement technique helps to circumvent this problem. A valve is attached to the airway to ensure that inspiration begins at a low lung volume, and the period of occlusion is standardized to 20 seconds. The resulting PImax values are about one-third more negative than those obtained with the nonstandardized approach. In healthy men, PImax and PEmax values are approximately 115 ± 27 (standard deviation) and 180 ± 40 cm H_2O. Values in women are approximately 25% lower. The PImax value is one of the standard measurements employed to determine a patient's ability to tolerate discontinuation of mechanical ventilation. Values that are more negative than −30 cm H_2O are considered to predict weaning success, while values that are less negative than −20 cm H_2O predict weaning failure. Although PImax is a "standard" weaning predictor, it performs poorly in this respect.

947 How important is respiratory monitoring? What parameters should be evaluated in patients receiving mechanical ventilation?

❑ Monitoring of mechanically ventilated patients is imperative because of their vulnerability to the sudden onset of a host of complications that might be life-threatening. Direct clinical observation remains an essential component that includes measurement of respiratory rate, detection of respiratory distress, and assessment of respiratory muscle performance in terms of accessory muscle use and paradoxical motion of the rib cage and abdomen. Laboratory evaluation includes measurement of ABGs and bedside spirometric measurements of vital capacity, minute ventilation, maximum voluntary ventilation, negative inspiratory pressure (as an indicator of respiratory muscle strength), and total thoracic compliance. In addition, continuous automated monitoring sensors are used to a varying extent with different ventilators. Many ventilators have alarms that are activated by predefined alterations in airway pressure, tidal volume, or FiO_2.

948 What major parameters should be monitored in patients receiving mechanical ventilation?

❑ Acutely ill, ventilator-dependent patients require close monitoring by members of the entire health care team including physicians, nurses, respiratory therapists, and others. Major aspects of patient monitoring include (1) evaluation of ventilator parameters, tracheal cuff pressure, and respiratory secretions; (2) blood gas analysis (including PO_2, PCO_2, and pH) and pulse oximetry; (3) frequent measurements of vital signs and continuous evaluation of ECG; (4) neurologic and mental status evaluation; (5) measurements of serum electrolytes, urine volume, fluid balance, and body weight; and (6) assessment of the integrity of mucous membranes and the skin. Effective and careful monitoring can help to prevent complications and facilitate their early detection, therefore augmenting the likelihood of a successful outcome.

949 What information on pulmonary mechanics can be obtained with the purpose of respiratory monitoring in ventilator-supported patients? Explain how static compliance (Cst) and dynamic compliance (Cdyn) are measured. What is the meaning of an *abnormal pulmonary compliance*?

❑ Important information on pulmonary mechanics can be obtained in patients receiving mechanical ventilation from simple calculations made at the patient's bedside. In ventilator-supported patients, dynamic respiratory compliance (Cdyn) is calculated as follows: Cdyn = delivered volume/(peak airway pressure − PEEP); in patients not receiving extrinsic PEEP but in whom auto-PEEP is present, the value of auto-PEEP must be subtracted when making this calculation. Cdyn is normally 50 to 80 mL/cm H_2O and is reduced by any of the factors that decrease Cst or by airway narrowing caused by bronchospasm, mucus plugging, or a kinked tube. The airway pressure at 1- to 2-second end-inspiratory pause, known as *plateau pressure,* is necessary to calculate the static respiratory compliance (Cst) as follows: Cst = delivered volume/(plateau pressure − PEEP). Cst is normally 60 to 100 mL/cm H_2O, and is decreased in patients with disorders of the thoracic cage or with a reduction in the number of functioning lung units caused by partial lung resection, bronchial intubation, pneumothorax, atelectasis, pneumonia, or pulmonary edema.

BLOOD GASES

950 How important are ABG measurements in respiratory monitoring? What are the limitations of this blood sampling assessment?

❑ ABG measurements remain the mainstay of respiratory monitoring. However, several problems exist with the use of ABG measurements alone for respiratory monitoring: Measurement requires an invasive procedure, intermittent sampling may miss sudden changes, the information obtained may not reflect systemic blood gas composition (which is better detected with mixed venous blood sampling), there may be a considerable lag time between ordering the test and obtaining the result, and deterioration in ABG measurements can occur relatively late in the evolution of respiratory failure.

951 What are the major drawbacks of ABG measurements in the assessment of pulmonary gas exchange?

❑ Although ABGs are an indispensable part of intensive care, they are not without their drawbacks. First, they are invasive, requiring an indwelling catheter or an arterial puncture. Second, inaccuracies can result from the manner of sampling. Introduction of air bubbles leads to inaccurate results. The use of excessive amounts of heparin (>0.2 mL) can lead to low PCO_2 and HCO_3^- readings due to a dilutional effect, and to artifactually high PO_2

values. Despite the acidity or heparin, pH is not affected because of the excellent buffering capacity of blood. These problems can be minimized by using large volumes of blood, small needles, and minimal amounts of heparin or by using syringes that contain lyophilized heparin. During transport, specimens should be stored in ice to minimize errors resulting from metabolism by white blood cells or platelets (low PO_2 and pH and high PCO_2), especially in patients with leukemia or thrombocytosis. Third, intermittent sampling may miss sudden changes, and frequently there is a considerable time lag between ordering an ABG analysis and obtaining the results. Fourth, ABG values in themselves do not provide a complete picture of the underlying pathophysiology, and are neither sensitive nor specific to changes in the efficiency of pulmonary gas exchange, being influenced by a number of nonpulmonary factors in addition to lung function. Fifth, although natural variability in the measurement is quite modest, with coefficient of variation of less than 5%, some stable patients display considerable fluctuations in PaO_2, more than 40 mm Hg, despite no other change in their condition. This emphasizes the need to base therapeutic decisions on trends in ABG values rather than on isolated measurements. Sixth, measurement of PaO_2 may not reflect oxygen transport; for example, PEEP may cause an increase in PaO_2 but a fall in cardiac output, with the result that oxygen transport is decreased. Finally, deterioration in ABG values can occur relatively late in the evolution of respiratory failure and so provide little advanced warning.

---

952 Briefly explain the use of PO_2 in arterial blood and mixed venous blood as well as other methods to monitor oxygenation (eg, oxygen saturation with fiberoptic catheters, pulse oximetry) in patients with acute and chronic respiratory failure.

❑ Adequate management of both acute and chronic respiratory failure requires close monitoring of oxygenation. PaO_2 is very valuable to assess pulmonary gas exchange but is not a reliable guide of tissue oxygenation. SaO_2 also falls short in properly assessing the level of oxygen at the tissue level. An estimation of the adequacy of overall tissue oxygenation is obtained with the measurement of the PO_2 in mixed venous blood ($P\bar{v}O_2$). Yet, this index might also be misleading under certain circumstances, including the presence of peripheral arteriovenous shunting and in high-cardiac-output states (eg, septic shock). The direct measurement of the oxygen saturation of mixed venous blood ($S\bar{v}O_2$) with fiberoptic flotation catheters using spectrophotometry can be most useful in the management of patients with hypoxemic respiratory failure. The noninvasive monitoring of oxygenation by the use of pulse oximetry is also generally reliable as long as blood flow is adequate, SaO_2 is higher than 60%, and a significant level of methemoglobin or carboxyhemoglobin is not present.

953 Is measurement of $S\bar{v}O_2$ useful in respiratory monitoring? What are the normal values?

❑ The development of a pulmonary artery catheter containing specially designed fiberoptic filaments makes it possible to monitor $S\bar{v}O_2$ continuously. In addition to measuring $S\bar{v}O_2$, fiberoptic catheters are capable of measuring all of the indices measured by a regular pulmonary artery catheter. An advantage of mixed venous oximetry over pulse oximetry is that $S\bar{v}O_2$ values fall on the steep portion of the oxyhemoglobin dissociation curve, where the relationship between $S\bar{v}O_2$ and $P\bar{v}O_2$ is linear. Healthy subjects have $S\bar{v}O_2$ values of 73% to 85%. An $S\bar{v}O_2$ value less than 50% is commonly associated with impaired tissue oxygenation. Since $S\bar{v}O_2$ is the weighted mean of venous blood from all the body, it can be also affected by alterations in the distribution of blood flow between organs with high and low ratios of oxygen consumption to perfusion.

954 What blood compartments must be sampled for the appropriate monitoring of acid-base composition and oxygenation in patients with circulatory failure? Compare the information obtained with arterial and venous blood gases.

❑ The appropriate monitoring of acid-base composition and oxygenation in patients with circulatory failure requires central venous blood sampling in addition to the sampling of arterial blood. Whereas arterial data provide an assessment of pulmonary gas exchange, central venous data gauge tissue acidity and oxygenation as determined by the relation between perfusion and prevailing metabolic demands. Patients with incipient circulatory compromise, especially those with even mild degrees of arterial acidemia, should also be assessed, if possible, by central venous blood sampling, for it may help detect critical hemodynamic deterioration. The standard practice of relying solely on arterial blood monitoring can lead to errors in diagnosis and might contribute to the high morbidity and mortality among patients treated in intensive care units.

955 What are the potential causes of an abnormal level of $S\bar{v}O_2$?

❑ The potential causes of an abnormal $S\bar{v}O_2$ can be readily observed by rearranging the Fick equation from $\dot{V}O_2 = \dot{Q}t\ (CaO_2 - C\bar{v}O_2)$, to $C\bar{v}O_2 = CaO_2 - (\dot{V}O_2/\dot{Q}t)$, where $\dot{Q}t$ indicates cardiac output; $\dot{V}O_2$, oxygen consumption; and $CaO_2 - C\bar{v}O_2$, the difference between arterial and mixed venous oxygen content. From the latter equation, it is apparent that the primary factors affecting $S\bar{v}O_2$ include $\dot{V}O_2$, $\dot{Q}t$, and CaO_2, which in turn is dependent on SaO_2 and the hemoglobin concentration. If $\dot{V}O_2$, SaO_2, and the hemoglobin concentration remain constant, changes in $S\bar{v}O_2$ should reflect changes in $\dot{Q}t$. Consequently, $S\bar{v}O_2$ has been used to evaluate changes in cardiac output in critically ill patients. In reality, the correlation between $S\bar{v}O_2$ and $\dot{Q}t$ is poor, indicating that changes in $\dot{Q}t$ are usually accompanied by simultaneous changes in $\dot{V}O_2$ and $S\bar{v}O_2$. Moreover, the interpretation of $S\bar{v}O_2$ should be made with caution because there are conditions (eg, sepsis) in which an increase in $S\bar{v}O_2$ does not necessarily signify an improvement in tissue oxygenation.

956 What clinical conditions are associated with a reduction in SvO_2?

❑ A reduction in $S\bar{v}O_2$ can occur as a result of (1) decreased cardiac output, (2) decreased SaO_2, (3) decreased hemoglobin concentration, and (4) increased oxygen consumption, if compensatory mechanisms (eg, increased tissue perfusion in response to augmented demand) fail to counterbalance the initial disturbance. In all of the previously mentioned conditions there may be a reduction in tissue oxygenation that can be recognized by the reduction in $S\bar{v}O_2$.

957 Name a condition in which the expected reduction in $S\bar{v}O_2$ that characterizes most states of circulatory failure is not observed.

❑ Sepsis is a state in which circulatory failure accompanied by abnormal tissue oxygenation is associated with an elevated $S\bar{v}O_2$. The high $S\bar{v}O_2$ in this instance may be due to several factors, including the perfusion of some vascular beds in excess of their metabolic demands, development of local arteriovenous shunting, and a reduction in oxygen extraction and consumption due to sepsis-induced cytotoxicity. Thus, $S\bar{v}O_2$ should not be employed as a sole guide to tissue oxygenation.

958 What clinical conditions are associated with an increase in $S\bar{v}O_2$?

❑ An increase in $S\bar{v}O_2$ can occur as a result of (1) increased oxygen delivery to the tissues (eg, augmented cardiac output), (2) decreased oxygen consumption, (3) decreased oxygen extraction by the tissues, (4) left-to-right intracardiac shunt, (5) severe mitral regurgitation, and (6) wedged pulmonary artery catheter (ie, artifactual increase in $S\bar{v}O_2$). Consequently, all these possibilities must be considered before concluding that the increased $S\bar{v}O_2$ expresses augmented oxygen delivery to the tissues caused by a higher cardiac output.

959 How reliable is the $P\bar{v}O_2$ as an indicator of effectiveness of oxygen delivery in satisfying tissue oxygen demands? Is a low $P\bar{v}O_2$ a reliable indicator of tissue hypoxia?

❑ A low $P\bar{v}O_2$ (eg, $<$20 mm Hg) is a reliable indicator of tissue hypoxia. Conversely, a normal or high $P\bar{v}O_2$ is not a reliable indicator of the absence of serious tissue hypoxia, since the opening of low-resistance systemic shunts may provide oxygen-rich blood into the venous circulation (eg, gram-negative septicemia) despite the presence of some severely underperfused capillary beds. In summary, tissue hypoxia is present if $P\bar{v}O_2$ is low irrespective of PaO_2 or cardiac output. Tissue hypoxia might be also present despite a normal $P\bar{v}O_2$ caused by arteriovenous shunting of oxygenated blood.

PULSE OXIMETRY

960 What is the basis of pulse oximetry? How accurate is this method?

❑ Pulse oximetry is based on two physical principles: (1) the different light absorption spectra of oxyhemoglobin and reduced hemoglobin, and (2) the presence of a pulsatile signal generated by arterial blood that is relatively independent of venous and capillary blood as well as from signals originated in other tissues. Currently available pulse oximeters use two wavelengths of light, 660 nm in the red region and 940 nm in the infrared region. The use of light-emitting diodes to generate red and infrared light has made it possible to use sensors that are lightweight and inexpensive or even disposable. With respect to the accuracy of the oximeters, they generally measure SaO_2 within 95% confidence limits of ±4% when SaO_2 is above 70%. Accuracy tends to decrease when SaO_2 is below 70%, probably due, at least in part, to the difficulty in obtaining reliable human calibration data during extreme hypoxemia. It must be recognized that several factors (described in the answer of another question) may decrease the accuracy of pulse oximeters. In general, ear probes have a faster response than do finger probes. Thus, the accuracy of oximeters varies with the type of probe and its location. Because pulse oximeters use only two wavelengths, these instruments can distinguish only between reduced hemoglobin and oxyhemoglobin.

961 What factors might contribute to inaccurate readings with pulse oximetry?

❑ The accuracy of oxygen saturation (SaO_2) measurements with pulse oximetry can be altered by multiple factors. Because the pulse oximeter does not differentiate oxyhemoglobin from carboxyhemoglobin, it overestimates the true SaO_2 in patients with high carboxyhemoglobin levels (reading represents the sum of the two forms of hemoglobin) such as fire victims. Nail polishes can produce false measurements; those black, blue, and green can lead to low oximeter readings. Dark skin pigmentation, some intravascular dyes, methemoglobinemia, a low perfusion state, and fluorescent and xenon arc surgical lights decrease the accuracy of readings.

962 Elaborate further on the factors that can impair the accuracy of noninvasive oximetry.

❑ Multiple factors can reduce the accuracy of noninvasive oximetry including ambient light, motion artifact, low tissue perfusion state, and the shape of the oxygen dissociation curve. Additional factors include the presence of carboxyhemoglobin, methemoglobin, intravascular dyes, skin pigmentation, and nail polish. Falsely high values are observed in patients with elevated carboxyhemoglobin (eg, smokers, victims of carbon monoxide poisoning), whereas falsely low values occur as a result of intravenous dyes (eg, indocyanine green, methylene blue), fluorescent and xenon arc surgical lights, and nail polish (eg, black, blue, green). Despite the existence of multiple factors that affect the accuracy of noninvasive oximetry, this technique is generally reliable and useful. It should be recognized, however, that oximetry is not a sensitive guide to changes in gas exchange in patients with high baseline PaO_2 values because of the peculiar shape of the oxyhemoglobin dissociation curve (ie, large changes in PaO_2 produce small changes in SaO_2 in the upper and flat portion of the dissociation curve).

963 What arterial oxygen saturation measured by pulse oximetry (SpO_2) should be aimed at when titrating FiO_2?

❑ If pulse oximetry is used to help titrate FiO_2 in a ventilator-dependent patient as well as during spontaneous respiration, the usual target of 90% of oxygen saturation of hemoglobin obtained with ABG analysis should not be used because it is insufficient and can be associated with significant hypoxemia. The oxygen saturation measured with pulse oximetry should be 92% and 95% in white and in black patients, respectively.

VITAL CAPACITY AND BREATHING PATTERN

964 How does evaluation of vital capacity help in respiratory monitoring? What conditions decrease vital capacity? Compare normal vital capacity to that indicative of a need to remain on ventilatory support.

❑ Vital capacity is an effort-dependent measurement of the greatest volume of gas a subject can exhale after maximum inspiration. It is reduced in patients with diseases involving the respiratory muscles or their neural pathways, in patients with obstructive and restrictive ventilatory impairment, and in patients who fail to cooperate fully. Vital capacity is normally 65 to 75 mL/kg, and a value of 10 mL/kg or higher is commonly considered a favorable predictor of weaning outcome. However, its predictive power is rather poor.

965 Is the assessment of ventilation a simple task in respiratory monitoring? Enumerate techniques that measure ventilation indirectly.

❑ Ventilation is easily measured in intubated patients using a spirometer attached to an endotracheal tube, but problems arise in attempting to monitor ventilation continuously in nonintubated patients. Critically ill patients have a low tolerance to devices that require the use of a mouthpiece or mask. Furthermore, these devices in themselves alter the breathing pattern. Consequently, several techniques have been developed to measure ventilation indirectly for the respiratory monitoring of patients. Most experience has been obtained with inductive plethysmography and magnetometry, both of which record motion of the rib cage and abdomen. Combined with breathing pattern analysis, this approach can provide information on the volume and timing of ventilation, the coordination of rib cage–abdominal motion, and changes in the FRC.

966 Explain the use of respiratory inductive plethysmography (RIP) to assess pulmonary ventilation.

❑ RIP is the most widely accepted indirect method for measuring ventilation in a noninvasive quantitative manner. The transducers consist of two coils of insulated wire sewn onto bands placed around the rib cage and abdomen. With proper calibration, RIP can provide accurate measurements of tidal volume and rib cage–abdomen coordination. Less commonly used methods to measure indirectly pulmonary ventilation include using mercury-in-Silastic strain gauges and magnetometers. These various methods that allow indirect measurement of pulmonary ventilation are used in sleep laboratories and in clinical research, but are not widely used for clinical purposes in the intensive care unit.

967 How can the patient's respiratory drive be monitored? Is this evaluation of clinical importance?

❑ Measurement of respiratory drive provides information on respiratory center function. Respiratory drive can be evaluated in patients on mechanical ventilation by measuring airway pressure at 0.1 second after initiating an inspiratory effort against an occluded airway ($P_{0.1}$). Another approach is to measure the mean inspiratory airflow, which is obtained by dividing tidal volume by inspiration time (V_T/T_I). Both $P_{0.1}$ and V_T/T_I can underestimate respiratory drive in the presence of deranged pulmonary mechanics, but an elevated value in this situation clearly represents increased drive. At the present time it is unknown whether monitoring the respiratory drive is helpful in the assessment and treatment of patients in the intensive care unit.

968 What techniques other than measuring maximum respiratory pressures can evaluate respiratory muscle function?

❑ A number of parameters or techniques are employed in the research setting to investigate respiratory muscle fatigue, such as maximum sustained ventilation, transdiaphragmatic pressure response to phrenic nerve stimulation, power spectral analysis of the electromyogram, and the relaxation rate of respiratory pressures. However, none of these have proved useful for the clinical diagnosis of fatigue, because of their dependence on patient motivation, their invasive nature, and their inability to diagnose fatigue at a single moment in time because of the requirement for comparison to measurements prior to the onset of fatigue.

969 Is paradoxical movement of the rib cage and abdomen a reliable indicator of respiratory muscle fatigue?

❑ Evaluation of the presence of paradoxical movement of the rib cage and abdomen has been suggested as a simple bedside indicator of respiratory muscle fatigue. However, muscle fatigue is neither a necessary nor a sufficient condition for the development of rib cage–abdominal paradox; instead, increased respiratory load is the major mechanism responsible for the development of abnormal motion of the chest wall and abdomen.

970 Explain the use of minute ventilation and breathing pattern in respiratory monitoring. How important is the presence of a high respiratory rate as a predictor of weaning failure and impending death?

❑ Minute ventilation is normally about 6 L/min, and in patients being considered for a weaning trial it should generally be less than 10 L/min (in the presence of normocapnia) and also less than 50% of maximum voluntary ventilation (which indicates a reasonable ventilatory reserve). However, these measurements have limited accuracy in predicting weaning outcome. In healthy subjects the tidal volume is approximately 400 mL, and the respiratory rate is approximately 17 breaths/min. In patients being considered for a weaning trial, a tidal volume of less than 300 mL and a respiratory rate of 25/min or higher predict an unsuccessful outcome. An elevated respiratory rate is often the earliest sign of an impending death caused by respiratory failure, and the degree of elevation is proportional to the severity of the underlying disease. Despite the simplicity of the measurement, nursing records of the respiratory rate are commonly inaccurate, contributing to an underappreciation of its clinical value.

971 How useful is the evaluation of breathing pattern in respiratory monitoring?

❑ Assessing the patient's breathing pattern is one of the most valuable methods of respiratory monitoring. An elevated respiratory rate (>22 breaths/min) is often the earliest sign of respiratory failure and the degree of elevation is proportional to the severity of the patient's condition. In one study, most patients who had a cardiopulmonary arrest developed an increased respiratory rate lasting several hours before the arrest; conversely, other tests, including the ECG, did not show a consistent abnormality that helped as a warning sign. With respect to qualitative changes in the breathing pattern, it must be recognized that the rib cage and abdomen normally move in synchrony in which the chest and abdomen expand on inspiration and contract on expiration. However, abdominal paradox is detected in many patients with respiratory failure. Paradoxical motion (one compartment moving in the opposite direction to the other) is an indicator of either increased respiratory load or diaphragmatic paralysis but does not accurately signify respiratory muscle fatigue.

972 How is patient's monitoring performed during a weaning trial from a ventilator while breathing spontaneously either through a T-tube circuit or through the ventilator circuit?

❑ The patient's general clinical status should be closely observed by a physician or nurse during a weaning trial from a ventilator, with frequent measurements of the respiratory rate, accessory muscle activity, rib cage and abdominal motion, heart rate, and blood pressure. If the patient's condition is satisfactory, the trial should be continued for 20 to 30 minutes, at which time ABGs may be analyzed. If the patient's performance is satisfactory, the patient can be immediately extubated. If the patient's condition is borderline, the weaning trial may continue for up to 1 hour, but prolonged T-tube trials should be avoided.

973 What are the limitations of simple visual inspection in the evaluation of breathing pattern?

❑ Clinical examination of breathing pattern has generally consisted of counting the respiratory rate over a 15- to 60-second period, assessing whether abnormally deep or shallow respirations were present, and establishing the presence of abnormal patterns such as Cheyne-Stokes or Kussmaul's breathing. In addition, a more detailed analysis of breathing pattern can provide valuable information regarding respiratory system performance. Yet, simple visual inspection has serious limitations. Many clinicians measure respiratory frequency by observing chest wall motion over 15 seconds and multiplying the resulting value by 4. With this approach, an error of 4 breaths/min or more can easily occur, a rather large error for a parameter that is normally 16 to 20 breaths/min. The limitation of this approach is due to the technique of evaluation (ie, a 15-second period of observation) and is not due to an intrinsic limitation of the usefulness of respiratory rate measurements. Assessment of tidal volume is also made during bedside examination and clinicians commonly report on the depth or shallowness of breathing. However, a very poor correlation exists between subjective estimations of tidal volume made by intensive care unit personnel (including physicians) and objective measurements. Furthermore, the discontinuous nature of bedside evaluations may miss sudden changes in critically ill patients.

974 How can breathing pattern be monitored with a noninvasive technique?

❑ Impedance pneumography is the technique most often used to noninvasively monitor breathing pattern. Two standard ECG electrodes placed on the chest wall serve to pass an alternating current through the chest, allowing measurement of the electrical impedance. The waveform tracing obtained with this device is qualitatively similar to that obtained with spirometry. Calibration of this instrument to obtain quantitative volume measurements is not possible and measurement of respiratory frequency may be inaccurate.

PULMONARY ARTERY CATHETERIZATION

975 What is the most common indication for pulmonary artery catheterization in critically ill patients? What hemodynamic parameters can be evaluated with this technique?

❑ Measurement of wedge pressure is the most common indication for the insertion of a pulmonary artery catheter. Pulmonary artery wedge pressure is used as an indirect measure of left ventricular preload. For accurate measurements of pulmonary artery wedge pressure, the catheter tip should be located in a dependent region of the lung (ie, zone 3), where pulmonary artery pressure is higher than pulmonary venous pressure, and the latter is higher than alveolar pressure. Because of marked changes in intrathoracic pressure during spontaneous and mechanical ventilation, the pressure level displayed on a digital monitor can be misleading, and the assessment should be made on an actual tracing at the end of spontaneous and mechanical expiration. In addition, pulmonary artery catheterization can be performed with the purpose of measuring cardiac output and obtaining a mixed venous sample for measurement of blood gases.

---

976 What information should be used for hemodynamic monitoring of patients with marked respiratory variations of pulmonary pressure level?

❑ Patients in respiratory distress or receiving mechanical ventilation may display marked respiratory variation in the blood pressure tracings obtained with a pulmonary artery catheter. The marked variation in the blood pressure is caused by the combined effect of large fluctuations in intrathoracic pressure (secondary to spontaneous or mechanical ventilation) and the fact that vascular pressure is referenced to the atmospheric level. However, it must be recognized that hemodynamic function depends on transmural pressures that are obtained by subtracting intrathoracic pressure from measured intravascular pressure. Because most recording systems employed for clinical purposes do not correct for the effect of intrathoracic pressure on the level of intravascular pressure, the measurements obtained from a digital display of data arising from a Swan-Ganz catheter may be very misleading. The circulatory pressures recorded at end-expiration (both in spontaneously breathing and mechanically ventilated patients) are, in general, least affected because at end-expiration intrathoracic pressure is predictably near the atmospheric level.

---

977 How can pulmonary artery catheterization in patients with respiratory failure help to recognize the presence of mitral regurgitation, cardiac tamponade, and constrictive pericarditis? What is the square root sign in pulmonary artery monitoring?

❑ Insertion of a pulmonary artery catheter is helpful to reach a diagnosis in several conditions, as follows: (1) in mitral regurgitation, in which giant V waves can be detected, especially on the wedge tracing; (2) in cardiac tamponade, in which equalization of pressures on the right side of the circulation (right atrial, right ventricular end-diastolic, pulmonary artery diastolic, and pulmonary artery wedge pressure) can be observed with values of approximately 20 mm Hg; and (3) in constrictive pericarditis, which produces a characteristic early diastolic dip and late diastolic plateau (square root sign) in the right ventricular pressure tracing.

978 What errors with the interpretation of data from pulmonary artery catheterization might be encountered?

❑ The inflated balloon of the catheter should impact and wedge in a small-caliber pulmonary artery, to collect the necessary information. For the pulmonary artery wedge pressure to reflect left atrial pressure, the vascular system distal to the catheter tip (ie, the pulmonary capillaries and veins) must be freely patent and must provide a direct, blood-filled vascular connection between the catheter tip and the left atrium. Obstruction of the pulmonary veins will cause the pulmonary artery wedge pressure to be significantly higher than the left atrial pressure. High alveolar pressures interfere with the measurement of pulmonary arterial wedge pressure because the alveolar vessels are quite collapsible and major variations in blood flow between different regions of the lung develop in this condition. With respect to the location of the catheter in the lung fields, zone 3 at the base of the lungs (in which pulmonary artery pressure is higher than pulmonary venous pressure and the latter is higher than the alveolar pressure) is the only region where a pulmonary aterial wedge pressure can reflect left atrial pressure. Fortunately, most balloon-tipped catheters, because they are flow directed, tend to position toward the dependent portions of the lung, usually at or below the mid atrial level and thus, are positioned in zone 3. However, hypovolemia, PEEP, and gas trapping secondary to airway obstruction predispose to the development of zone 1 or 2 conditions even though the catheter is anatomically positioned in zone 3. An additional problem with the interpretation of data derived from a pulmonary artery catheter relates to the presence of marked variations in the tracing during the respiratory cycle (see answer to pertinent question).

979 What is the rationale for monitoring cardiac output with the use of a pulmonary artery catheter in critically ill patients?

❑ A pulmonary artery catheter can be inserted to measure cardiac output in conjunction with a therapeutic regimen aimed at optimizing oxygen delivery. Markedly increasing oxygen delivery with the intention of augmenting oxygen uptake by the tissues has been advocated on the belief that critically ill patients have pathologic supply dependency for oxygen consumption; that is, oxygen uptake is directly related to oxygen delivery. However, this approach has been abandoned because the studies on which this concept was based had serious flaws.

980 Outline the most important potential problems associated with pulmonary artery catheterization.

❑ The major potential problems of pulmonary artery catheterization can be separated into (1) equipment errors, (2) complications arising during insertion of the catheter and while the catheter is in place, and (3) inadequate interpretation of the data collected. Equipment errors include those derived from calibration, zeroing, frequency response, and balloon inflation; all of them lead to the collection of unreliable data. Complications arising from insertion of a pulmonary artery catheter might include venous air embolism, pneumothorax, hemorrhage, catheter malposition as well as knotting and fragmentation of the catheter, arrhythmias, and cardiac conduction abnormalities. Complications that can occur while the catheter is in place are venous thrombosis, pulmonary infarction, endocardial damage, balloon rupture, pulmonary artery perforation, hemothorax, hemomediastinum, and infection. Problems of interpretation are examined in the answers to other questions.

CAPNOGRAPHY

981 What methods for PCO_2 monitoring can be used in addition to ABG measurements?

❑ The patient's PCO_2 level can be monitored continuously with noninvasive techniques, which measure PCO_2 on the skin or the airway. The transcutaneous PCO_2 determination is much more reliable in neonates than in other patient populations. The PCO_2 in the airway is measured either by infrared spectrophotometry or mass spectrometry. Whereas the transcutaneous PCO_2 level is higher than the $PaCO_2$, the end-tidal PCO_2 value is lower than the latter. In the normal state, the end-tidal PCO_2 is 1 to 4 mm Hg lower than the $PaCO_2$, but in pulmonary diseases this difference can increase up to 10 mm Hg or more.

982 What is capnography and how does this method help respiratory monitoring?

❑ Measurement of expired carbon dioxide represents a noninvasive method of continuously monitoring alveolar and arterial PCO_2. A capnometer is a device that measures and displays the breath-by-breath numerical values of carbon dioxide concentration, while a capnograph also displays the carbon dioxide waveform. In the pulmonary function laboratory, sleep laboratory, and intensive care unit, the infrared absorption technique is usually employed to measure expired carbon dioxide. It operates on the principle that carbon dioxide is able to absorb infrared light within a narrow wavelength range. Infrared absorption of expired gas can be measured with either side-stream or mainstream sensors. Side-stream monitors have a low-negative-pressure pump that aspirates a small sample of expired gas through a capillary tube and transmits it to the infrared absorption chamber. A major problem with side-stream systems is condensation of water and mucus, which can occlude the tubing, causing erroneous measurements. Mainstream sensors, which are incorporated into the breathing circuit, contain a special insert that allows infrared light to pass through the airway. Mainstream sensors are heated to approximately 40°C to prevent condensation on the sensor window, which might lead to a falsely elevated carbon dioxide reading. The mainstream sensor is interposed between the endotracheal tube and the ventilator circuit. The side-stream sample is aspirated from the airway and carried via capillary tubing to a distant infrared absorption chamber.

983 How useful and reliable is capnography in respiratory monitoring?

❑ Noninvasive measurement of end-tidal carbon dioxide tension ($P_{ET}CO_2$), taken as the plateau value of an exhaled sample, approximates $PaCO_2$ (within 1 mm Hg) in healthy subjects. However, in patients with lung disease, large and unpredictable differences (10 to 20 mm Hg) between $PaCO_2$ and $P_{ET}CO_2$ occur because of uneven distribution of ventilation with respect to pulmonary perfusion. $P_{ET}CO_2$ is therefore misleading in patients with significant pulmonary disease.

984 What is the cause for failure to measure $P_{ET}CO_2$ following intubation? What clinical conditions can produce sudden or gradual decreases in this parameter?

❑ Failure to detect $P_{ET}CO_2$ following intubation indicates misplacement of the tube in the esophagus (ie, esophageal intubation). Consequently, this finding facilitates the immediate recognition and correction of a potentially lethal error with airway intubation. Conditions leading to a sudden decrease in $P_{ET}CO_2$ include sudden hyperventilation, a brisk decrease in cardiac output, massive pulmonary embolism, air embolism, disconnection of the ventilator, obstruction of the endotracheal tube, and leakage in the ventilatory circuit. A gradual decrease in $P_{ET}CO_2$ is observed in the presence of hyperventilation, decrease in oxygen consumption, and reduced pulmonary perfusion.

HEMODYNAMIC PARAMETERS

985 What are the standard goals or desired levels for the various hemodynamic parameters (ie, PCWP, systemic vascular resistance, right atrial pressure, systolic blood pressure) when monitoring the response to therapy with intravenous vasodilators and diuretics in patients with cardiorespiratory failure?

❑ The hemodynamic goals during treatment of cardiorespiratory failure with vasodilators (eg, nitroprusside) and diuretics are (1) PCWP of 15 mm Hg or less, (2) systemic vascular resistance of 1200 dyn · sec · cm^{-5} or less, (3) right atrial pressure of 8 mm Hg or less, and (4) systolic blood pressure of 80 mm Hg or higher, and (5) cardiac output of 2.3 L/min/m^2 of body surface area or higher.

986 Describe a commonly used approach to evaluate ventricular performance (ie, right and left ventricles) in the intensive care unit.

❑ Examination of the responses of cardiac output, arterial pressure, and PCWP to rapid expansion of blood volume in patients with low cardiac output or hypotension provides information about myocardial performance. If the abnormal hemodynamic status is due to hypovolemia, an elevated preload will increase cardiac output, cardiac work (ie, product of cardiac output and the difference between arterial and atrial pressures), and the slope of the relationship between cardiac work and filling pressure. None of these changes will be observed if the patient's abnormal hemodynamic condition is due to decreased myocardial contractility.

987 What measures might be helpful in the management of mechanically ventilated patients who develop severe arterial hypoxemia and abnormal hemodynamics status?

❑ Insertion of a flow-directed, right-sided heart, balloon-tipped (Swan-Ganz) catheter to monitor pulmonary arterial and capillary wedge pressures and measuring cardiac output by the thermodilution technique can be of significant help in the assessment and management of these patients.

988 What are the optimal levels of PCWP in the management of ARDS?

❑ Considering that the alveolar-capillary membrane of ARDS patients is leaky (ie, increased permeability), efforts should be made to maintain the PCWP as low as possible. PCWP should be the minimum that maintains adequate blood pressure, cardiac output, and urine volume. The judicious prescription of inotropic and vasoactive agents (eg, dopamine) might help to achieve the goal of maintaining an adequate hemodynamic condition and a relatively low PCWP.

989 Is the demonstration of a normal cardiac output (eg, in the intensive care unit, cardiac catheterization laboratory) during the resting state evidence of normal cardiac function?

❑ No. Many patients with cardiac diseases leading to low-output heart failure, particularly at early stages, develop effective compensatory mechanisms such that cardiac outputs during the resting (basal) state are normal. The expanded plasma volume due to salt and water retention augments ventricular end-diastolic pressure, allowing for preservation of near-normal stroke volume and cardiac output. Nevertheless, this failing heart produces less cardiac output for a given ventricular end-diastolic volume. In other words, the cardiac output is kept at the normal level due to increased end-diastolic ventricular volume and pressure. Furthermore, the failing heart is less able to increase cardiac output in response to exercise, even if its output is normal at rest.

---

990 A 32-year-old woman develops a gastrointestinal hemorrhage that is complicated by aspiration pneumonia and shock unresponsive to conventional therapy. A pulmonary artery catheter is inserted and the following hemodynamic data are obtained:

Cardiac output ($\dot{Q}t$)	3.2 L/min
Systolic arterial pressure	88 mm Hg
Diastolic arterial pressure	64 mm Hg
Mean arterial pressure (MAP)	72 mm Hg
Mean pulmonary artery pressure (MPAP)	32 mm Hg
Pulmonary capillary wedge pressure (PCWP)	19 mm Hg
Right atrial pressure (RAP)	10 mm Hg

What are the estimated levels of systemic vascular resistance and pulmonary vascular resistance of this patient?

❑ Measurement of systemic vascular resistance (SVR) is helpful in the differential diagnosis and management of patients with circulatory collapse (also known as *profound circulatory failure* or *shock*). Vascular resistance is calculated by dividing mean pressure difference between two points in the vascular system by the blood flow between them (ie, mean amount of blood passing from one point to the other per unit of time). Calculation of vascular resistance in R units (also known as *Wood's units*) requires expression of the pressure gradient (in mm Hg) and blood flow (in L/min); this unit may be converted to CGS (cm-gm-sec) units by multiplying its value times 80, resulting in vascular resistance (expressed in dyn · sec · cm^{-5}). Thus,

$$\begin{aligned} \text{SVR} &= (\text{MAP} - \text{RAP})/\dot{Q}t \\ &= (72 - 10)/3.2 \\ &= 19.4 \text{ R units (Wood units)} \\ &= 19.4 \times 80 = 1552 \text{ dyn} \cdot \text{sec} \cdot \text{cm}^{-5} \end{aligned}$$

Since the normal SVR is 770 to 1500 dyn · sec · cm^{-5}, the patient's level was slightly above the upper-normal level. Pulmonary vascular resistance (PVR) is calculated from hemodynamic monitoring data as follows:

$$\begin{aligned} PVR &= (MPAP - PCWP)/\dot{Q}t \\ &= (32 - 19)/3.2 \\ &= 4.1 \text{ R units (Wood units)} \\ &= 4.1 \times 80 = 328 \text{ dyn} \cdot \text{sec} \cdot \text{cm}^{-5} \end{aligned}$$

Considering that the normal PVR is 20 to 120 dyn · sec · cm^{-5}, the patient's level was severely augmented by the aspiration pneumonia and possibly other factors.

Selected Readings

1. Adrogué HJ, Wesson DE. Acid-Base. Boston, MA: Blackwell Scientific Publications, 1994.

2. Tobin MJ, ed. Respiratory Monitoring. New York, NY: Churchill Livingston, 1991.

3. Tobin MJ, ed. Principles and Practice of Mechanical Ventilation. New York, NY: McGraw-Hill, 1994.

4. Murray JF, Nadel JA, eds. Respiratory Medicine. Philadelphia, PA: W.B. Saunders Company, 1994.

5. Nunn JF. Nunn's applied respiratory physiology. Oxford: Butterworth-Heinemann, 1993.

Index

Numbers after index entries indicate question numbers.